VITAMIN A AND BETA-CAROTENE ARE MIRACLE WORKERS

Vitamin A and Beta-Carotene are Miracle Workers

Frank Murray

Foreword by

Richard A. Passwater, Ph.D.

GYAN

Vitamin A and Beta-Carotene are Miracle Workers

ISBN: 978-81-212-1138-3

Published in 2012 in India by
Gyan Publishing House
23, Main Ansari Road
New Delhi-110002
Phones : 23282060, 23261060
Fax : 011-23285914
E-mail: books@gyanbooks.com
Website: www.gyanbooks.com

Laser Typesetting : Quick Media, Delhi
Printed at : Chawla Offset Printers, Delhi

CONTENTS

FOREWORD

The importance of vitamin A—and its precursor beta-carotene—to life has been known for nearly a hundred years. Perhaps the fact that we have known about its critical role to health for so long is a contributing factor in why so many people today seem to have lost tract of this fact.

Indeed, it was the importance of vitamin A to general health that led to its early discovery. It was the first fat-soluble vitamin identified, and the second vitamin overall, just after vitamin B1.

So critical, so inexpensive, and yet hundreds of thousands of children die each year or are blinded because they are deficient in vitamin A.

According to the World Health Agency, vitamin A deficiency is estimated to affect approximately one-third of children under the age of five around the world (World Health Organization, Global Prevalence of Vitamin A Deficiency in Populations At Risk, 1995-2005, WHO Global Database on Vitamin A Deficiency).

A vitamin A deficiency is estimated to claim the lives of 670,000 children under the age of five. (Black, R. E., Allen, L. H., Bhutta, Z.A., Caulfield, L. E., De Onis, M., Ezzati, M., Mathers, C., Rivera, J., et al. "Maternal and Child Undernutrition: Global and Regional Exposures and Health Consequences," Lancet 371(960):243-260, 2008).

Approximately 250,000 to 500,000 children in developing countries become blind each year owing to a vitamin A deficiency, with the highest prevalence in Southeast Asia and Africa. ("Office of Dietary Supplements, Vitamin A," National Institutes of Health; http;//www.dietary-supplements.info.nih.gov/factsheets/vitamina.asp), Yet, the problem with an inexpensive solution goes on apparently without much concern, since 670,000 young children a year is more than 1,800 each day.

What would your reaction be if you read that four or five 747 planes carrying 400 young children crashed every day and killed every child aboard?

Would you call for immediate action to stop these flights?

Why don't we call for immediate action to eradicate vitamin A deficiency?

One inexpensive, high-dose vitamin A pill per child every six months will go a long way in halting these endless deaths and blindness.

Vitamin A deficiency hampers the immune system and greatly increases the likelihood of contracting diseases, including measles, malaria, diarrhea, respiratory tract infections, and blindness. According to Vitamin Angels, a charitable group with the mission of reducing child mortality worldwide, vitamin A supplementation could reduce the mortality for children under five years of age by 23%.

In Vitamin A and Beta-Carotene Are Miracle Workers, Murray points out that, in addition to the role of vitamin A in the general health of children, it is important in saving children from measles. This disease is still killing about 500 young children a day—a full 747-load of children. He explains how vitamin A improves resistance against measles, and thus spares many children, but in those who do contract the disease, vitamin A supplements reduce deadly complications in severe cases and hastens recovery.

Vitamin A is not just for children. Vitamin A deficiency is rampant, and this impacts health care costs in every nation.

People today seem to remember that vitamin A is needed for "good eyesight" (actually to prevent night blindness), but they seem unaware of the role of the vitamin in the immune system, and in the reduction in risk of many diseases.

Fortunately, Frank Murray has written a book that should overcome this lack of awareness.

Murray points out that, in addition to the diseases of childhood, vitamin A supplements are life-saving for adults as well—especially against the scourages of malaria, cancer, and HIV/AIDS. He discusses the extensive research showing that vitamin A, through its role in immunity, lessens HIV/AIDS incidence and mortality.

Murray discusses why the actual number of deaths from malaria may be under-reported and actually may be invisible to health-care systems. He reviews the considerable evidence that vitamin A supplementation is associated with up to a 35% reduced risk of malaria, and that it is important for the recovery of patients.

The teachings of this book can save the lives of millions worldwide. It should be read by all.

Richard A. Passwater, Ph.D.

INTRODUCTION

It has been known for over 50 years—some have said 100 years—that vitamin A can jump-start the immune system, thereby protecting us from cancer and other life-threatening illnesses.

For cancer alone, this suggests that, if people had been ingesting more vitamin A and beta-carotene—in foods and supplements—the cancer rates might have dropped precipitously.

The importance of vitamin A to health and visual acuity in children has been known since the 1920s.

More recently, doctors and researchers have determined that vitamin A and beta-carotene are necessary for treating measles, blindness, malaria, HIV/AIDS, skin problems, pneumonia, diarrhea, Cystic fibrosis, lung diseases, diabetes, asthma, and numerous other health problems.

In December 2008, the World Health Organization in Geneva, Switzerland, predicated that cancer will overtake heart disease as the World's No. 1 killer shortly.

Unfortunately, vitamin A has always had a bad press. How often have you heard someone—even professionals—say that "vitamin A is very dangerous". So is water if you ingest too much of it.

The problem may have arisen because vitamin A, like the other fat-soluble vitamins—D, E, and K—is stored in the liver, where it becomes a miraculous reservoir to protect against possible vitamin A deficiencies.

It's possible that some wag—not knowing his elbow from his clavicle—theorized that, if you are consuming a lot of vitamin A, you are bound to become sick. Fortunately, that rarely happens.

In all of the medical literature, there may be 20 cases of people getting too much vitamin A. I recall a bloke in England, who consumed nothing but carrot juice for an extended period. Naturally, he was not getting essential amounts of vitamins, minerals, protein, etc., and he turned a bright orange from the carotene in the carrots before he kicked the bucket.

If you were to eat at one meal a 3 oz. serving of cooked beef liver (30,325 International Units of vitamin A); one-half cup of carrots (1,793 IU); one-half cup of spinach (1,572 IU); and one medium cantaloupe (1,555 IU); you will have ingested over 35,000 IU of the vitamin. This healthful meal will hardly have you carted off to the hospital, even though the vitamin A amount is way above the Recommended Dietary Allowance of 5,000 IU.

Pregnant women should have their vitamin A intake—from foods and supplements—monitored by their doctor so as not to harm the fetus. This is of little concern to the mother, but, of course, the liver of a fetus is very small.

By the same token, children should have their vitamin A intake evaluated by a health-care provider. However, as you will read later in this book, children are being prescribed 100,000 IU and more of vitamin A to rid them of life-threatenging illnesses. The dosage is tailored to the age and size of the child, and the length of the treatment is determined by their doctor.

As you read through the book, I suspect you will be astonished that vitamin A and beta-carotene are so important to your health, since you may have been brainwashed into hearing that the two essential vitamins are something you should avoid.

I am hopeful that this book will be widely circulated, especially in developing countries, since it is scandalous that millions of adults and children die unnecessarily each year when inexpensive supplements and lifestyle modifications are so readily available.

In addition, hopefully, the book will encourage more researchers to undertake studies to highlight the importance of vitamin A and beta-carotene. As you will see, the two vitamins are truly miracle workers.

FRANK MURRAY

New York

1
THE IMPORTANCE OF VITAMIN A

In 1913, vitamin A was discovered by Elmer V. McCollum and Marguerite Davis at the University of Wisconsin at Madison, and simultaneously by Thomas B. Osborne and Lafayette B. Mendel of the Connecticut Experiment Station, according to Foods & Nutrition Encyclopedia.[1]

While working independently, the research teams discovered the presence of an essential dietary substance in fatty foods. McCollum and Davis found it in butterfat and egg yolks, while Osborne and Mendel located it in cod-liver oil.

They felt that it was only 1 factor, which they called fat-soluble vitamin A, and that it was needed to supplement purified diets, and might defend an infectious eye disease, which was prevalent in undernourished animals. In 1915, McCollum and Davis reported that a deficiency in the vitamin caused night blindness.

In 1919, the encyclopedia continued, Steenbock and co-workers at the University of Wisconsin noted that an unknown substance found in sweet potatoes, carrots, and corn—later identified as carotene—could support normal growth and reproduction.

In 1920, an English scientist, Drummond, suggested that the compound be called vitamin A, and, in 1930, Moore, another Englishman, demonstrated that this substance is provitamin A (beta-carotene).

"In 1931, P. Karrer, a Swiss researcher, isolated the active substance in halibut liver oil, and determined the chemical formula of vitamin A, the first vitamin to have its chemical structure determined," the publication added. "For this, and his work on riboflavin (B2), he received the Nobel Prize." (In 1911, Dr. Casimir Funk, a Polish-American scientist, then working at the Lister Institute in London, England, isolated the first vitamin from rice polishings that prevented beriberi. This turned out to be thiamine (B1).

However, vitamin A was not produced by Karrer in crystalline form from fish liver oils until 1937, and it did not become available in a synthetic form until Isler found out how to do it in Switzerland in 1947.

Vitamin A is available in several forms, with each one possessing different degrees of activity. Two forms are retinol and dehydroretinol. Retinol—formerly called vitamin A—is found as an ester—retinyl palmitate—in ocean fish oils, other fats, liver, butterfat, and egg yolk. It is biologically active as an alcohol, an aldehyde, and an acid.

"The alcohol, the most common form, is usually referred to as retionol, the aldehyde as retinal or retinene, and the acid as retinoic acid," the publication added.

Dehydroretinol, or vitamin A2, differs from retinol in that: (1) it has an extra double bond; and (2) it has about 40 per cent the biological activity. It is found only in freshwater fish and in birds that eat these fish; hence, it is of limited interest in nutrition. The general term vitamin A is used for both retinol and dehydroretinol.

In addition to the actual forms of vitamin A, related compounds, known as carotenes, are found in several fruits and vegetables, the publication said. Carotene is also called: (1) provitamin A, because it can be converted to vitamin A in the body; and (2) a precursor of vitamin A, because it procedes vitamin A. At least 10 of the carotenoids—of over 600 so far isolated—found in plants can be converted with varying efficiencies into vitamin A. Four of these carotenoids—alpha-carotene, beta-carotene, gamma-carotene, and cryptoxanthine (the main carotenoid in corn)—are of especial importance, due to their provitamin A activity. However, beta-carotene has the highest vitamin A activity, and provides about two-thirds of the vitamin A necessary for human nutrition.

Vitamin A values in animal foods vary according to the vitamin A value of the feed of the animals that produced them. As an example, livers from older animals and from animals eating green grass are higher in vitamin A than the livers of younger animals on dry, bleached foods, and the butterfat in milk is usually yellower and higher in vitamin A when the cows are grazing on green pastures.

Fish liver oils are the richest natural sources of vitamin A. Fish eat smaller fish or crustaceans, which, in turn, have fed on marine plants that contain provitamin A.

Foods, such as yellow fruits and vegetables, supply vitamin A in the form of vitamin A, vitamin A esters, and carotenes. Virtually no absorption of vitamin A occurs in the stomach. Storage of vitamin A is largely in the liver, although small amounts are stored in the lungs, body fat, and kidneys. From the liver, vitamin A enters the bloodstream as a free alcohol, there it travels to the tissues for use. Since vitamin A is not water-soluble, none is excreted in the urine, but considerable unabsorbed carotene is normally found in the feces, the publication continued.

"In the small intestine, vitamin A and beta-carotene are emulsified with bile salts and products of fat digestion, and absorbed in the intestinal wall", the publication said. "This is where much of the conversion of beta-carotene to vitamin A (retinol) takes place."

The absorption is influenced by several factors, including the presence in the small intestine of bile, dietary fat, and antioxidants. Bile acids emulsification and fat must be absorbed simultaneously, and antioxidants—vitamin E and lecithin—decrease the oxidation of carotene.

In addition, the presence of protein enhances the conversion of carotene to vitamin A. The absorption of vitamin A is adversely affected by the presence of mineral oil in the intestinal tract. Since mineral oil is not absorbed, and since it holds carotene and vitamin A in solution, carotene and vitamin A are lost through excretion. Thus, mineral oil should never be used as a substitute for regular fats in food preparation.

It is also noted that intestinal parasites affect the absorption of vitamin A and carotenes, and the conversion of carotene to vitamin A. This is especially critical in tropical regions where intestinal parasites are common.

"In the blood, vitamin A esters are transported in association with a retinol-binding protein, whereas the carotenoids are associated with the lipid/fat-bearing protein," the publication added. The amount of storage of vitamin A in the body tends to increase with age, but this depends on the quantity in the diet and the amount absorbed. A normal adult may store sufficient vitamin A in the liver to meet the needs for 4 to 12 months. Infants and children, however, do not build these resources, therefore, they are more susceptible to deficiencies.

Writing in the landmark publication, "Food—the Yearbook of Agriculture, 1959," Ernestine B. McCollum and Elmer V. McCollum, reported that an eye disease, xerophthalmia, or dry dyes, a result of too little vitamin A, was observed in Japan in 1904, and children in Denmark in 1917.[2]

A deficiency of vitamin A injures the epithelial cells throughout the body, causing them to become dry and flatten, and slough off when the vitamin is lacking. The cells, instead of being soft and moist, become hard and dry like the scales of dry skin.

"The mucous membranes are barriers against many kinds of bacterial invasion, and impairment of their structure and function when vitamin A is deficient lowers resistance to respiratory and other infections," the authors said.

Vitamin A is necessary for vision, and the retina of the eye contains a pigment, visual purple, which is composed of vitamin A and protein.

"Visual purple is converted first to visual yellow and then to visual white when the eye is exposed to light," the authors added. "Vitamin A is lost in this conversion, but visual purple is regenerated if a fresh supply of vitamin A is available. Without this regeneration, vision in subdued light is impaired following exposure to bright light, a condition known as night blindness."

The authors went on to say that night blindness has a long medical history, in which it is associated with diet. It was common in Newfoundland among fisherman, who worked in open boats in bright sunshine and exposed their eyes to the glare on the water. There was an old belief that if a man could not see at night, his vision would be restored by the next night if he ate the liver of a codfish or a seagull. (As early as 1850 B.C., the Egyptians were aware that liver is beneficial to those with night blindness).

"If a child gets too little vitamin A when his teeth are developing, the enamel-forming cells become abnormal and lose their effectiveness in forming enamel prisms," the authors continued. "Some prisms in the finished enamel may be missing, and pits are formed. Such pits may later harbor food deposits, which may ferment and form acids that etch the enamel and lead to decay."

The biological activities of vitamin A and carotene are expressed in International Units (IU) or United States Pharmacopoeia (USP Units). These units have the same value, and the terms are used interchangeably. They are defined in terms of standardized, pure, crystalline vitamin A, or beta-carotene. Three-tenths of a gram of crystalline vitamin A or six-tenths of a gram of pure beta-carotene is equal to 1 unit. A unit is very small, and there are 1 million grams in a gram and about 30 grams in an ounce. An ounce of pure, crystalline vitamin equals 30 million units.

Various dietary factors influence the requirement for vitamin A. For example, vitamin E protects carotene and vitamin A against oxidative destruction within and outside the body. The livers of animals deprived of vitamin E are rapidly depleted of vitamin A. The store of vitamin A in the liver can then increase when vitamin E is provided again.

Carotene and vitamin A are insoluble in water, thus there is no loss by extraction during cooking. Exposure to air or oxygen, especially in the presence of heat, however, causes destruction of vitamin A and the presence of heat, however, causes destruction of vitamin A and carotene. Air drying of such foods as eggs and vegetables results in a significant loss of vitamin A value, however, vacuum drying prevents this loss.

As has been reported, vitamin A is essential for the promotion of general health, the maintenance of visual function, the regulation of differentiation of epithelial tissues, the embryonic development[3], according to Guangwen Tang, and colleagues at the Jean Mayer USDA Human Nutrition Research Center on Aging at Tufts University in Boston, Massachusetts.[4]

"Vitamin A deficiency can cause visual malfunction such as night blindness and xerophthalmia[5], and reduce immune responsiveness (6), which results in an increased incidence or severity of respiratory infections, gastrointestinal infection[7], and measles[8]," the researchers said.

The research team added that it is estimated that some 250 million preschool children, mostly in developing countries, have some level of vitamin A deficiency.

According to the U.S. National Academy of Sciences, the retinol equivalent of carotenoids in foods is 12 mcg all-trans beta-carotene, or 24 mcg of other provitamin A carotenoids, equivalent to 1 mcg of retinol, the researchers said.

"Although factors such as the food preparation method, the fat content of a meal, or the relative bioavailability of carotenoids from mixed vegetables and fruit have been investigated, the bioavailability of carotenoids and their conversion to vitamin A from single vegetable sources has not been extensively studied because of the limited availability of isotopically labeled foods that can be fed to humans. This is unfortunate because estimates from some previous studies suggest that the conversion of beta-carotene to retinol is as high as 26 to 1," the researchers said.[9]

To achieve an accurate assessment of carotenoid bioavailability from an individual plant food and its subsequent vitamin A value, one can use foods in which the carotenoids have been endogenously or intrinsically labeled with a low-abundance stable isotope, the researchers continued. This method allows presentation of the carotenoids in their normal cellular compartments, and the isotopic tag enables identification of serum carotenoids (or derived retinol and other metabolites), which come from the specific food being tested.

"Determinations of the efficiency of absorption of plant provitamin A carotenoids and their conversion to vitamin A are needed to make sound recommendations on which plant foods can provide vitamin A to humans," the researchers said.[10]

As a result of their study, the researchers added that spinach and carrots can provide a significant amount of vitamin A, even though the amount is not as great as previously thought.

They said that it is worth mentioning that the conversion factor for spinach or carrot beta-carotene to vitamin A might be different (that is, less efficient) for populations with poorer general nutritional status or Helicobacter pylori). Conversely, people with a marginal vitamin A status might have improved (i.e., become more efficient) conversion of beta-carotene to vitamin A.

While carrots contain both beta-carotene and alpha-carotene, the blood response to each mole of carrot beta-carotene was significantly higher—almost double—relative to equal moles of carrot alpha-carotene, the researchers continued.

"Although vegetable beta-carotene is a safe form of provitamin A and can provide substantial amounts of vitamin A to humans, the use of plant provitamin A as a sustainable and effective strategy for combating vitamin A deficiency in various parts of the world, from an array of plant sources, needs continued scientific and quantitative evaluation," the researchers concluded.

In a lengthy article in Cancer and Nutrition, Jae Ho Kim, M.D., and colleagues, of Henry Ford Hospital in Detroit, Michigan, detailed the many uses of antioxidants in cancer treatments. Here are their notations on vitamin A.[11]

1. Retinoids/vitamin A have been shown to have antitumor activity against acute polymorphocytic leukemia, as well as chemopreventive effects of second malignancies of the aerodigestive tract.
2. Combining cis-retinoic acid and interferon is an effective regimen against skin and cervical carcinoma.
3. Radiotherapy may be enhanced by the combination of interferon and cis-retinoic acid.
4. Vitamins C, E, and retinoic acid have reduced bleomycin-induced lung cancer.
5. A mixture of vitamins A, C, E, and beta-carotene have been shown to be more effective than individual vitamins

in reducing the growth of some human cancer cells in culture.

6. Individually, vitamins A, C, and E can enhance the growth inhibition effect of radiation.
7. Vitamin A and beta-carotene, in conjunction with cyclophosphamide or radiation, has produced more than 90 per cent cure rate in rats transplanted with adenocarcinoma of the breast, whereas animals who received vitamins, drug, or radiation alone died.
8. Local administration of vitamin E and beta-carotene near tumors has caused regression of oral tumors in hamsters.
9. High doses of individual vitamins, such as vitamin C, retinoids, and beta-carotene, have resulted in varying degrees of regression of pre-neoplastic lesions, and certain well-established cancers in humans.

Based on this and other evidence not mentioned, the authors recommend that patients undergoing chemo- and/or radiotherapy follow special dietary and behavioral modifications and use high-dose vitamins.

The vitamin doses are vitamin C as calcium ascorbate at 10 g/day in divided doses; vitamin E as d-alpha-tocopherol succinate at 800 IU/day; and mixed carotenoids at 60 mg/day. (A gram is 1,000 mg).

Also, multivitamins should be utilized that contain appropriate minerals. Dietary modifications consists of reducing fat intake to 10-15% of total calories, and increasing fiber to 25-30 g/day.

High fiber can be obtained from diets containing fruits, vegetables, and cereals. There should be no smoking, caffeine, alcohol, moderate exercise, and some form of meditation.

Twenty people with brittle asthma had significantly lower median dietary intakes of vitamin A and vitamin E than 20 nonbrittle asthmatics and 20 healthy controls with a mean age of 49.5 years, according to Thorax. Night blindness, alcoholic liver disease, and hypogonadism are frequently seen in chronic alcoholic patients, reported the International Journal of Vitamin and Nutrition Research. In 23 men and 2 women, with a mean age of 43.8 years, 3 of the 25 patients had deficient vitamin A levels.[12]

When given 2,500 IU/day of vitamin A as retinol orally for 5 days, there was improvement of blood levels of the vitamin, except for a 61-year-old man.

Researchers recommend vitamin A supplementation, along with other vitamins, during conventional detoxification therapy for alcohol withdrawal in order to prevent the manifestation of hypovitaminosis A.

There are certain drugs whose absorption is enhanced by foods or nutrients, and there is a whole classification of drugs whose absorption is delayed by foods or nutrients, according to John A. Thomas, of the University of Texas Health Science Center in San Antonio.[13]

He added that there are also drugs whose absorption can be retarded or decreased by foods or nutrients. Some drug-food/drug-fluid interactions affect the absorption process, including indirect mechanisms such as drug-induced changes in gastrointestinal motility (anticholinergic), and drug-induced malabsorption syndromes (neomycin).

Alcohol definitely has an effect on the biotransformation of drugs, and some drug nutrient interactions include a variety of vitamins.

Fat-soluble vitamins have a reduced absorption with mineral oil, cholestyramine retards the absorption of vitamins A, D, and E. Neomycin retards the absorption of vitamin A.

Nutrition plays an important role in a drugs pharmacologic response, and some disease states may affect both nutrient conditions and a drug's therapeutic efficacy, the authors said. While a drug's pharmacokinetics can be predicted, nutrients can modify this particular profile as well as certain other pathophysiologic conditions.

Plastic jugs which contain milk expose vitamin A and vitamin B2 in milk to light, which reduces their content, according to Environmental Nutrition. Light can also trigger "off" flavors.[14]

A translucent plastic bag of skim milk in a lighted dairy case for just 1 day can lose up to 70 per cent of its vitamin A and B2. Milk in a cardboard carton loses only 2 per cent of its B2, and 15 per cent of its vitamin A.

In a laboratory animal test, dietary vitamin A at 250 mcg (750 IU) protected the animal against 100 mg of aspirin toxicity, reported the Journal of the American College of Nutrition.[15]

In 37 vitamin A-deficient stable alcoholic cirrhosis patients, 11 had low blood levels of zinc, which ranged from 45 to 63 mcg/dl. Initial taste and olfaction mean detection thresholds for all the test substances were significantly higher in all patients compared with 21 sex-matched healthy people of the same age range.[16]

Of the patients, 27, including the 11 patients with low levels of zinc, were given oral vitamin A at 10,000 mcg/day for 4 weeks.

In those who were vitamin A deficient, there was a significant improvement following vitamin A treatment in the mean detection and mean recognition thresholds for bitter and salty tastes, and for pyridine olfaction, regardless of zinc status. Pyridine is a liquid used in analytical chemistry and for denaturing alcohol.

With improvement in vitamin A status, there was an improvement in taste and olfaction, and ark adaptation toward normal, according to Giampaolo Bianchi, M.D. Ark in this instance refers to offering protection.

As reported by researchers at Michigan State University at Lansing, it is noted that polyhalogenated aromatic hydrocarbons are ubiquitous pollutants, which can alter vitamin A metabolism by accelerating the breakdown of vitamin A and its metabolites, as well as causing depletion of vitamin A body stores.[17]

Polyhalogenated aromatic hydrocarbon intoxication presents as a vitamin A deficiency-like syndrome. This intoxication probably affects enzymes that are involved with vitamin A metabolic pathways.

For those exposed to polyhalogenated aromatic hydrocarbons, inadequate vitamin A function will ensue, which may cause multiple health problems, reported Maija H. Zile.[17]

It was Umberto Saffiotti, M.D., of the National Cancer Institute in Washington, D.C., who reported to the 9th International Cancer Congress that vitamin A can prevent lung cancer, according to Ruth Adams in The Complete Home Guide to All the Vitamins. The story was reported in the October 25, 1966 issue of the *New York Times*.[18]

Saffiotti had worked out elaborate experiments with hamsters in which he induced lung cancer by blowing into their lungs some of the same chemical particles that are found in urban air pollution and in cigarette smoke.

"Hamsters, like human beings, do not develop lung cancer unless they are exposed to some cancer-causing agent or carcinogen," Adams said. "Saffiotti was in the news in 1969 as to whether or not cyclamates were cancer-causing."

In his research, Saffiotti noted that the changes which occurred in the cells of the hamsters' lungs are changes that precede cancer, Adams continued. Eventually, up to 100 per cent of the animals developed lung cancer, depending on how much of the cancer-producing chemical they were given. Giving the animals vitamin A prevented these changes in lung cells and hence prevented the lung cancers.

At the above-named Congress, Sir Alexander Haddow, a British scientist, announced that "as many as 80% of all human cancers may be due to environmental causes, and, that if that is true, the implications for prevention are immense and exciting."

Studies of large populations make it clear that vitamin A has anti-cancer effects, reported Sheldon Saul Hendler, M.D., Ph.D. In one study of 8,000 men who were monitored for over a 5-year period, those with the lowest intake of beta-carotene were found to be at the greatest risk of getting lung cancer.[19-24]

"In an even longer term study of 2,000 men, it was shown that smokers with the lowest intake of beta-carotene were several times more likely to develop lung cancer than smokers with the highest intake of beta-carotene," he added.

Other studies have suggested that the cancer-protective effects of beta-carotene are related to numerous cancers, including those of the bladder, larynx, esophagus, stomach, colon/rectum, and prostate.

In addition to the population studies, there are literally hundreds of papers demonstrating that vitamin A in the preformed variety, can suppress the malignant behavior of cultured cells adversely transformed by radiation, chemicals, or viruses, and can delay the development of transplanted tumors, and can even completely prevent malignancy in animals exposed to various potent cancer-causing substances, he added.

"Some of these results, it should be noted, have been obtained with doses of preformed vitamin A far too high and too toxic for general, preventive care," Hendler continued. "Experiments of the same sort with the far less toxic beta-carotene, meanwhile, appear promising, but are still few in number."

He went on to say that drug derivatives of vitamin A are also showing promise in the fight against cancer. Accutane, for example, has been shown to be of benefit in the treatment of cutaneous T-cell lymphoma, a blood cancer that affects the skin. There is also emerging of Accutane's usefulness in the treatment of myelodyspastic syndrome, a premalignant condition with leukemia-like characteristics. Accutane, in addition, has been able to shrink dramatically and, in some cases, completely eradicate oral leukoplakia, which are precancerous lesions found on the lips and inside the mouth.

"The same vitamin A derivative that is used in Retin-A has been used in experiments that suggest this substance may help prevent cervical cancer," Hendler said. "In one study, 50 per cent possible precancerous cervical lesions disappeared completely after treatment with a vitamin A derivative Tretinoin."

The role of vitamin A in the control and regulation of epithelial cell growth has been long appreciated, reported F.L. Meyskins, Jr., of the University of California at Irvine. Synthetic derivatives of vitamin A (retinoids) have potent effects on malignant cells as well.[25]

"I and my colleagues have investigated the role of retinoids in the prevention and therapy of human cancer for the past decade," he told the 30th Annual Meeting of the American College of Nutrition, September 23-25, 1989 in Norfolk, Virginia.

He added that, "a number of trials by him and his colleagues and others have been initiated to determine whether retinoids can block the primary development of cutaneous lung cancers."

"We have documented keratoacanthomas, epithelial dysplasia verruciformix, cervical dysplasia, and oral leukoplakia," he said.

Surprisingly, he continued, we have also found considerable activity of beta-carotene against oral leukoplakia as well. We have also documented considerable activity of 13-cis-retinoic acid against advanced squamous cancer of the skin and T-cell lymphoma of the skin (mycosis fungoides), topical retinoic acid but not oral 13-cis-retinoic acid caused regression of dysplastic nevi and established melanoma.

"These and other results indicate that vitamin A derivatives have a role in the control of certain cancers," he continued.

Symptoms of both vitamin A deficiency and toxicity were known long before vitamins were recognized, according to Abram Hoffer, M.D., Ph.D.[26]

Night blindness, xerophthalmia, and keratomalacia were described over a century ago, because Arctic explorers knew that polar bear liver was dangerous, since explorers in the 16th century lost their skin after eating polar bear liver—one pound would contain over 30 million IU of vitamin A.

For cancer, Willett and MacMahon, in 1984; Nettesheim in 1980; and Prasad and Rama in 1985; reviewed the relationship between vitamin A, vitamin A analogues (retinoids), carotene, and cancer, Hoffer reported.

"These compounds have inhibited tumor induction, inhibited the promotion phase, and caused some tumors to regress," he said. "Some of the synthetic retinoids are most potent in prevention and treatment of cancer."

As reported in Cancer Research, in 2,440 men, ages 50 and older, who were followed for 10 years, it was found that 84 men developed prostate cancer.[27]

The mean serum vitamin A levels were significantly lower in the prostate cancer patients than in the non-cases. Also, there was an increased risk of prostate cancer with decreasing levels of serum vitamin A.

The inverse relationship between serum vitamin A and prostate cancer incidence was independent of age at examination or other variables.

The authors added that this was the first prospective study of blood levels of vitamin A and prostate cancer, which included a large number of patients.

Animal Sources of Vitamin A

Food	*IU*	*%DV**
Liver, beef, cooked, 3 oz.	30,325	610
Liver, chicken, cooked, 3 oz.	13, 920	280
Egg substitute, fortified, ¼ cup	1, 355	25
Cheeze pizza, 1/8 of a 12-in. diameter pie	380	8
Cheddar cheese, 1 oz.	300	6
Whole egg, 1 medium	280	6
Milk, whole, 1 cup	305	6
Fat-free milk, fortified with Vitamin A, 1 cup	500	10

* DV-Daily Value. DVs are reference numbers based on the Recommended Dietary Allowance (RDA). They were developed to help consumers determine if a food contains a lot or a little of a specific nutrient. The DV for vitamin A is 5,000 IU (1,500 micorograms retinol). Most food labels do not list a food's vitamin A content. The percent DV (%DV) Listed on the above table indicates the percentage of the DV provided in one serving. Percent DVs are based on a 2,000-caloric diet. Your Daily Values may be higher or lower, depending on your calorie needs. Foods that provide lower percentages of the DV also contribute to a healthful diet.

Source: "Vitamin A and Carotenoids," Clinical Nutrition Service, Warren Grant Magnuson Clinical Center, Office of Dietary Supplements, National Institutes of Health, Bethesda, Maryland, October 6, 2003.

Recommended Dietary Allowance (RDA) for Vitamin A as Preformed Vitamin A (Retinol Activity Equivalents)

Life Stage	*Age*	*Males: mcg/day (IU/day)*	*Females: mcg/day (IU/day)*
Infants	0-6 months	400 (1,333 IU)	400 (1,333 IU)
Infants	7-12 months	500 (1,667 IU)	500 (1,667 IU)
Children	1-3 years	300 (1,000 IU)	300 (1,000 IU)
Children	4-8 years	400 (1,333 IU)	400 (1,333 IU)
Children	9-13 years	600 (2,000 IU)	600 (2,000 IU)
Adolescents	14-18 years	900 (3,000 IU)	700 (2,333 IU)
Adults	19 and older	900 (3,000 IU)	700 (2,333 IU)
Pregnancy	18 and younger	—	750 (2,500 IU)
Pregnancy	19 and older	—	770 (2,567 IU)
Breast-feeding	18 and younger	—	1,200 (4,000 IU)
Breast-feeding	19 and older	—	1,300 (4,333 IU)

Source : "Vitamin A", Linus Pauling Institute at Oregon State University, Corvallis, October 20, 2008.

Tolerable Upper Level of Intake for Preformed Vitamin A (Retinol)

Age Group	*UL in Mcg/Day (IU/Day)*
Infants 0-12 months	600 (2,000 IU)
Children 1-3 years	600 (2,000 IU)
Children 4-8 years	900 (3,000 IU)
Children 9-13 years	1,700 (5,667 IU)
Adolescents 14-18 years	2,800 (9,333 IU)
Adults 19 years and older	3,000 (10,000 IU)

Source: "Vitamin A," Linus Pauling Institute at Oregon State University, Corvallis, October 20, 2008.

References

1. Ensminger, Audrey, et al. Foods & Nutrition Encyclopedia. Clovis, CA: Pegus Press, 1983, pp. 2225ff.
2. McCollum, Ernestine B., and McCollum, Elmer V. "Vitmains A, D, E, K." In Food: The Yearbook of Agriculture. Washington, D.C.: Department of Agriculture, 1959, pp. 130ff.
3. Tang, Guangwen, et al. "Spinach or Carrots Can Supply Significant Amounts of Vitamin A as Assessed by Feeding with Intrinsically Deuterated Vegetables," American Journal of Clinical Nutrition 82:821-828, 2005.
4. Underwood, B.A., and Arthur, P. "The Contribution of Vitamin A to Public Health," FASEB Journal 10:1040-1048, 1996.
5. Sommer, A. "Nutritional Blindness: Xerophthalmia and Keratomalacia," Oxford University Press, New York, 1982.
6. Ross, A., et al. "Vitamin A and Retinols in Antiviral Responses," FASEB Journal 10:979-985, 1996.
7. Usha, N., et al. "Assessment of Preclinical Vitamin A Deficiency in Children with Presistent Diarrhoea," Journal of Pediatric and Gastroenterology and Nutrition 13:168-175, 1991.
8. Sommer, A., et al. "Vitamin A Deficiency, Health Survival, and Vision." Oxford University Press, New York, 1996.
9. de Pee, S., et al. "Orange Fruit Is More Effective Than Are Dark-Green, Leafy Vegetables in Increasing Serum Concentrations of Retinol and Beta-Carotene in School children in Indonesia," American Journal of Clinical Nutrition 68:1058-1067, 1998.

10. West, C.E., et al. "Consequences of Revised Estimates of Carotenoid Bioefficiency for Dietary Control of Vitamin A Deficiency in Developing Countries," Journal of Nutrition 132:2920S-2926S, 2002.
11. Kim, Jae Ho, M.D., et al. "The Use of High Dose Vitamins As An Adjunct to Conventional Cancer Treatment," Cancer and Nutrition 205:212, 1998.
12. Majumder, S.K., et al. "Vitamin A Utilization Status in Chronic Alcoholic Patients," International Journal of Vitamin and Nutrition Research 53(3):273-279, 1983.
13. Thomas, John A., and Tschanz, Christian. "Nutrient-Drug Interactions," Nutrition Technology, Raven Press, New York, 1994, pp. 139-148.
14. Environmental Bulletin 19(9):7, September 1996.
15. Rettura G., et al. "Vitamin A Protects Against Aspirin Toxicity," Journal of the American College of Nutrition 3:291-292, 1984.
16. Garrett-Laster, M., et al. "Impairment of Taste and Olfaction in Patients with Cirrhosis: Role of Vitamin A," Human Nutrition, Clinical Nutrition 380:203-214, 1984.
17. Zile, Maija H. "Vitamin A Homeostasis Endangered by Environmental Pollutants," Proceedings from the Society for Experimental Biology and Medicine 201:141-153, 1992.
18. Adams, Ruth. The Complete Home Guide to All the Vitamins. Atlanta, GA: Larchmont Books, 1984, pp. 73ff.
19. Hendler, Sheldon Saul, M.D., Ph.D. The Doctors' Vitamin and Mineral Encyclopedia. New York: Simon & Schuster, 1990, pp. 39ff.
20. Hong, W.K., et al. "13-cis-retinoic Acid in the Treatment of Oral Leukoplakia," New England Journal of Medicine 315:1501-1505, 1986.
21. Kune, G.A., et al. "Serum Levels of Beta-Carotene, Vitamin A and Zinc in Male Lung Cancer Cases and Controls," Nutrition and Cancer 12:169-176, 1980.
22. Menkes, M.S., et al. "Serum Beta-Carotene, Vitamin A and E, Selenium and the Risk of Lung Cancer," New England Journal of Medicine 315:1250-1254, 1986.
23. Ziegler, R.G. "A Review of Epidemiologic Evidence that Carotenoids Reduce the Risk of Cancer," Journal of Nutrition 119:116-122, 1989.

24. Micksche, M., et al. "Stimulation of Immune Response in Lung Cancer Patients by Vitamin A Therapy," Oncology 34:234-238, 1977.

25. Meyskins, F.L., Jr. "Prevention and Therapy of Human Cancers with Vitamin A Derivatives." Paper read at the 30th annual meeting of the American College of Nutrition, September 23-25, 1989, Norfolk, Virginia.

26. Hoffer, Abram, M.D., Ph.D. Orthomolecular Medicine for Physicians. New Canaan, CT: Keats Publishing, Inc., 1989, pp. 29ff.

27. Reichman, E., et al. "Serum Vitamin A and Subsequent Development of Prostate Cancer in The First National Health and Nutrition Examination Survey Epidemiologic Follow-up Study," Cancer Research 50:2311-2315, April 15, 1990.

2

WHAT IS BETA-CAROTENE?

Plants and algae synthesize beta-carotene that contributes to their color, and it may confer health benefits as part of diets rich in fruits and vegetables, according to a research team at the University of California at Davis.[1]

About 600 carotenoids are found naturally in foods, however, less than 60 are found in foods commonly consumed by humans.[2] Of these, beta-carotene is the best known because, pursuant to its central cleavage to retinol and oxidation to retinol, it serves as an important source of vitamin A.

"Excentral cleavage of beta-carotene to retinols and apo-carotenoids has been shown in a variety of in vitro systems and animal models," the researchers said. "Whether excentral cleavage occurs in vivo in humans, and, if so, to what extent, is unclear."

In the study, a healthy man was given an oral dose of all-trans beta-carotene, and its fats and that of its metabolites, were measured in plasma samples. Its formation in the feces and urine was also measured.

It was found that 65% of the substance was absorbed, and 15.7% was eliminated in urine during the first 21 days after dosing.

"These data suggest that excentral cleavage (splitting) of ingested beta-carotene occurs in vivo (in the body) in humans," the researchers added. "However, confirmation of that possibility requires further study."

The reason that beta-carotene is such an efficient producer of vitamin A is that the body splits a molecule of it exactly in half to produce 2 molecules of vitamin A, according to Richard A. Passwater, Ph.D. The other carotenoids yield at most only 1 molecule of vitamin A, and not all carotenoids can be converted to vitamin A because of differences in chemical structure.[3]

"Beta-carotene is converted into vitamin A in the body by the enzyme beta-carotene-15,15'-dioxygenase," Passwater said. "An enzyme is a compound that helps reactions occur without entering into the reaction itself—a reusable catalyst that controls a reaction. When vitamin A levels in the body fall, more dioxygenase is produced to increase the conversion of beta-carotene into vitamin A."

He went on to say that, when vitamin A levels in the body are restored, the amount of dioxygenase is diminished. Excess beta-carotene does not produce vitamin A toxicity, because no more of it is converted to vitamin A than the body requires at the moment. However, excess vitamin A in the bloodstream—as from animal sources or excessive supplementation—is eventually stored in the liver, with potential toxic effects.

Some people appear to have a reduced ability to convert beta-carotene into vitamin A, and genetic differences and chronic conditions such as diabetes or thyroid disease may impair the conversion.

"Beta-carotene not converted into vitamin A during absorption is stored until needed," Passwater continued. "The principal storage site for beta-carotene is fat tissue, but significant quantities circulate in the blood and are present in fatty areas of all cells. An excess of beta-carotene—which is not harmful—can be recognized as a yellowish cast to the skin, especially in the palms of the hands, resulting from its storage in fat just beneath the skin."

Vitamin A is essential for life, and a severe deficiency of the vitamin causes blindness and mortality, reported researchers at the National Institute for Nutrition and Food Safety in Beijing, China, and colleagues at other institutions in China, Massachusetts, Switzerland, and Texas.[4,5,6,7,8]

As observed in various studies, beta-carotene is an effective and safe source of vitamin A and is referred to as provitamin A. High doses of 180 mg/day of beta-carotene were given to people for several months without any observed adverse effects, other than changes in skin color.

In many countries, plant foods rich in beta-carotene are major sources of vitamin A. As an example, in China, 59% of vitamin A comes from vegetables.

Their study was to determine the vitamin A equivalent of spirulina beta-carotene in humans. Spirulina is an alga that is rich in protein and carotenoids, mainly beta-carotene. In one study, the incidence of a symptom of vitamin A deficiency, Bitot's spot, decreased from 80% to 10% after 1 gram spirulina/day was provided for over 150 days to 5,000 preschool-age children in Madras, India.

The study also involved 10 healthy Chinese men who consumed 5.8 micromole of retinyl acetate in oil as a reference dose with a breakfast containing 13 grams of fat. A micromole is one-millionth of a mole.

A week later, the volunteers consumed 7.9 micromole of trans-beta-carotene in spirulina with a breakfast containing 22 grams of fat. All of the men followed diets low in both vitamin A and carotenoid.

"In a group of well-nourished, normal-weight Chinese men following low-vitamin A diets, 4.5 mg of spirulina-beta-carotene, consumed with 22 grams of fat, has the same vitamin A activity as does of 1 mg of retinyl acetate," the researchers reported.

Vitamin A deficiency results in growth retardation, anemia, reduced resistance to infection, impaired cellular differentiation, xerophthalmia (dry eyes), and, ultimately, blindness and death, reported Judy D. Ribaya-Mercado, and colleagues at the Jean Mayer U.S. Department of Agriculture Human Nutrition Research Center, Tufts University, in Boston, Massachusetts.[9,10]

Plant foods containing provitamin A often are the primary sources of vitamin A in some populations in whom vitamin A deficiency is prevalent.[11] Thus, strategies for improving the absorption and bioconversion of plant carotenoids are essential.

"In certain groups, the concomitant consumption of plant carotenoids and dietary fat enhances serum (plasma) retinol concentrations," the researchers said. "However, because serum retinol is subject to homeostatic control over the physiologic range of liver vitamin A concentrations, serum retinol could remain unchanged with dietary intervention."

Their study was designed to assess the influence of amounts of dietary fat on: (1) the bioavailability (i.e., change in serum concentrations) of provitamin A carotenoids in yellow and green leafy vegetable meals; and (2) the effectiveness of plant carotenoids in improving the vitamin A status of marginally nourished school-age children as assessed by the deuterated-retinol-dilution (DRD). Deuterate refers to introducing deuterium into a compound. Duterium is an isotope of hydrogen.

The DRD techniques that use deuterium-labeled vitamin A have been used to assess the total-body vitamin A pool size (referred to as total-body vitamin A stores) in adults and children in the United States, Bangladesh, Gautemala, Philippines, China, Peru, and Nicaragua, researchers said.

In the study, in the Philippines, school children, ages 9 to 12, were fed standardized meals 3 times/day, 5 days/week, for 9 weeks. The meals provided 4.2 mg of provitamin A carotenoids/day (mainly from beta-carotene) from yellow and green leafy vegetables (carrots, bok choy, spinach, and swamp cabbage), and 7, 14, or 29 g fat/day (2.4, 5 or 10 g fat/meal) in Groups A, B, and C, which represented 39, 39, and 38 children, respectively.

Before and after the intervention, total-body vitamin A pool sites and liver vitamin A concentrations were measured, with the deuterated-retinol-dilation method. Blood levels of retinol and carotenoid concentrations were measured by high-pressure liquid chromatography (HPLC).

After 9 weeks, similar increases in mean serum beta-carotene, alpha-carotene, and beta-cryptoxanthin concentrations; total body vitamin A pool size; and liver vitamin A concentrations were observed in all 3 study groups. However, mean serum retinol concentrations did not change appreciably.

The researchers added that the total beta-carotene intake from the study meals, plus self-selected foods, was similar between the 3 groups, and was 14 times the usual intake.

They went on to say that carotene-rich yellow and green

leafy vegetables, when ingested with animal fat, enhance serum carotenoids and the total-body vitamin A pool size, and can restore low liver vitamin A concentrations to normal concentrations.

"Data from the present study indicate that it is possible to improve the total-body vitamin A pool size and restore low liver vitamin A concentrations to normal concentrations by eating sufficient amounts of carotene-rich yellow and green leafy vegetables and minimal amounts of dietary fat," the researchers added. "Thus, carotene-rich plant foods can effectively meet vitamin A needs."

They added that this finding is important, especially in developing countries, where health professionals and policymakers can promote the use of carotene-rich vegetables for combating vitamin A deficiency in vulnerable groups.

"In the United States and other countries, where school feeding and other food programs are in place, this information is useful for formulating dietary guidelines for inclusion of carotene-rich vegetables in meals," the researchers concluded.

In 8 people with Barrett's esophagus, daily supplements of 25 mg of beta-carotene were given for 8 months. Six of the patients had striking improvements in their gastroesophageal reflux. Symptom scores decreased from 7 to 2.7, and there was also histologic improvement, according to Family Practice News.[12] Histology is concerned with the minute structure of cells, tissues, and organs.

At the University of Michigan in Ann Arbor, and the University of California at Los Angeles, a research team evaluated the effects of dietary fiber on the absorption of beta-carotene. The researchers studied the effects of 12 g/day of citrus pectin on blood levels of beta-carotene.[13]

The volunteers consumed a diet containing 25 g of beta-carotene, while plasma samples were collected at 0, 8, 30, 48, and 192 hours after the meals.

The researchers reported that pectin reduced plasma beta-carotene levels at 30 and 192 hours postmeal. The average percentage increase in plasma beta-carotene following a meal was decreased by more than one-half when pectin was added to the meal. Pectins are water-soluble substances that bind adjacent cell walls in plant tissues, yielding a gel which is the basis of fruit jellies.

A number of studies have said that greater increases in plasma beta-carotene are noted when a purified supplement is consumed as opposed to carrots as a dietary source of provitamin A.

The study, as reported in the American Journal of Clinical Nutrition, support these findings and provide evidence that certain soluble fibers, such as pectin, might reduce blood levels of beta-carotene following ingestion of carotenoid-rich foods as compared with supplements.[13]

Beta-carotene, and to some extent other carotenoids, may play a significant role in preventing disease at its earliest stages, reported the European Journal of Nutrition.[14]

In the study, a research team invited 8 healthy men and women to take supplements of natural beta-carotene, lutein, and lycopene, all carotenoids. Each supplement was taken alone at a dosage of 15 mg/day for 1 week, followed by a 3-week "washout" (no supplement) period between each supplementation regimen.

The researchers exposed white blood cells from the patients to hydrogen peroxide, a potent generator of free radicals. They then compared levels of DNA strand breaks and their repair before and after supplementation.

The rejoining or repair of broken DNA strands occurred rapidly when the people had been taking natural beta-carotene supplements, however, no such benefit was seen after lutein supplementation. When the white blood cells were exposed to air, DNA breaks were reduce by supplementation with beta-carotene and lycopene.

Although carotenoids are well-established antioxidants, the research team reported that natural beta-carotene was especially important in preventing DNA damage.

Writing in The Nutrition Report, Thomas E. Edes, M.D., of the Harry S. Truman Memorial V.A. Hospital in Columbia, Missouri compared and contrasted the biological effects of beta-carotene and vitamin A, with emphasis focusing on beta-carotene.[15]

Vitamin A can be derived from beta-carotene in mammals, but, by this mechanism, toxicity to vitamin A does not occur. Of all the carotenoids, beta-carotene has the highest provitamin A activity, while canthaxanthin is a carotenoid that does not have any vitamin A activity.

Beta-carotene appears to have a more pronounced anticancer effect than vitamin A, Edes continued. It also has anticancer properties such as inhibiting squamous cell carcinoma in cell cultures. In animal models, beta-carotene supplements have reduced the incidence of mammary tumors, he said.

In addition, beta-carotene's antioxidant properties may help to prevent against tissue or DNA damage, which is a prerequisite for carcinogenesis. Beta-carotene may also stimulate carcinogen metabolizing enzymes such as hydrocarbon hydroxylase in the small intestine in animal models. Vitamin A has no effect in this instance, he added.

Edes went on to say that exposure to the carcinogen benzopyrene in cigarette smoke depletes tissues of vitamin A. Tissue enzymes induced by exposure to carcinogens may degrade vitamin A, and high-dose vitamin A may help to prevent the depletion caused by these enzymes, he continued.

Aside from the carotenoids' antioxidant effects and carcinogen metabolizing enzyme induction, the carotenoids may also enhance immune function and metabolic degradation, Edes concluded.

Foods rich in beta-carotene have been reported to counteract the carcinogenic effects of cigarette smoke, reported Medical Tribune. Beta-carotene may also counter the effects of charcoal-broiled meats and industrial waste.[16]

People are exposed to benzopyrenes in cigarette smoke, industrial exposure, and charcoal-broiled meats, and smokers are known to have low levels of vitamin A, the publication added.

Tobacco products reduce the body's levels of many nutrients, including antioxidants, and, at the same time, the liver needs higher levels of some of these nutrients to promote the detoxification or breakdown of hazardous compounds in tobacco smoke, according to the Journal of Nutritional Biochemistry.[17]

A combination of beta-carotene, vitamin C, and vitamin E

boosted levels of protective antioxidant enzymes in male smokers, who also have elevated levels of free radicals.

The study involved 42 male smokers, all of whom had elevated blood levels of cholesterol and triglycerides. They were given a combination of antioxidant supplements daily for 6 weeks. One group took 15 mg of beta-carotene, 500 mg of vitamin C, and 400 IU of vitamin E 30 minutes before breakfast. The other group took the same supplements at 2 meals daily, thus consuming twice the amount of the supplements.

The researchers reported that blood levels of key antioxidant enzymes—catalase, glutathione peroxidase, and superoxide dismutase—increased significantly in both groups. Also, oxidized (free-radical damaged) fats in cholesterol decreased significantly. Levels of iron, which are known to promote free-radical reactions, also went down.

The vitamin A content in plant foods is usually given as Retinol Equivalents (RE), that is, the amount of vitamin A that could be derived from the carotene content, according to Robert A. Ronzio, Ph.D.[18]

One RE is defined as 1 mcg of (trans) retinol (vitamin A), 6 mcg of (trans) beta-carotene; or 12 mcg of other carotenoids that can be converted to vitamin A.

The other way of expressing the activity of carotenoids is in terms of International Units (IU). One IU of vitamin A is equivalent to 0.3 mcg, and 1 IU of beta-carotene is equivalent to 0.6 mcg of beta-carotene. Thus, 1 mg of beta-carotene represents 1,667 IU, Ronzio said.

The optimum intake of beta-carotene and natural carotenoids to afford maximum protection is not known, he continued. According to the National Cancer Institute and the Food and Drug Administration, the beta-carotene intake should be the equivalent to about 6 mg daily, however, actual consumption is around 1.5 mg/day. Therefore, the average American consumes only 25% of the amount estimated to lower cancer risks.

"This means that most Americans should increase their daily intake of foods containing the most beta-carotene," Ronzio added. "One sweet potato contains 5 to 10 mg of beta-carotene, representing 2,500 RE. About 15 mg/day may be recommended if the diet is compromised by processed food, or in cases of infection or diabetes."

Epidemiologic studies suggest that a vegetable intake is associated with reduced risk of free-radical mediated degenerative diseases, such as epithelial cancers, cardiovascular disease, and age-related eye diseases, according to Karin H. von het Hof, and colleagues at Wageningen Agricultural University in the Netherlands, and colleagues in other facilities in that country.[19]

"Various studies have shown a significant correlation between habitual vegetable intake and plasma carotenoid concentrations," the researchers said. "In addition, increased vegetable consumption results in increased blood carotenoid concentrations. However, the effectiveness of vegetables as a source of carotenoids has been questioned because studies show that the bioavailability of beta-carotene from vegetables is less than previously thought. This was shown conclusively for green leafy vegetables."

The researchers added that the bioavailability of beta-carotene may, however, vary among types of vegetables because a difference was also found between fruit and green leafy vegetables.

In the study, over 4 weeks, 22 healthy adults consumed a high-vegetable diet (490 g/day), 22 consumed a low-vegetable diet (130 g/day), and 10 consumed a low-vegetable diet supplemented with pure beta-carotene (6 mg/day) and lutein (9 mg/day).

It was reported that plasma concentrations of vitamin C and carotenoids—alpha-carotene, beta-carotene, lutein, zeaxanthin, and beta-cryptoxanthin—were significantly higher after the high-vegetable diet than after the low-vegetable diet.

In addition to an increase in blood levels of beta-carotene and lutein, the pure carotenoid-supplemented diet induced a significant decrease in plasma lycopene concentration. The responses of plasma beta-carotene and lutein to the high-vegetable diet were 14 and 67%, respectively, of those to the pure carotenoid-supplemented diet. Conversion of beta-carotene to retinol/vitamin A may have attenuated its plasma response compared with that of lutein. There was no significant effect on the resistance of LDL-cholesterol oxidation, the researchers added.

"Increased vegetable consumption enhances blood levels of vitamin C and carotenoid concentrations, but not resistance of LDL to oxidation," the researchers said. "The relative bioavailability of lutein from vegetables is higher than that of beta-carotene." (LDL cholesterol is the bad kind.)

The bioavailability of carotenoids is determined by characteristics of the food source and interactions with other dietary constituents, according to Garry J. Handelman and colleagues at the Jean Mayer USDA Human Nutrition Research Center on Aging at Tufts University in Boston, Massachusetts.[20]

Studies with beta-carotene and lycopene have shown that association with a lipid (fat) matrix increases the bioavailability of these carotenoids.

"Localization within a plant—in chloroplasts or chromoplasts and compounds that interfere with intestinal micelle formation, that is, pectin—can decrease carotenoid bioavailability," the researchers added. "To some extent, the inhibitory effects of the plant matrix can be overcome by cooking to break down the plant cell wall and by decreased food particle size—chopping and pureeing. And mineral oil, which is not digestible, can interfere with the absorption of carotenoids."

In the study, 11 moderately hypercholesterolemic (high cholesterol) men and women consumed 2 separate diets, which contained 29-33% of energy as total fat, with 20% of energy as either beef tallow or corn oil. The diets were supplemented with cooked chicken egg yolks (1.3 egg yolks/day).

Each volunteer consumed each diet for 4.5 weeks, with a washout period of over 2 weeks between diet phases. At the end of each diet phase, fasting morning plasma samples were collected and stored for carotenoid analysis by high-pressure liquid chromatography. Egg yolks were analyzed for carotenoids and cholesterol.

Egg yolk supplementation of the beef tallow diet increased plasma lutein by 28% and zeaxanthin by 142%, the researchers said. Supplementation of the corn oil diet increased plasma lutein by 50% and zeaxanthin by 114%.

Changes in plasma lycopene and beta-carotene were variable, with no consistent trend. However, egg yolk supplementation increased plasma LDL-cholesterol concentrations by 8-11%.

"Lutein and zeaxanthin have been identified as carotenoids that accumulate in the macular region of the human retina, which may play a role in the prevention of age-related macular degeneration, and some forms of cancer," the researchers continued. "However, like many dietary carotenoids, lutein and zeaxanthin are not converted to vitamin A by human metabolism.

They went on to say that egg yolks produced in the United States contain large amounts of lutein and zeaxanthin when compared with other common dietary sources of carotenoids, and the chicken egg yolk is a matrix composed of digestible lipids, i.e., cholesterol, tryacylglycerol, and phospholipids. The 2 carotenoids are dispersed in this matrix along with other fat-soluble micronutrients such as vitamins A, D, and E.

"Egg yolk is a highly bioavailable source of lutein and zeaxanthin," the researchers added. "The benefit of introducing these carotenoids into the diet with egg yolk is counterbalanced by potential LDL-cholesterol elevation from the added dietary cholesterol."

A number of studies have demonstrated that beta-carotene can enhance some aspects of immunity, reported Biological and Pharmaceutical Bulletin. One study found that carrots inhibited an early step in the immune response to lab animals sensitized to an allergen, which suggests the potential benefits of nutrients in preventing or easing allergies.[21]

The research team tested the immune-modulating effects of beta-carotene in mice immunized with egg albumin to develop sensitivity to this egg white protein. The sensitized animals consumed food without added beta-carotene or with one of three different levels of beta-carotene.

It was reported that beta-carotene had significantly lower levels of two allergy-related antibodies—IgE and IgG1—than the mice not given beta-carotene. The mice fed beta-carotene had increased levels of IgG2a antibodies.

In addition, the mice consuming beta-carotene in their chow did not suffer a shock-like decrease in body temperature after exposure to an allergen.

The researchers also reported that the mice given beta-carotene altered the cytokine production in spleen cells, shifting the chemical signals associated with a specific type of allergic reaction that produces hypersensitivity to foods or airborne allergens.

The research team concluded that dietary beta-carotene could be helping in preventing allergies, especially during infancy, through suppression of the antigen-specific IgE antibody response.

Between 1983 and 1984, 6 hospitals in southwestern France were sources of 106 cases of epidemoid lung cancer and compared with 212 controls, according to the European Journal of Clinical Epidemiology.[22]

Daily intakes of vitamin A and beta-carotene were computed, and it was reported that lower consumption of preformed vitamin A and beta-carotene were independently and significantly correlated with epidemoid lung cancer.

The researchers, at the University of Bordeaux in France, confirmed the protective role of beta-carotene against lung cancer, and gave evidence that preformed vitamin A may also have a protective effect. Vitamin A is thought to inhibit tumor promotion, while beta-carotene tends to inhibit tumor initiation.

Oxidative stress contributes to brain aging, and antioxidant supplements, especially over the long term, are thought to confer cognitive benefits, according to F. Grodstein, et al., in Archives of Internal Medicine.[23]

Among 1,904 newly recruited volunteers, who had been treated for 1 year, cognition was similar across treatment assignments. Also, among 4,052 continuing participants from the Physicians' Health Study, with a mean treatment of 18 years, the mean global score was significantly higher in the beta-carotene group than in those given a placebo.

In the study, beta-carotene was given at 50 mg on alternative days. On verbal memory, the men given long-term beta-carotene supplements performed significantly better than the placebo group.

"We did not find an impact on short-term beta-carotene supplementation on cognitive performance, but long-term supplementation may provide cognitive benefits", the researchers said.

In one clinical study, it was reported that during the year prior to being diagnosed with cancer, men who got less than 1.7 mg (about 2,000 IU) of beta-carotene a day—the amount in about an inch of carrot—were twice as likely to develop the disease as men who got more than 2.7 mg (about 4,400 IU) daily, reported Prevention's Healing with Vitamins.[24]

In another study, breast cancer risk almost doubled in postmenopausal women who ate the fewest carotene-rich foods, compared with women who ate more of these foods. The risk was said to drop off sharply once women reached a beta-carotene intake of more than 5,824 IU per day. That is the amount in about a third of a carrot or 36-oz, glasses of vegetable juice cocktail.

"Laboratory studies support beta-carotene's anti-cancer role," commented Norman Krinsky, Ph.D., of Tufts University School of Medicine in Boston, Masachusetts. "Animals given large doses of beta-carotene prior to being exposed to a cancer-causing chemical are less likely to develop cancerous tumors."

In a study by Abram Hoffer, M.D., Ph.D., and Linus Pauling, Ph.D., they evaluated people with cancer who were receiving state-of-the-art treatment, such as chemotherapy and radiation.

"Those who continued eating as they had before they found out they had cancer had an average life span of 5.7 months," the researchers said. "Of those receiving nutritional therapy—high-dose vitamins and minerals as well as information on food selection—20% were considered poor responders. Still, their survival time was almost twice that of the patients not receiving nutritional support. The 80% considered good responders had an average life span of 6 years."

This group included those with tough-to-treat cancers—lung, pancreas and liver—commented Patrick Quillin, Ph.D., of the Cancer Treatment Centers of America in Arlington Heights,

Illinois. Women with cancer of the breast, overies, cervix or uterus did the best. Their life span was 10 years, a 21-fold improvement over those who did not get nutrition therapy.

In a study at West Virginia University School of Medicine in Morgantown, men with bladder cancer who took mega-doses of vitamin A (40,000 IU); vitamin B6 (100 mg); vitamin C (2,000 mg), vitamin E (400 IU), and zinc (90 mg), in addition to a multivitamin/mineral that provided the RDA and their regular therapy, had a 40% reduction in tumor recurrence compared with those getting only the RDA of these nutrients. The study reported that after 5 years, the men taking large amounts of nutrients went for a significantly longer time without tumor recurrence.

For those who have had lung cancer, some doctors may recommend up to 500,000 IU of beta-carotene, added Quillin. While this amount is considered non-toxic, you should review it with your doctor.

Reduced blood levels of beta-carotene are associated with an increased incidence of cancer in humans, according to Richard P. Huemer, M.D.[25,26]

Beta-carotene is a powerful photochemical quenching agent of the oxidant species singlet oxygen. If not quenched, singlet oxygen, which is 22 kal/mole above the ground-state energy of normal molecular oxygen, can react with unsaturated lipids (fats) to yield hydroperoxides.

"These hydroperoxides can then initiate free-radical damage to DNA, resulting in mutagenesis or possibly carcinogenesis," Huemer said. "Singlet oxygen is produced in cellular systems by dismutation of superoxide anion, either enzymatically or chemically."

Singlet oxygen can also be produced by photodynamic action, which is the transfer of sun energy through a photosensitizer such as hemoglobin to the oxygen molecule, he continued. Much of the sun-induced damage to skin, with associated potential for skin cancer, may be due to the secondary effects of photodynamically produced singlet oxygen, which induces DNA alteration.

"By quenching singlet oxygen, beta-carotene has the same protective role against this peroxidizing agent as the enzyme superoxide dismutase (SOD) does with superoxide anion," he added. "Bland, et al. have demonstrated that singlet oxygen is one of the major oxidant species responsible for oxidation of the erythrocyte membrane when the red cell is exposed to light and oxygen."

The intake of antioxidants, which can neutralize reactive oxygen species (ROS) generated endogenously or exogenuously, has been extensively investigated to relation of DNA damage and cancer risk, reported Lee C. Yong and colleagues at the National Institute for Occupational Safety and Health in Cincinnati, Ohio.[27-31]

The information is of special interest to airline pilots, astronauts in space flight, flight crews, and frequent fliers.

"Ionizing radiation (IR) is an established human carcinogen and an efficient inducer of chromosome aberration, which have also been shown to be associated with increased cancer risk in prospective studies," they said.

They went on to say that, in addition to causing direct damage to DNA, IR exposure is an exogenous source of a wide range of reactive oxygen species, including the superoxide anion and hydroxyl radicals and other nonradical species such as hydrogen peroxide.

Their study indicates that high intakes of vitamin C, beta-carotene, beta-cryptoxanthin, and lutein-zeaxanthin from food, especially their combined intakes that include vitamin E, are significantly associated with a decrease in the translocation frequency of airline pilots with ionizing radiation exposure.

"These findings suggest that a diet containing a variety of fruit and vegetables that provide a natural source of these antioxidants, as well as other potential protective factors, may offer the best protection against cumulative DNA damage associated with ionizing radiation exposure," they continued.

They added that their results may be applicable to flight crews worldwide, astronauts in space flight, and frequent fliers in the general population. Studies involving larger IR-exposed populations and their intake of these antioxidants are needed to determine any possible cancer risk, they added.

Selected Plant Sources of Vitamin A (From Beta-Carotene)

Food	*IU*	*% DV*
Carrot, 1 raw, 7 1/2 in. long	20,250	410
Carrots, boiled, 1/2 –cup slices	19,150	380
Carrot juice, canned, 1/2 cup	12,915	260
Sweet potatoes, canned drained solids, 1/2 cup	7,015	140
Spinach, frozen, boiled, 1/2 cup	7,395	150
Mango, raw, 1 cup sliced	6,425	130
Vegetable soup, canned, chunky, ready-to-serve, 1/2 cup	5,880	115
Cantaloupe, raw, 1 cup	5,160	105
Kale, frozen, boiled, 1/2 cup	4,130	80
Spinach, raw, 1 cup	2,015	40
Apricot nectar, canned, 1/2 cup	1,650	35

*DV - Daily Value. DVs are reference numbers based on the Recommended Dietary Allowance (RDA). They were developed to help consumers determine if a food contains a lot or a little of a specific nutrient. The DV for vitamin A is 5,000 IU (1,500 mcg retinol). The percent DV (% DV) listed on the nutrient facts panel of food labels tells adults what percentage of the DV is provided in one serving. Percent DVs are based on a 2,000 calorie diet. Your Daily Value may be higher or lower depending on your calorie needs. Foods that provide lower percentages of the DV also contribute to a healthful diet.

Source: "Vitamin A and Carotenoids," National Institutes of Health, Bethesda, Maryland, October 6, 2003.

Retinol Activity Equivalents (RAE) Ratios for Beta-Carotene and Other Provitamin A Carotenoids

Quantity Consumed	*Quantity Bioconverted to Retinol*	*RAE Ratio*
1 mcg of dietary or supplemental vitamin A	1 mcg of retinol*	1:1
2 mcg of supplemental beta-carotene	1 mcg of retinol	2:1
12 mcg of dietary beta-carotene	1 mcg of retinol	12:1
24 mcg of dietary alpha-carotene	1 mcg of retinol	24:1
24 mcg of dietary beta-cryptoxanthin	1 mcg of retinol	24:1

*One IU is equivalent to 0.3 microgram (mcg) of retinol, and 1 mcg of retinol is equivalent to 3.33 IU of retinol.

Source: "Vitamin A," Linus Pauling Institute at Oregon State University, Corvallis, October 20, 2008.

Selected Plant Sources of Vitamin A (From Beta-Carotene)

Food	*IU*	*%DV**
Oatmeal, instant, fortified, plain, prepared with water, 1 packet	1,510	30
Tomato juice, canned, 6 oz.	1,010	20
Apricots, with skin, juice pack, 2 halves	610	10
Pepper, sweet, red, raw 1 ring, 3 in. in diameter by 1/4 in. thick	570	10
Peas, frozen, boiled, 1/2 cup	535	10
Peach, raw, 1 medium	525	10
Peaches, canned, juice pack, 1/2 cup halves or slices	470	10
Papaya, raw, 1 cup cubes	400	8

*DV-Daily Value. DVs are reference numbers based on the Recommended Dietary Allowance (RDA). They were developed to help consumers determine if a food contains a lot or a little of a specific nutrient. The DV for vitamin A is 5,000 IU (1,500 mcg retinol). The percent DV (%DV) listed on the nutrition facts panel of food labels tells adults what percentage of the DV is provided in one serving. Percent DVs are based on a 2,000 calorie diet. Your Daily Values may be higher or lower depending on your calorie needs. Foods that provide lower percentages of the DV also contribute to a healthful diet.

Source: "Vitamin A and Carotenoids," National Institutes of Health, Bethesda, Maryland, October 6, 2003.

References

1. Ho, Charlene C., et al. "Excentral Cleavage of Beta-Carotene in Vivo in a Healthy Man," American Journal of Clinical Nutrition 85:770-777, 2007.

2. Khachik, F., et al. "Separation, Identification, and Quantification of Carotenoids in Fruits, Vegetables and Human Plasma by High Performance Liquid Chromatography," Pure Applied Chemistry 63:71-80, 1991.

3. Passwater, Richard A., Ph.D. "Beta-Carotene and Vitamin A." The Nutrition Superbook: The Antioxidants. New Canaan, CT: Keats Publishing, Inc., 1995, pp. 50 ff.

4. Wang, Jie, et al, "Vitamin A Equivalence of Spirulina Beta-Carotene in Chinese Adults as Assessed by Using a Stable-Isotope Reference Method," American Journal of Clinical Nutrition 87:1730-1737, 2008.

5. Ross, A.C., et al. "Vitamin A and Retinoids in Antiviral Responses," FASEB Journal 10:979-985, 1996.
6. Goodman, D.S. "Vitamin A and Retinoids in Health and Disease," New England Journal of Medicine 310:1023-1031, 1984.
7. Weld, G. "Molecular Basis of Visual Excitation," Science 162:230-239, 1968.
8. Hathcock, J.N., et al. "Evaluation of Vitamin A Toxicity," American Journal of Clinical Nutrition 52:183-202, 1990.
9. Ribaya-Mercado, Judy D., et al. "Carotene-Rich Plant Foods Ingested with Mineral Dietary Fat Enhances the Total-Body Vitamin A Pool Size in Filipino School Children as Assessed by Stable-Isotope-Dilution Methodology," American Journal of Clinical Nutrition 85:1041-1049, 2007.
10. Sommer, A., et al. "Vitamin A deficiency. Health, Survival and Vision. New York: Oxford University Press, 1966.
11. Roels, O.A., et al. "Carotene Balances on Boys in Rawanda Where Vitamin A Deficiency is Prevalent," Journal of Nutrition 65:115-127, 1958.
12. Sherman, Carl. "Beta-Carotene Aids Barrett's Esophagus Symptoms," Family Practice News, December 15, 1995, p. 13.
13. Rock, C., et al. "Plasma Beta-Carotene Response in Humans After Meals Supplemented with Dietary Pectin," American Journal of Clinical Nutrition 55:96-99, 1992.
14. Torbergsen, A.C., and Collins, A.R. "Recovery of Human Lymphocytes from Oxidative DNA Damage: The Apparent Enchancement of DNA Repair by Carotenoids is Probably Simply An Antioxidant Effect," European Journal of Nutrition 39:80-85, 2000.
15. Edes, Thomas E., M.D. "Beta-Carotene and Vitamin A: Casting Separate Shadows," The Nutrition Report 10(2):9, 16, February 1992.
16. Hurley, Dan. "Beta-Carotene May Detoxify Carcinogens," Medical Tribune, August 20, 1992, p. 24.
17. Chao, J.C.J., et al. "Effects of Beta-Carotene, Vitamin C and E on Antioxidant Status in Hyperlipidemic Smokers," Journal of Nutritional Biochemistry 13:427-434, 2002.
18. Ronzio, Robert A., Ph.D. The Encyclopedia of Nutrition and Good Health. New York: Facts on File, Inc., 1997, pp. 47-48.
19. Van het Hof, Karin H., et al. "Bioavailability of Lutein from Vegetables is 5 Times Higher Than That of Beta-Carotene," American Journal of Clinical Nutrition 70:261-268, 1999.

20. Handelman, Garry J., et al., "Lutein and Zeaxanthin Concentrations in Plasma After Dietary Supplementation with Egg Yolk," ibid, pp. 247-251.
21. Sato, Y., et al. "The Feeding of Beta-Carotene Down-Regulates Serum IgE levels and Inhibits the Type 1 Allergic Response in Mice," Biological and Pharmaceutical Bulletin 27:978-984, 2004.
22. Dargigues, J.F., et al. "Dietary Vitamin A, Beta-Carotene and Risk of Epidermoid Lung Cancer in Southwestern France," European Journal of Clinical Epidemiology 6(3):261-265, 1990.
23. Grodstein, F., et al. "Randomized Trial of Beta-Carotene Supplementation and Cognitive Function in Men: The Physicians' Health Study II," Archives of Internal Medicine 167(20):2184-2190, 2007.
24. Feinstein, Alice, managing editor, Prevention's Healing with Vitamins. Emmaus, PA: Rodale Press, Inc., 1996, pp. 143ff.
25. Bland, Jeffrey, Ph.D. "Lipid Peroxidation-Induced Diseases: A Model of Molecular Disease." In Huemer, Richard P., M.D. The Roots of Molecular Medicine. A Tribute to Linus Pauling. New York: W.H. Freeman and Co., 1986, pp. 62ff.
26. Rosenbaum, Michael, M.D. "Nutrients and the Immune System," *ibid*, p. 162.
27. Yong, Lee C., et al. "High Dietary Antioxidant Intakes are Associated with Decreased Chromosome Translocation Frequency in Airline Pilots," American Journal of Clinical Nutrition 90:1402-1410, 2009.
28. Diplock, A.T., et al. "Functional Food Science and Defense Against Reactive Oxygen Species," British Journal of Nutrition 80(Supp.1): S77-S112, 1998.
29. Machlin, L.J., and Bendich, A. "Free Radical Tissue Damage: Protective Role of Antioxidant Nutrients," FASEB Journal 1:441-445, 1987.
30. Rao, A.V., and Rao, L.G. "Carotenoids and Human Health, Pharmacological Research 55:207-216, 2007.
31. Lin, J., et al. "Vitamins C and E and Beta-Carotene Supplementation and Cancer Risk: A Randomized Controlled Trial," Journal of the National Cancer Institute 101:14-23, 2009.

3

HIV/AIDS

HIV / AIDS

Acquired Immunodeficiency Syndrome (AIDS) was initially recognized in 1981 by experts from the Centers for Disease Control and Prevention in Atlanta, Georgia, according to Medical and Health Annual. The earliest patients were homosexual men in New York and California, but, within a short time, as cases were recognized in intravenous drug users and in blood-transfusion and blood-product recipients, it became clear that the disease affected a wide range of the population, explained Julia Heptonstall, M.Sc.[1]

In 1983, the virus that causes AIDS, named human immunodeficiency virus (HIV), was isolated, and blood tests for the diagnosis of HIV infection were in widespread use by the end of 1985.

"During the mid-1980s, the worldwide spread of AIDS became evident, and the rapidly increasing rate of HIV infection in Africa was revealed," Heptonstall said. "By 1990, health officials had become concerned about the growing number of HIV-positive people in Asia."

The initial stages of HIV infection may be completely asymptomatic, and those infected with the virus may remain perfectly well for many years. During this time, however, they are capable of transmitting the virus to others. Once AIDS has been diagnosed, average survival is between 2 and 3 years. Actually, more than 50% of AIDS patients will not survive 5 years.

"Between 13 and 48% (the figures vary widely between) countries) of babies born to infected women acquire HIV before, during, or after birth," Heptonstall continued.

Two types of HIV, with different patterns of geographic distribution, are known to exist. Type 1, called HIV-1, is the predominant virus, having spread rapidly worldwide from the mid- to late 1970s onward. The World Health Organization estimated that by mid-1993, 14 million people were infected with HIV-1, and the number was expected to rise.

The second type, HIV-2, appears to be both less infectious and less virulent than HIV-1. Although occasional cases of HIV-2 have been reported from outside Africa, at present the virus is largely confined to West Africa.

HIV has been transmitted by the use of inadequately sterilized needles, syringes, and other medical equipment, as well as unprotected sex. In addition to injections and vaccines, traditional healing practices, acupuncture, tattoing, and ear or body piercing may carry a risk of HIV infection.

"Even such seemingly innocuous activities as getting a shave in a barber shop or a manicure or pedicure in a beauty saloon could carry a risk of infection, if razors and other implements are not scrupulously cleaned after each use," Heptonstall added.

At the XVII International AIDS Conference in Mexico City, Mexico, in August 2008, there were an estimated 33 million people living with HIV worldwide, of whom 2.7 million became infected in 2007, and 2 million died from AIDS in 2007.[2]

However, in general, fewer children, who account for about 15% of the totals and fewer adults became infected, reported Robert Steinbrook, M.D.

In sub-Saharan Africa, most national epidemics have stabilized or—in Zimbabwe, for example—have begun to diminish, as measured by annual determinations of HIV prevalence among women given prenatal care. However, in Kenya, infections are on the rise, as they are in Russia and Ukraine, which have the largest epidemics in Eastern Europe and Central Asia. In Russia, injection-drug users lack access to methadone and to large-scale programs providing clean needles and syringes.

"Highly active antiretroviral therapy is remarkably effective for infected people who can receive treatment on an ongoing basis," Steinbrook added. "Indeed, many people with HIV infection can now look forward to achieving nondetectable viral loads and relatively normal lives and life spans—developments that were once hard to imagine."

There are 25 approved antiretroviral drugs, and more are on the way, but poverty, stigma, discrimination, inadequate health care systems, and other social problems remain powerful barriers to treatment and prevention programs.

"The search for an effective AIDS vaccine, the holy grail of biomedical HIV-prevention research, remains unsuccessful, in large part because there is insufficient understanding of the critical immune responses for controlling the virus," Steinbrook continued.

Although mother-to-child transmission has been almost entirely preventable for years, only a third of infected pregnant women receive antiretroviral drugs to prevent transmission, and even fewer receive medications for their own health.

Steinbrook went on to say that the Swiss National AIDS Commission recently concluded that those with HIV infection cannot transmit the virus through sexual relations if they are receiving effective treatment, take their medications as prescribed, have had undetectable virus in plasma (less than 40 copies per milliliter) for at least 6 months, and have no additional sexually transmitted diseases.

The Centers for Disease Control and Prevention in Atlanta, Georgia, estimates that the one quarter of HIV-infected people in the United States who are unaware that they are infected account for more than half of all new infections. The CDC has yet to update its estimate that roughly 1 million people were infected as of the end of 2003.

"Now that the world is gaining ground against the AIDS epidemic, the challenge is to sustain and accelerate the progress before the XVIII International AIDS Conference convenes in Vienna, Austria, in July 2010," Steinbrook concluded. "The message from Mexico City was that individuals and societies must implement effective and multifaceted treatment and prevention programs, advance human rights, and invest in AIDS and health-care systems."

While we have seen dramatic successes in the treatment of HIV-infected people in the United States and many other countries, the pandemic still rages, with 2.7 million new infections in 2007, reported Margaret I. Johnston, Ph.D., and Authony S. Fauci, M.D., in the August 28, 2008 issue of the New England Journal of Medicine.[3]

However, for every infected person who began receiving antiretroviral therapy in 2007, 2.5 people were newly infected with HIV. Historically, vaccines have been among the most effective public health interventions, preventing the spread of viral infections, but an HIV vaccine has thus far been elusive and the quest disappointing and frustrating, prompting some to wonder whether an effective vaccine will ever be added to the HIV-prevention toolbox, the authors said.

Concerning an HIV infection, the natural immune response against HIV is completely inadequate and, once primary infection is established, fails to eradicate the virus. With uncommon exceptions, HIV disease is relentlessly progressive, and virtually no one has a spontaneous recovery. Unlike other viruses for which we have successful human vaccines, HIV quickly integrates itself into the DNA of the host cell, where, in some cells, it remains latent and essentially invisible to the immune system.

"Because latency is established very early—within days to weeks after infection—the window of opportunity wherein HIV remains vulnerable to eradication through the immune response is very short," the authors continued. "Once latency is established, it has not yet been possible to eradicate the virus, even in patients receiving highly active antiretroviral therapy for extended periods."

The authors added that by the time the body produces antibodies directed at the outer HIV envelope protein, which is the key target for neutralizing antibodies, the protein has mutated in such a way that the circulating antibodies cannot neutralize it. New antibodies are induced, but new mutations repeatedly enable the virus to evade the immune system.

A lack of vitamin A is known to increase the risk of many infections, and it has been associated with a greater risk of HIV in underdeveloped countries, according to the Journal of Acquired Deficiency Syndrome. The susceptibility may be due, in part, to weakened mucosal epithelial lining around tissues, whose integrity depends on vitamin A.[4]

In the study, a research team evaluated men and women who were treated at 2 clinics in India, which specialized in sexually transmitted diseases. Because of their lifestyle, these patients have an above-average risk of contracting HIV.

The research team measured blood levels of antioxidants in 44 men and women who were diagnosed with the HIV infection, and compared them with 44 men and women who had not contracted HIV.

The researchers found that most of the micronutrients measured in the volunteers were lower than the normal range for healthy adults in the United States. While there was no difference between average micronutrient levels of patients who contracted the virus, compared with those who did not, people with low blood levels, of either beta-carotene or vitamin A, were more likely to contract HIV infection than patients with high levels.

Those with low levels of beta-carotene, which, as we know, is converted into vitamin A in the body, were 21 times more likely to acquire the HIV infection.

At Johns Hopkins Hospital in Baltimore, Maryland, Richard D. Semba, M.D., and colleagues, evaluated vitamin A levels, helper cells, complete blood count, and serologic markers of liver disease in 179 HIV-1 infected people.[5]

More than 15% of the HIV-1 positive people had plasma vitamin A levels less than 1.05 micromol/1. This level is consistent with a vitamin A deficiency.

The HIV-1 seropositive people had lower mean plasma vitamin A levels than the HIV-1 seronegative people. A vitamin A deficiency was associated with lower CD4 helper cell levels among both seronegative and seropositive patients.

Semba added that, in the HIV-1 seropositive patients, vitamin A deficiency was associated with increased mortality. Therefore, a vitamin A deficiency appears to be an important risk factor for disease progression in HIV-1 infection.

As reported in Medical Tribune, 21 HIV-infected patients, most of whom were taking the drug AZT, were given either 180 mg/day of beta-carotene or a placebo for 4 weeks. This was followed by 4 weeks of the opposite therapy.[6]

Blood samples were taken after 2, 3, 6, and 8 weeks, and it was found that CD4 helper cells in some people improved after 4 weeks. CD4 is a large glycoprotein that is found on the surface of T4 cells, and is the receptor for HIV.

Those given beta-carotene had average elevations in their CD4 cells of about 17%. Total white blood cell counts also increased with beta-carotene but not with placebo. There were no side effects on the vitamin therapy, and nobody died.

Gregg O. Coodley, M.D., who discussed the research at the Oregon Health Sciences Center in Portland, noted the possibility that beta-carotene supplemented HIV-infected patients would not be susceptible to opportunistic infections, and the progression from HIV to full-blown AIDS may even be delayed.

By applying techniques from molecular biology to the quantification of HIV, scientists have developed assays based on detection of the virus's Ribonucleic Acid (RNA), its genetic material. Like all retroviruses, HIV carries its genetic information in the form of RNA, rather than DNA, according to Daniel R. Kuritzkes, M.D.[7]

It is the eventual depletion of HIV T-helper cells, also known CD4 + lymphocytes (which, along with monocytes, are the immune system cells targeted by the virus), that leads to immunodeficiency and AIDS.

"As the immune system deteriorates, the rate of virus production increases, and the plasma levels of HIV RNA rise," Kuritzkes said. "Thus the lowest levels of virus are found in relatively healthy patients with normal CD4-lymphocyte counts. Slightly higher levels are found in patients with lower CD4 + counts, and mild symptoms of HIV infection, and the highest levels of virus are found in patients with nearly depleted CD4+ lymphocytes and AIDS."

Healthy people have 800 to 1,200 CD4+lymphocytes per cubic millimeter of blood. A CD4+ count of 200 or less is diagnostic of AIDS.

In a study of 60 AIDS patients with retinol (vitamin A) status, who were not taking vitamin supplements, and who were not pregnant, 22% had low levels of retinol in their blood, according to Dennis L. Karter, M.D., and colleagues, St. Vincent's Hospital in New York.[8]

There was a 241-fold greater prevalence of low retinol levels than that of the normal U.S. population. Also, there was a positive association between serum retinol and dietary intake, but 27% of those who had adequate intake had blood levels of the vitamin below the normal range.

These results suggest that, regardless of intake, patients with AIDS may be a population at risk for vitamin A deficiency, Karter added. Actually, absorption and utilization of vitamin A may be as important as dietary intake in this population.

The link between dietary serum vitamin A levels with oxidative stress, helper T-cell counts, vertical transmission of HIV, the progression of AIDS, the mortality shown in previous studies suggest that an investigation on the value of vitamin A supplemention on the clinical progression of AIDS is warranted, Karter added.

Beta-carotene appeared to have immunostimulatory effects in not only HIV-infected patients, but also healthy people as well, according to the American Journal of Clinical Nutrition.[9]

The study evaluated lymphocyte subsets before and after 44 weeks of beta-carotene supplementation at 60 mg/day in 10 patients with HIV and 10 controls.

The researchers reported an increase in plasma and mononuclear cell beta-carotene levels to 4 and 3 times the baseline (beginning) values after 2 and 4 weeks, respectively.

It was also reported that CD4/CD8 (helper suppressor ratio) increased after 9 months of beta-carotene supplementation, although natural killer cells, virgin T cells, memory T cells, and cytotoxic T cells remained unchanged. No side effects were recorded.

The CD4/CD8 count is the ratio of the number of helper-induced T lymphocytes to cytotoxic-suppressor T lymphocytes, as measured by monoclonal antibodies to the CD4 surface antigen found on helper-inducer T cells, and the CD8 surface antigen found on cytotoxic-suppressor T cells, according to Stedman's Medical Dictionary.[10]

The publication added that, "when the body mounts an immune response, as against a virus or a transplant, the ratio is almost always reduced because of a decrease in the number of circulating helper-inducer cells, and an increase in suppressor cells."

The CD4/CD8 count has been used to monitor signs of organ rejection after transplantation, and more recently has become a tool for assessing the relative condition of HIV patients, the publication continued. With the CD4 absolute count, and the CD4 lymphocyte percentage, it provides a way of gauging the progression from HIV to AIDS.

In studying 84 HIV positive patients, researchers in Brooklyn, New York, found 31% of the patients were carotene deficient and an additional 40% of the population were in the lower quartile of the normal range. This indicates more than 70% of the patients were either carotene deficient or in the low-normal range.[11]

The cause of carotene deficiency is not known, but it may be due to decreased absorption or increased metabolic use of carotenes in HIV-infected patients.

HIV-infected patients have selenium and vitamin A deficiencies, compared with unaffected controls, and they may benefit from supplementation, according to a research team at the University of Bordeaux in France.[12]

At the University of Natal in South Africa, a randomized, placebo-controlled trial of vitamin A supplementation was carried out in 118 offspring of HIV-infected women in Durban, South Africa. The infants were given a supplement of 50,000 IU of vitamin A at 1 and 3 months of age; 100,000 IU at 6 and 9 months; and 200,000 IU at 12 and 15 months of age.[13]

Among all the children, the supplemented group had a lower overall morbidity than the placebo group, reported Anna Coutsoudis, Ph.D.

Among the 85 children of known HIV status, morbidity associated with diarrhea was significantly reduced in the supplemented affected children, whereas there was no effect on supplementation on diarrheal morbidity noted among the unaffected children.

In a population that is not generally vitamin A deficient, vitamin A supplementation for children with HIV-infected women appeared to be beneficial, reducing morbidity. The benefit was especially observed for diarrhea among HIV-infected children.

It is noted that vitamin A is inexpensive, and it can be expected to benefit infected children by reducing the incidence and severity of diarrhea and, therefore, the burden on health care services, not less, by improving the quality of life for children and their caretakers, Coutsoudis added.

As reported in The Lancet, 10 to 40% of HIV-positive women who give birth will infect their children with the virus, according to Richard D. Semba, M.D. A vitamin A deficiency is common among pregnant women with HIV, and nutritional intervention may be a practical and inexpensive way of reducing mother-to-child transmission of HIV.[14]

A number of nutritional abnormalities in HIV infection include vitamins A, E, B6, B12, B2, copper and zinc deficiencies, Semba said.

In the study, mother-to-child transmission in 338 HIV-positive women was 21.9% among mothers whose infants survived to 12 months of age. Mean vitamin A concentrations in 74 mothers who transmitted HIV to their infants was lower than the 264 who did not transmit to their infants.

It was also reported that there was an inverse relationship between vitamin A concentrations in the mother and the risk of HIV transmission. Maternal helper cell counts, percent helper cells, and the helper/suppressor ratio were associated with an increased risk to mother-to-child transmission.

The authors added that maternal vitamin A deficiency contributes to mother-to-child transmission of HIV.

The presence of hyporetinemia in HIV virus-infected diseases is 29%, according to Clinical Infectious Diseases. These patients have a 3.5-5-fold increased risk of death.[15]

HIV-infected people with very low or very high intakes of vitamin A and beta-carotene have greater rates of diseases progression than do those with intermediate intakes, reported Ajani Nimmagadda and colleagues.

In the developing countries, 1½ up to 60% of HIV-infected pregnant women are hyporetinemic. And in these patients, the relative risk of perinatal HIV transmission may be increased more than 4-fold.

A vitamin A deficiency is common in HIV-infected patients in developed countries, and supplementation with the vitamin may be especially beneficial as an adjunctive therapy for HIV-infected pregnant women living in developing countries, the researchers added.

In evaluating 687 children, ranging in age from 6 months to 5 years, they were admitted to hospital with pneumonia, reported Pediatric and Infectious Disease Journal.[16]

The older children were given a placebo or 400,000 IU of vitamin A, given in 2 divided doses of 200,000 IU, while those under 1 year of age received half that amount. The children were given additional doses utilizing the same regimen 4 and 8 months after hospital discharge. Of the 648 children who were evaluated, 9% were HIV-infected.

Compared with uninfected children, all-cause mortality was higher among HIV-infected children, as was mortality caused by pneumonia or diarrhea.

Overall, vitamin A supplementation results in a 49% reduction in mortality, the researchers said. And vitamin A supplementation reduced all-cause mortality by 63% among HIV-infected children.

The researchers added that vitamin A supplements were also associated with a 68% reduction in AIDS-related deaths, and a 92% reduction in diarrhea-related deaths.

Research conducted at the Tucson Veteran's Administration Medical Center and the University of Arizona Health Sciences Center in Tucson, found that those with confirmed HIV infection showed improved immune response as a result of increasing their beta-carotene intake.[17]

Each of the patients was given 60 mg/day of beta-carotene for 4 months. Clinical data was collected at the beginning of the study, during the study, and 2 months following supplementation.

Following 3 months of beta-carotene supplementation, increases were found in natural killer cell and lymphocyte activity, in spite of no changes in total lymphocyte numbers. No toxicity symptoms were reported.

The research team added that beta-carotene might enhance certain aspects of immune function in HIV-infected people, just as this provitamin A has been shown in other studies to stimulate immunocompetence in healthy people.

Serum vitamin A and beta-carotene concentrations were measured in 74 pregnant seropositive females with AIDS, and 148 pregnant seronegative controls, reported researchers at Mahidol University in Bangkok, Thailand.[18]

Both parameters were decreased in HIV-1 infected women in the first trimester with CD4 counts lower than 200 cells/mcg/l. Beta-carotene and vitamin A correlated with CD4 counts, reported Winit Phuapradit, M.D.

In evaluating 108 HIV-1 seropositive men, researchers found a deficiency in vitamin A and vitamin B12 was associated with a decline in CD4-helper cell counts, while normalization of vitamin A, vitamin B12, and zinc was associated with higher CD4 counts, according to Marianna K. Baum, M.D., and colleagues at the University of Miami School of Medicine in Florida. Zidovudine (AZT) an inhibitor of in vitro replication of the HIV virus, the causative agent of AIDS and AIDS-related complex (ARC), used in the management of these diseases, did not affect any of these values.[19]

Low levels of vitamin B12 at the beginning of the study predicted accelerated HIV-1 disease progression. This data suggests that micronutrient deficiencies are associated with HIV-1 progression, and raises the possibilities that normalizing these micronutrient levels may increase symptom-free survival, the researchers said.

Urine and blood samples of vitamin A were evaluated in AIDS patients, and those who were not experiencing acute infection had small amounts of retinol excreted in the urine, reported AIDS magazine.[20]

Exacerbation of AIDS may result in vitamin A depletion, according to a research team at the University of Alabama in Birmingham. A lower dose of vitamin A (13,000 to 20,000 IU/day), rather than a higher dose of more than 20,000 IU/day may cause slower progression of AIDS, the researchers said.

Fifty adults who died of AIDS infections were matched with 227 controls who survived, reported Richard D. Semba, M.D., in the Journal of Infectious Diseases. At a mean length of follow-up of 2.4 years, vitamin A deficiency occurred in 50% and wasting occurred in 38% in the last visit before death.[21]

A CD4 cell count less than 200 mcg/1, wasting, and vitamin A deficiency were associated with mortality.

Semba and his colleagues added that there was a higher risk of death in HIV-infected patients with vitamin A deficiency and wasting. The latter refers to a disease characterized by emaciation and becoming abnormally thin. These conditions are common during HIV-infection, and are independent predictors of mortality in HIV-infected injection drug users.

In 449 HIV-seriopositive pregnant women, who were evaluated at entry, 25 and 34 weeks gestation, and in delivery, the women were enrolled in an HIV multicenter cohort study, reported Clinical Infectious Diseases.[22]

Results showed that during the third trimester 29.6% of the women had low and 11.1% had very low vitamin A levels. Women with low and very low vitamin A levels before the third trimester were more likely to deliver infants with low-birth weight (less than 2,500 mg), than were the women with higher levels. But there was no statistically significant association between vitamin A levels and mother-to-infant transmission of HIV.

However, anemia and low body mass index before the third trimester were associated with an increased risk of HIV transmission from mother to infant.

In evaluating serum and urinary retinol in 26 patients from an AIDS clinic (non-acute illness) or hospital (acute illness), it was found that mean serum retinol levels were lower in hospitalized patients than in clinic patients, reported Pauline E. Jolly, Ph.D.[23]

Urinary retinal loss was significantly higher in hospitalized patients than clinic patients, and there were significant correlations between urinary retinol excretion and body weight loss in clinic patients, and between urinary retinol loss and high serum bilirubin levels in hospital patients. An excess of bilirubin is associated with jaundice.

It was also reported that a significantly greater proportion of those who lost weight subsequently died versus those who survived. Urinary loss of retinol was significantly predicted by increased body temperature and by decreased CD4 counts in clinic patients.

In addition, the presence of acute illness in hospitalized patients with AIDS appeared to increase the risk for low serum retinol, and increased urinary excretion of retinol/vitamin A. Greater urinary retinol loss and more severe illness are associated with body weight loss and death, Jolly added.

An estimated 17 million women, ranging in age from 15 to 49 worldwide, are HIV-infected (HIV-positive), and 77% of them reside in sub-Saharan Africa, according to the American Journal of Clinical Nutrition.[24]

In many areas of southern Africa, the prevalence of HIV is over 40% in women attending antenatal clinics. In spite of concern about the risk of transmitting HIV to infants via breastfeeding, and the suggestion that breastfeeding may have an adverse effect on the nutritional status of HIV-positive women, the use of replacement milks for infant feeding is often unacceptable, unaffordable, or unsafe, commented Peggy C. Papathakis at the Africa Centre for Health and Population Studies in Somekele, South Africa, and colleagues in the United States and United Kingdom.

Complex bi-directional relations exist between HIV infection, nutrition, and immune function, the researchers added. In HIV-negative adults, inadequate micronutritional intake and mild deficiency are associated with altered immune function. Zinc, selenium, iron, copper, folic acid (a B vitamin), and vitamins A, C, E, and B6 all have important roles in immune function.

"Several studies in industrialized countries have found an association between HIV disease progression and low blood concentrations of copper, zinc, and vitamins A, E, B2, B6, and B12, although the causal direction of the relation is uncertain. Nevertheless, there is concern that inadequate diets may compound the susceptibility to secondary infection and thereby cause a further worsening of immune function of HIV-positive people," the researchers continued.

Articles in the November 2008 issue of Scientific American are devoted to whether or not there will ever be a cure for HIV/AIDS, and whether or not an AIDS vaccine can be developed, since there have been repeated failures.[25,26]

The editors reported that, "HIV has so far defeated the best efforts of vaccine scientists, because the virus evades and undermines the immune system."

Ironically, there was no mention of vitamin A, which we have found out in this book, can strengthen the immune system and help to fight the infection.

Why doesn't the Bill and Melinda Gates Foundation, the National Institutes of Health, and others, use some of their extensive budgets to investigate this inexpensive approach?

While it is not the purview of this book, in addition to vitamin A, a variety of other inexpensive nutrients should be investigated for jump-starting the immune system, such as mixed carotenoids, vitamins C, D, and E, the B Complex, zinc, selenium, magnesium, fish oil, and others. This is certainly more cost-effective than the millions of dollars being spent on questionable drugs and vaccines. Obviously, drugs and vaccines need to be developed, but so should these other sensible approaches.

Both HIV and Ebola have documented primate origins, and a paper published in the February 2008 issue of Nature noted that 60% of emerging human pathogens came from animals, reported Elizabeth Svoboda in the October 21, 2008 issue of the New York Times.[27]

"We are starting to expand the watershed of global disease control," said Nathan Wolfe, M.D., of Stamford University in Palo Alto, California. "Before, the best thing you could do was develop a vaccine, but now people are recognizing that's not going to be enough."

While studying primate hunters in Cameroon, Wolfe hopes to persuade the hunters to supply him with blood samples, so that he can form a better idea of which new animal diseases they are exposed to, and, by extension, which emerging viruses could pose the biggest threat to humans.

In studying the "bushmeat" hunters, Wolfe faces a singular occupational hazard in that their blood often mingles with that of their prey, Svoboda said. Because animals like chimpanezees and orangutans are genetically similar to humans, the likelihood of virus transmission between species is very high.

Since beginning his hunter studies, Wolfe has identified several viruses never before seen in humans, including retroviruses from the same family as HIV.

With the goal of identifying more of these new disease-causing pathogens—and checking them off—Wolfe started the Global Viral Forecasting Initiative. If new disease strains could be culled before they had a chance to take hold in humans, health organizations would have to spend less money and energy in developing expensive vaccines and treatment drugs, Svoboda continued.

"Thanks to new techniques of sequencing DNA in the viruses they find, epidemiologists can quickly identify the most virulent new pathogens—the ones that have high mutation rates or lend themselves to recombination—in which strands of DNA are broken and then joined to other genetic material," Svoboda said. "A new variant of influenza, for example, could be dangerous, but it could cause epidemics only if it were genetically capable of staying one step ahead of the immune system's defenses."

Once a harmful virus has been located, the next step is to determine how quickly it can spread. Wolfe and his colleagues have developed computer simulations that can be customized to take account of population size and density, family size, and transportation patterns.

So far, simulations show that for all but the most virulent new pathogens there is a reasonable combination of policy options well within the range of the health authorities that, if prepared in advance and implemented quickly, could stop a global disaster, added Donald S. Burke, M.D., of the University of Pittsburgh in Pennsylvania.

Wolfe acknowledged that the task of preparing for the next pandemic is gargantuan—"far too big for his team alone," Svoboda said.

Speaking of the Ebola virus, a series of outbreaks of the infection in central Africa appears to be the result of separate introductions of the pathogen from different animal sources involving several different viral strains, according to a study from the Institute of Research and Development in Franceville, Gabon, and other institutions.[28]

The outbreaks were apparently touched off by hunters handling carcasses of infected animals.

Villagers reported an unusually large number of chimp, gorilla, and antelope carcasses in nearby areas before and during the outbreaks. Tests of the remains showed that most of the animals were positive for the virus, reported Joan Stephenson, Ph.D., in the February 18, 2004 issue of the Journal of the American Medical Association.

One virus, causing agonizing pain, kills in less than 2 weeks, while another virus, stealthily weakens its host's immune defenses, which can take years to causes death, reported John Travis in Science News.[29]

These killers are variola, the virus that causes smallpox, which may have taken more lives of more people than any other infectious agent in history, and HIV, the virus that causes AIDS.

"Researchers found that HIV and a member of the poxvirus family, which includes variola, infect cells by using some of the same cell-surface proteins," Travis said. "This unexpected finding, if extended to variola, may help biologists develop a better smallpox vaccine and design antiviral drugs in case smallpox emerges or is used as a biological weapon by extremists."

The discovery raises a fascinating conjecture, Travis added. Some people with natural resistance to the AIDS virus may owe their good fortune to a genetic mutation handed down to them by survivors of ancient smallpox outbreaks.

A lymph node biopsy removed in 1960 from a woman living in what is now Kinshasa, Democratic Republic of Congo, contained traces of the HIV-1 genome, reported Philip Yam in the December 2008 issue of Scientific American.[30]

In comparing the biopsy with existing HIV sequences suggests that the virus surfaced in 1908, pushing back by a decade an earlier estimate based on an infected blood sample collected from the same city in 1959.

Trade routes may have contributed to the emergence of the

virus, which probably originated among chimpanzees in Cameroon, which is hundreds of kilometers (a kilometer is equal to 0.62 mile) from Kinshasa, reported the original article in the October 2, 2008 issue of Nature.

In countries with a high prevalence of HIV-1, a HIV infection contributes significantly to infant mortality, according to Avy Violari at the University of Witwaterstrand in Johannesburg, South Africa, and colleagues at other facilities in South Africa, England, and the United States.[31]

In the study, HIV-infected infants 6 to 12 weeks of age with a CD4 lymphocyte percentage—the CD4 percentage—of 25% or more were randomly assigned to receive antiretroviral therapy—lopinavir—ritonavir, zidovudine, and lamivudine—when the CD4 percentage decreased to less than 20% (25% if the child was younger than 1), or clinical criteria were met—the deferred antiretroviral-therapy group—or to immediate initiation of limited antiretroviral therapy until 1 year of age or 2 years of age—the early anti-retroviral therapy group.

The study was conducted at 2 centers in South Africa; the Perinatal HIV Research Unit, Chris Hani Baragwanath Hospital in Soweto, and the Children's Infectious Disease Clinical Research Unit at Tygerberg Children's Hospital in Cape Town.

The researchers reported that early HIV diagnosis and early antiretroviral therapy reduced early infant mortality by 70% and HIV progression by 75%.

"These data provide strong support for the initiation of antiretroviral therapy from an early age, regardless of the CD4 percentage or count," the researchers said. "A good program for the prevention of mother-to-mother transmission of HIV-1, encompassing early diagnosis in infants, is fundamental to the success of any early antiretroviral-therapy strategy."

A study by researchers at Harvard University in Boston, Massachusetts, has concluded that the South African government in Johannesburg could have prevented the premature deaths of 365,000 people earlier if it had provided antiretroviral drugs to AIDS patients, and widely administered drugs to help prevent pregnant women from infecting their babies, reported Celia W. Dugger in the November 26, 2008 issue of the *New York Times*.[32]

For years, the South African government did not provide antiretroviral medicines, even as Botswana and Nambia, neighboring countries with epidemics of similar scale, took action, Dugger said.

The Harvard researchers estimated that, by 2005, South Africa could have been helping half those in need but had reached only 23%, Dugger added. By comparison, Botswana was already providing treatment to 85% of those in need, and Nambia to 71%.

The study concluded that the 330,000 South Africans who died for lack of treatment, and the 35,000 babies who perished because they were infected with HIV, together, lost at least 3.8 million years of life.

Thousands of people are dying needlessly of AIDS in Myanmar (formerly Burma) each year, because the government allocates too little money for treating them, reported Donald G. McNeil, Jr., in the December 2, 2008 issue of the *New York Times*.[33]

About 240,000 in the country are infected with HIV, and about 76,000 are ill enough to need antiretroviral treatment. However, only 15,000 are said to be getting treatment, and Doctors Without Borders is paying for 11,000 of those.

Many Burmanese cannot afford the $30 a month for the cheapest drugs from private physicians.

"According to Doctors Without Borders, the Myanmar junta spends only 70 cents per capita for health care each year," McNeil added. "Money for AIDS drugs is available from the Global Fund to Fight AIDS, Tuberculosis, and Malaria, but governments, not charities, must apply for it, and they must prove that the money will not be diverted to corrupt ends."

The Joint United Nations Programme on HIV/AIDS (UNAIDS) and the World Health Organization recommend safe, voluntary male circumcision as an additional, important strategy for the prevention of heterosexually acquired HIV infection in men in areas with high HIV prevalence and low levels of male circumcision, according to Lawrence O. Gostin, JD, and Catherine A. Hankins, M.D., of Georgetown University in Washington, D.C., and the UNAIDS program in Geneva, Switzerland.[34]

According to a number of observational studies, 3 randomized controlled trials in Africa have shown that circumcision reduced the likelihood of female-to-male HIV transmission by 50 to 60%. However, there is no comparable evidence that male circumcision protects against male-to-female transmission, or male-to-male transmission, the researchers added.

"Male circumcision will have to be acceptable, available, and safe; sensitive to cultural and religious values; respectful of patients' rights to consent and confidentiality; and defend human rights of girls and women," the researchers said.

Referring to an article by S.A. Strathdee and C. Magis-Rodriguez in a previous issue of JAMA, Jose R. Castillo-Mancilla, M.D., of the University of Colorado at Denver, said that a relevant point the authors did not discuss was transfusion-associated HIV infection (TAHI) is still a latent concern in some developing countries.[35,36]

In spite of the goal set by the WHO in 1997 for all blood donations to come from unpaid volunteer donors, as of 2006, only 49 of 124 countries surveyed had established this as a standard and may still rely heavily on paid and unsafe donors," the author said.

"An estimated 77% of donations in developing countries are from voluntary unpaid donors, compared with 92% in developed countries, and more than 1 million blood units were collected from paid donors in 2006," the author continued.

He went on to say that Mexico is an example of how responsible public health measures can have positive results, even in economically restricted environments.

"Similar actions could have a major effect on the HIV epidemic of many other developing countries," he added. "Adequate supply of safe blood can be assured only by regular donations from voluntary unpaid donors, which should continue to be a major focus for the prevention of HIV transmission worldwide."

An estimated 50 million women in Asia are at risk of acquiring the HIV infection from their husband or long-time partner, reported Joan Stephenson, Ph.D., in the September 16, 2009 issue of the Journal of the American Medical Association.[37]

The report was released in August 2009 by the Joint United Nationals Programme on HIV/AIDS or UNAIDS.

"Evidence from many countries in Asia indicate that most women are acquiring HIV, not because of their own sexual behavior, but because their partners engage in unsafe behaviors," Stephenson reported.

It is estimated that over 90% of approximately 1.7 million women in Asia are currently living with HIV acquired from their partners.[38]

The report urged preventive programs that are aimed at men who engage in unsafe behaviors, including drug use or with men or female prostitutes.

In two studies at the University of Minnesota in Minneapolis, a research team reported that, despite a substantial and sustained increase in the CD4+ cell count, as compared with antiretroviral therapy alone, interleukin-2 plus antiretroviral therapy yielded no clinical benefit in either study.

Writing in the New England Journal of Medicine, Aaron A.R. Tobian, M.D., and colleagues, at the National Institutes of Health in Bethesda, Maryland, reported that male circumcision has been shown to decrease the rates of HIV, herpes simplex virus type 2 (HSV-2) and human papillomavirus (HPV) infection in men, and of trichomoniasia and bacterial vaginosis in their female partners.[39-41]

They added that circumcision also reduces symptomatic ulceration in HIV-negative men and women, and HIV-positive men.

"Therefore," they continued, "male circumcision reduces the risk of several sexually transmitted infections in both sexes, and these benefits should guide public health policies for neonatal, adolescent, and adult male circumcision programs."

Commenting on the study, Renee Ridzon, M.D., and Kanwarjit Singh, M.D., of Bill and Melinda Gates Foundation in Seattle, Washington, said that in sub-Saharan Africa, about 30 million men are uncircumcised, and it is not clear how to scale up circumcision where health care providers are scarce.

Lacking from this discussion, they continued, are male-circumcision devices to reduce operation times, complication rates, and time to wound healing.

"With disposable devices that remain on the penis for several days, sutures for hemostasis and skin closure—which are time-consuming parts of the operation—are unnecessary," they added.

Male-circumcision devices are used successfully in infants and young boys, and several devices are available in adult sizes. Research to assess the reliability, safety, acceptability, and cost effectiveness of such devices for use in settings where there is a high prevalence of HIV infection should be a priority, they concluded.

Michelle R. Storms, M.D., of Michigan State University College of Human Medicine, in Marquette, commenting on the Tobian, et al., study, said that uncircumcised men with HIV have the virus on the glans 65% of the time, whereas circumcised men with HIV have the virus on the glans 48% of the time.

"Consequently," she continued, "sampling only the glans will underestimate the risk of HIV among circumcised men by about 35%. If the numbers reported by Tobian, et al. are adjusted for the sampling bias, the odds ratio 0.83 (95% confidence interval (CI), 0.56 to 1.24), which is no longer statistically significant."

Similarly, men in the intervention study were instructed to abstain from sex until healing took place, but no adjustment was made for the difference in exposure when the risk of HIV infection was determined.

Wound healing was certified in 85.05% of men 4 weeks after surgery, and in 95.8% of men 6 weeks after surgery. Men were urged to refrain from intercourse until certification of wound healing, so adjusting for this period of sexual abstinence, they estimated that the incidence of HIV-2 infection would be 4.2 per 100 person-years in the intervention group and 5.4 per 100 person-years in the controls.

The HIV/AIDS epidemic in South Africa appears to have stabilized at a prevalence of about 11%, reported Joan Stephenson, Ph.D., in the July 15, 2009 issue of the Journal of the American Medical Association. This was the gist of a report from the Human Sciences Research Council.[42]

While the overall prevalence has shown little change since the Council's initial 2 surveys in 2002 and 2005, the latest report shows a substantial decrease in HIV prevalence among young South Africans 15 to 24, from 10.3% in 2005 to 8.6% in 2008. HIV incidence also decreased among children 2 to 14, from 5.6% in 2002 to 2.5% in 2008.

"These promising trends appear to reflect successful implementation of prevention efforts, including programs to prevent mother-to-child transmission, and promotion of increased condom use," Stephenson added.

Unfortunately, the overall situation remains "dire," including the high level of HIV prevalence among women 25 to 29—33%—that has persisted since the previous 2 surveys.

Women infected with HIV face a combination of health threats along with immunodeficiency, including compromised nutrition and adverse gynecological conditions, according to Beth C. Tohill, M.D., of the Centers for Disease Control and Prevention in Atlanta, Georgia, and colleagues at other institutions. The relation among HIV, nutrition, and adverse gynecological outcomes is complex and has rarely been studied.[43]

Those living with HIV, especially those with AIDS, have compromised nutritional status, including low blood concentrations of vitamin A, carotenoids, vitamin E, vitamin C, vitamin B12, folic acid, zinc, and selenium, the researchers said.

"Anemia is also common in HIV infection, and it is associated with increased risk of mortality," they added. "HIV-associated malnutrition is often the result of several factors, including HIV-related conditions that impair intake of nutrients such as loss of appetite, nausea, oral lesions, and those that affect nutrient absorption, such as persistent diarrhea, impaired nutrient storage, and altered nutrient metabolism."

Some nutritional deficiencies are themselves associated with adverse gynecological outcomes irrespective of HIV status, they added. Low concentrations of folic acid (a B vitamin) are associated with cervical dysplasia, cervical cancer, and human papillomavirus. Low concentrations of vitamin C and beta-carotene were associated with cervical dysplasia, cervical cancer, HPV, and ovarian cancer.

Higher concentrations of vitamins A, C, and E, and beta-carotene were associated with a lower risk of bacterial vaginosis. Recent research equates the latter problem with a vitamin D deficiency.

The researchers also reported that HIV-infected women had concentrations of albumin, hemoglobin, alpha-carotene, beta-carotene, lycopene, beta-cryptoxanthin, selenium, and zinc lower than the HIV-unaffected women in the same cohort. L. Belec, et al., reported that among women in Central Africa, vitamin A deficiency was associated with the number of genital tract infections diagnosed.[44]

Anemia is a frequent complication among HIV-infected people, and it is associated with faster disease progression and mortality, reported Wafie W. Fawzi, of the Harvard School of Public Health in Boston, Massaschusetts, and colleagues at Harvard and Muhimbili University College of Health Sciencies in Dar es Salaam, Tanzania.[45]

Their study examined the effect of multivitamin supplementation on hemoglobin concentrations, and the risk of anemia among HIV-infected pregnant women and their children.

Participants were given each day preformed vitamin A and beta-carotene,vitamins B, C, and E, plus preformed vitamin A and beta-carotene, plus multivitamins, or a placebo. All women were also given iron and folic acid supplements.

It was reported that blood concentrations among women who received multivitamins were 0.33 g/dl higher than among those who did not get supplements. Compared with placebo, multivitamin supplementation resulted in a blood increase of 0.59 g/dl during the first 2 years after enrollment.

In addition, compared to placebo, the children born to mothers who received multivitamins had a reduced risk of anemia. In this group, the risk of macrocytic anemia (folic acid deficiency) was 63% lower than in the placebo group.

The researchers concluded that, "multivitamin supplementation provided during pregnancy and in the postpartum period resulted in significant improvements in hemologic status among HIV-infected women and their children, which provides further support for the value of multivitamin supplementation in HIV-infected adults."

The interplay between nutrition and infection is well established, and poor nutrition predisposes to disease acquisition and progression, and disease leads to worsening nutritional status, explained Saurabh Mehta of the Harvard School of Public Health in Boston, Massachusetts, and colleagues at other facilities.[46,47]

"In the context of pregnancy and HIV infection, poor nutritional status, preexistent or as a result of HIV-induced wasting or weight loss, is likely to increase the risk of mother-to-child transmission of HIV," they said.

In addition, poor nutrition as reflected in short stature, low body mass index, poor weight gain during pregnancy, and a low hemoglobin concentration is an established risk factor for adverse pregnancy outcomes, such as low birth weight, fetal loss, preterm birth, and intrauterine growth retardation among HIV-infected women.

They went on to say that such interventions could include protein-energy and micronutrition supplementation and the treatment of infections such as malaria, intestinal parasitic infections, and other opportunistic infections—all cofactors in the etiology of malnutrition among HIV-infected women.

A research team in Harare, Zimbabwe, headed by Jean W. Humphrey, M.D., reported that early exclusive breastfeeding (EBF) is recommended by the World Health Organization in Geneva, Switzerland, but EBF rates remain low throughout the world.[48-51]

For infants born to breastfeeding HIV-positive mothers, early EBF is associated with a lower risk of postnatal transmission than is feeding breast milk together with other liquids or foods, the researchers said. However, studies in Africa have found no benefit of EBF for infants born to HIV-negative mothers.

The researchers referred to a Lancet series in 2003 on child survival, which identified the exclusive breastfeeding during the first 6 months of life, and continued breastfeeding to 12 months as the single most effective preventive public health intervention for reducing mortality among children less than 5 years of age.

"More recently," they continued, "the 2008 Lancet series on maternal and child undernutrition estimated that 1.06 million child deaths—10% of all mortality in children under 5 years of age—are attributable to nonexclusive breastfeeding in the first 6 months of life."

Most of the data came from studies in Africa and Latin America. In Africa, where over 40% of the world's deaths of children under 5 years of age occur each year, breastfeeding is nearly universal and prolonged, but early exclusive breastfeeding is rare.

"Our findings are especially notable because our study was conducted among relatively well-educated urban women, the vast majority of whom had access to tap water, toilet facilities, and electricity," the research team concluded.

Infections with the AIDS virus in China is spreading beyond the country's original high-risk groups—heroin addicts in the south and blood sellers in rural central counties, according to Donald G. McNeil, Jr., in the October 7, 2008 issue of the *New York Times*.[52]

While the number of estimated cases—700,000—is low in a population of 1.3 billion, it has risen 8% since 2005, McNeil said.

Scientists believe AIDS entered China in the 1980s with drug traffickers in Yunnan, which borders Southeast Asia's opium Golden Triangle. It increased in Henan, where illegal blood banks pooled blood from indigent farmers, spun it to remove clotting factors, and returned mixed red cells to all sellers.

"Tracking HIV subtypes suggests the virus has moved along drug-trafficking routes, creating an outbreak in western Xinjiang," McNeil added.

HIV and AIDS in the United States remain a major public health crisis, with over 1 million U.S. people estimated to be living with HIV, nearly a quarter of whom remain undiagnosed, reported John G. Bartlett, M.D., of Johns Hopkins University School of Medicine, Baltimore, Maryland, and colleagues at other facilities.[53]

On September 22, 2006, the Centers for Disease Control and Prevention in Atlanta, Ceorgia, published commendation for HIV testing in the United States that favored an opt-out strategy, meaning the test will be performed unless the patient declines. The World Health Organization issued similar recommendations in May 2007.

The CDC issued specific recommendations for HIV screening of those 13 to 64 in all health-care settings. The Agency's rationale is that treatment with highly active antiretroviral therapy is widely available, and it is more effective when started earlier in the course of HIV infection.

Concerns about the change include laws in some states that mandate signed consent and counseling, a perception that counseling is an effective prevention strategy, variability in payment coverage for the test, concerns that stigma and discrimination that may accompany the HIV diagnosis, and the possibility that other testing policies would be more effective.

Eleven of 16 states have changed legislation to reduce barriers to testing, 35 of 74 national professional societies have endorsed the new recommendations, and multiple demonstration projects have shown feasibility.

There is still the challenge of laws that preclude adoption of the recommendation of 9 states, the researchers said. Some third parties, including Medicare, still do not cover HIV as a screening test, and resource limitations are problematic for emergency departments.

"Issues of stigma and discrimination related to a diagnosis of HIV infection remain sources of continued debate," the researchers concluded. "Given the short interval since the CDC promulgated revised HIV testing recommendations for health care settings, it is too early to fully gauge the benefits and harms of these recommendations."

The availability of new antiretroviral drugs and formulations, including drugs in new classes, and recent data on treatment choices for antiretroviral-naïve and-experienced patients warrant an update of the International AIDS Society-USA guidelines for the use of antiretroviral therapy in adult HIV infection, reported Scott M. Hammer, M.D., et al., of Columbia University College of Physicians and Surgeons in New York.[54]

The rational for the current update of the 2006 International AIDS Society-USA (IAS-USA) antiretroviral treatment recommendations[55] is based on: (1) the recent approval of 3 novel agents, maraviroc, a CC chemokine receptor 5 (CCR5) antagonist; raltegravir, an integrase strand transfer inhibitor; and etravirine, a second-generation nonnucloside reverse transcriptase inhibitor (NNRT1); (2) new data that better inform the choice of drugs for initial therapy, and the management of treatment failure; and (3) new pathogenic insights into the role of human HIV in disease processes previously considered non-AIDS-related conditions.

"The 21 years since zidovudine (AZT) was approved for the treatment of HIV infection have witnessed remarkable advances in the understanding of disease pathogenesis, translation of that knowledge into practical therapeutics, continued discovery of complications or disease states associated with HIV, or its treatment that increase the complexity of management, and a dynamic drug development process that has led to the current availability of over 30 individual drugs and fixed-dose combinations to treat HIV infection," the researchers said.

In spite of these advances, they continued, disease management remains challenged by toxicities, maintenance of adherence, clinical manifestations related to both the drugs and the HIV infection itself, and the threat of drug resistance. Sustainability and expansion of the progress achieved will depend on maintaining a robust drug development pipeline, and the ability to deliver effective therapy and monitoring tools to the worldwide affected populations.

"With creativity and political will, the progress and individualized approach to antiretroviral therapy evident in the developed world can be adapted to the public health approach in the developing world, where 90% of the world's HIV-infected population lives," they concluded.

Tactical approaches to outmaneuvering the HIV virus include prevention programs, and an array of agents to counteract the progression of HIV disease, reported Gianna Zuccotti, M.D., and Jeanette M. Smith in the November 25, 2009 issue of the Journal of the American Medical Association.[56]

"Much effort has been applied to improving access to treatment, and an estimated 4 million people were receiving antiretroviral therapy in low-income and middle-income countries by December 2008," they said.

However, they continued, an estimated 33 million people are infected with HIV worldwide, leaving no doubt as to remaining challenges. In the U.S., the estimates of new cases suggest that messages about risk of HIV infection may require renewed force and clarity.

In July 2010, the Journal of the American Medical Association published an issue featuring HIV/AIDS research. This coincides with the 18th International AIDS Conference in Vienna, Austria.

At the University of Washington at Seattle, researchers reported in the February 4, 2010 issue of the New England Journal of Medicine that their study of heterosexual HIV-1 serodiscordant couples showed that, among the partners who were infected with both HIV-1 and HSV-2, who had CD4 counts of 260 or more cells per cubic millimeter, treatment with standard doses of acylovir (zovirax) for the suppression of HSV-2 infection did decrease the incidence of transmission of HIV-1 to the uninfected partners, in spite of significant reductions in HIV-1 blood levels, and in the incidence of genital ulcer disease.[57]

The seroprevalence of herpes simplex virus type 2 (HSV-2), the most common cause of genital ulcer disease, is 60 to 90% in populations with human immunodeficiency virus type 1 (HIV-1).

The clinical manifestations of HSV-2 range from unrecognized or mild genital symptoms in most people with HIV-1 infection to severe genital ulcer disease in those with advanced HIV-1 disease, the researchers said.

Writing in the July 15, 2010 issue of the New England Journal of Medicine, Patrice Severe, M.D., of Groupe Haitien d'Etude du Sarcome de Kaposi et des Infections Opportunistes in Port of Prince, Haiti, and colleagues at other facilities, reported that early antiretroviral therapy decreased the rate of death by 75% in HIV-infected adults with a CD4+ T-cell count greater than 200 and less than 350/cubic millimeter.[58]

They added that access to antiretroviral therapy should be expanded to all HIV-infected adults with CD4+ T-cell count of less than 350/cubic millimeter, especially those who live in locations with limited resources.

Following WHO guidelines, the first-line regimen of antiretroviral therapy consists of zidovudine/AZT, lamivudine, and efavirenz. Of those treated with this therapy, about 85% were alive in 5 years, the researchers said.

However, the research team admitted that there is limited data on the optimal time to start antiretroviral therapy in those who live in locations with limited resources, where high rates of TB, malnutrition, and coinfection with tropical diseases may alter the natural history of HIV disease, and the optimal time to initiate therapy.

"The median time to the initiation of antiretroviral therapy in our standard-treatment group was 2 years," the researchers added. "At current pricing, 2 years of antiretroviral drugs will cost about $400 per person, the rate of death can be decreased by 75%, and the incidence of active tuberculosis by 50%."

A study jointly undertaken by the Tamil Nadu State AIDS Control Central Society (TNSACS) in India, and Duke University in Durham, North Carolina, has found that nutritional supplements greatly improved the health and quality of life for people living with HIV/AIDS, according to the HIV/AIDS Information Gateway on November 4, 2010.[59]

The 18-month study of over 10,500 people with HIV/AIDS in Tamil Nadu may be the biggest of its kind in India. The study began in September 2005, in 3 centers that provide antiretroviral therapy (ART), as well as those who did not need it.

Macronutrient supplements—calories, protein, carbohydrates, fat, and fiber were given to 10,780 adults and children, who were part of the ART project. They were also given supplements of vitamin A, B Complex (including folic acid), vitamin C, etc., in the form of tablets, to 11,109.

The most dramatic improvement was recorded in the CD4 count of those being treated. Those affected with HIV were provided ART only when his/her CD4 count fell below 200. Those on ART had a CD4 count of 113. This went up to 309, 6 months into the study, and reached 402 by the end of the study.

"The improvement was marginal for those not on ART, increasing their count from 494 to 515 at the end of the study.

"The study confirms that good nutrition helps to delay the progression of the disease," said Supriya Sahu, project director of TNSACS. "The advantage is that, with good nutrition, a person will take longer to reach a stage when he/she needs ART, and those on ART will live healthier lives."

The study also confirmed that good nutrition helped patients to gain weight—5 kg in men and 4 kg in women on ART. For those who did not need treatment, the weight gain was 4 kg in men and 2 kg in women.

The study also found that, as the health of patients improved, the rate of tuberculosis dropped. For those on ART from 25% coinfected with TB at the start of the study to 5% at the conclusion of the trial.

For those who did not need treatment, TB rates went down from 10% to 3% after 18 months.

For the other opportunistic infections affecting AIDS patients, this showed a drop from 46% to 10% at the study's end. For those who did not need ART, the reduction was 20% to 10%.

The researchers added that the results of the study are so encouraging that they have introduced the program to all ART centers in the state. The ART project was begun in Tamil Nadu in March/April 2007, and it affects 21,000 people.

The cost of the nutritional treatment is 90 rupees per person per year. This is significant because of the savings realized from the delayed ART, as well as reducing the cost of medications for TB and other opportunistic infections.

With improved nutrition, the patients are now working, and children's attendance at school has improved, the researchers said.

Where AIDS Began

Acquired immunodeficiency syndrome (AIDS) was coined in 1982, a year after doctors in the United States recognized an epidemic of pneumonias, rare cancers, and assorted bacterial infections among mostly young males, and mostly previously healthy adults, reported Christine Soares in the September 2009 issue of Scientific American.

In 1983, French researchers isolated the cause of the immune system collapse that defined the syndrome, which was a virus that selectively infects and destroys immune cells.

The HIV virus currently resides in over 30 million people, and seemed to come out of the blue in the early 1980s, but it is now known to have been infecting humans for at least a century, she said.

"Recent studies of preserved tissue samples show that HIV was present in the former Belgian Congo (now the Democratic Republic of the Congo) in 1959; in Haiti in 1966; and possibly the United States as early as 1969," she continued.

Analysis of these early specimens place the emergence of the most virulent HIV strain, known as Group M, in southern Cameroon around 1908.

Its ancestor was most likely a virus that has been infecting West African chimpanzees since 1492.

If this is true, she added, many rural people were exposed to simian immunodeficiency syndrome (SIV) over the centuries through live chimps or in bush meat before the infection caught hold in the human population.

"AIDS researchers are studying the behavior of SIV in its native host because, although the simian virus is nearly identical to HIV, in wild chimps it is generally benign," Soares continued.

She went on to say that the human cells of our closest primate cousins get infected also, but they eventually manage to rally and reconstitute their numbers. The origin of AIDS, therefore, lies in some combination of minute changes in HIV itself—and the body's responses to it—and remains a mystery.

Source: "AIDS and HIV—The Viral Infection's Origin Among Apes Might Hold a Key for Someday Taming It," Scientific American 301(3): 91, September 2009.

HIV/AIDS in India

Previously it was thought that about 5 million people were living with HIV in India, more than in any other country, according to AVERT/International HIV and AIDS Charity.

A better national household survey conducted in 2005-2006, and an estimate released in 2007, found 2.3 million people living with HIV in India. Of these, 39% are females and 3.5% are children.

Across India, the prevalence of HIV seems to be low among the general population, but disproportionately high among high-risk groups, such as intravenous drug users, prostitutes, men who have sex with men, and workers at sexually transmitted disease clinics.

At the end of 2005, the number of HIV cases that had progressed to full-blown AIDS was 116,905, of which 34,177 were women. About one-third of these patients were under 30.

In many cases, a patient will die without HIV having been diagnosed, with death attributed to opportunistic infections such as TB.

Source: "India HIV and AIDS Statistics," AVERT/International HIV and AIDS Charity, updated.

Research and Development Funding by Disease

Disease	Amount in US. $
HIV/AIDS	1.1 billion
Malaria	468.4 million
Tuberculosis	410.4 million
Kinetoplastid diseases	125.1 million
Diarrheal diseases	113.9 million
Dengue fever	82.0 million
Helminth infection	51.6 million
Bacterial pneumonia and meningitis	32.5 million
Typhoid and paratyphoid fever	9.1 million
Leprosy	5.8 million
Buruli ulcer	2.4 million
Trachoma	1.7 million
Rheumatic fever	1.7 million

Source: JAMA 301(17): 1755, 2009.

References

1. Heptonstall, Julia, M.Sc. "HIV/AIDS," Medical and Health Annual. Chicago, IL: Encylopaedia Britannica, Inc., 1995, pp. 52 ff.
2. Steinbrook, Robert, M.D. "The AIDS Epidemic—A Progress Report from Mexico City," New England Journal of Medicine, August 28, 2008, pp. 885-887.
3. Johnston, Margaret I., Ph.D., and Fauci, Anthony S., M.D. "An HIV Vaccine—Challenges and Prospects," *ibid*, pp. 888-889.
4. Mehendale, S.M., et al. "Low Carotenoid Concentrations and the Risk of HIV Seroconversion in Pune, India," Journal of Acquired Immune Deficiency Syndrome 26:352-359, 2001.
5. Semba, Richard D., M.D., et al. "Increased Mortality Associated with Vitamin A Deficiency During Human Immunodeficiency Virus Type 1 Infection," Archives of Internal Medicine 153:2149-2154, 1993.
6. McKeown, L.A. "Beta-Carotene Lifts CD4 Counts at Dose of 180 Mg. Study Found 17% Increase in HIV-Infected People," Medical Tribune, 4(34):1, February 25, 1993.
7. Kuritzkes, Daniet R., M.D. "AIDS Update." Medical and Health Annual. Chicago, IL: Encyclopaedia Britannica, Inc., 1997, pp. 164ff.
8. Karter, Dennis L., et al. "Vitamin A Deficiency in Non-Vitamin-Supplemented Patients with AIDS: A Cross-Sectional Study," Journal of Acquired Immune Deficiency Syndrome and Human Retrovirology 8:199-203, 1995.
9. Murata, Tajuji, et al. "Effect of Long-Term Administration of Beta-Carotene on Lymphocyte Subsets in Humans," American Journal of Clinical Nutrition 60:597-602, 1994.
10. Spraycar, Marjory, editor. Stedman's Medical Dictionary, 26th Edition. Baltimore, MD: Williams & Wilkins, 1995, p. 297.
11. Branowitz, S.A., et al. AIDS 16(1): 115, 1996.
12. Delmas-Beauvieus, Marie-Christine, M.D., et al. "The Enzymatic Antioxidant System in Blood and Glutathione Status in Human Immunodeficiency Virus (HIV-Infected) Patients: Effects of Supplementation with Selenium and Beta-Carotene," American Journal of Clinical Nutrition 64:101-107, 1996.
13. Coutsoudis, Anna, Ph.D., et al. "The Effects of Vitamin A Supplementation on the Morbidity of Children Born to HIV-Infected Women," American Journal of Public Health 85(8): 1076-1081, August 1995.

14. Semba, Richard D., M.D., et al "Maternal Vitamin A Deficiency and Mother-to-Child Transmission of HIV-1," The Lancet 343:1593-1597, June 25, 1994.

15. Nimmagadda, Ajani, et al. "The Significance of Vitamin A and Carotenoid Status in Persons Infected by the Human Immunodeficiency Virus," Clinical Infectious Diseases 26:711-718, 1998.

16. Fawzi, W.E., et al. "A Randomized Trial of Vitamin A Supplements in Relation to Mortality Among Human Immunodeficiency Virus-Infected and Uninfected Children in Tanzania," Pediatric and Infectious Disease Journal 18(2):127-133, February 1999.

17. Garewal, H., et al. "A Preliminary Trial of Beta-Carotene in Subjects Infected with the Human Immunodeficiency Virus," Journal of Nutrition 122:728-732, 1992.

18. Phuapradit, Winit, M.D., Ph.D., et al. "Serum and Vitamin A and Beta-Carotene Levels in Pregnant Women Infected with Human Immunodeficiency Virus-1," Obstetrics and Gynecology 87(4):564-567, April 1996.

19. Baum, Marianna K., M.D., et al. "Micronutrients and HIV-1 Disease Progression," AIDS 9:1051-1056, 1995.

20. Jolly, Pauline E., Ph.D. et al. "Vitamin A Depletion in HIV Infection and AIDS," AIDS 10(1):14, 1996.

21. Semba, Richard D., M.D., et al. "Vitamin A Deficiency and Wasting As Predictors of Mortality in Human Immunodeficiency Virus-Infected Injection Drug Users," The Journal of Infectious Diseases 171(5): 1196-1202, 1995.

22. Burns, D.N., et al. "Vitamin A Deficiency and Other Nutritional Indices During Pregnancy in Human Immunodeficiency Virus Infection: Prevalence, Clinical Correlates, and Outcome," Clinical Infectious Diseases 29:328-334, August 1999.

23. Jolly, Pauline E., Ph.D. "Vitamin A Depletion in Hospital and Clinic Patients with Acquired Immunodeficiency Syndrome: A Preliminary Report," Nutrition Research 17(9): 1427-1441, 1997.

24. Papathakis, Peggy C., et al. "Micronutrient Status During Lactation in HIV-Infected and HIV-Uninaffected South African Women During the First 6 months After Delivery," American Journal of Clinical Nutrition 85:182-192, 2007.

25. Watkins, David T. "The Vaccine Search Goes on," Scientific American, November 2008, pp. 69ff.

26. Stevenson, Mario. "Can HIV Be Cured?" *ibid*, pp. 78ff.

27. Svoboda, Elizabeth. "Deep in the Rain Forest, Stalking the Next Pandemic," The New York Times, October 21, 2008, pp. D5, D9.

28. Stephenson, Joan, Ph.D. "Ebola Virus Transmission," JAMA 291(7):813, 2004.

29. Travis, John, "Survivors' Benefit? Some AIDS Resistance May Stem from Ancient Smallpox Epidemics," Science News 157(4):63, January 22, 2000.

30. Yam, Philip. "Longtime Companion," Scientific American, December 2008, p. 20.

31. Violari, Avy, et al. "Early Antiretroviral Therapy and Mortality Among HIV-Infected Infants," New England Journal of Medicine 359:2233-2244, 2008.

32. Dugger, Celia W. "Study Cites Toll of AIDS Policy in South Africa," New York Times, November 26, 2008, pp. Al, All.

33. McNeil, Donald G., Jr. "Thousands Die Needlessly Because Junta Spends Too Little on AIDS, Group Says," New York Times, December 2, 2008, p. D6.

34. Gostin, Lawrence O., JD, and Hankins, Catherine A., M.D. "Male Circumcision As An HIV Prevention Strategy in Sub-Saharan Africa," JAMA 300 (21):2539-2541, 2008.

35. Castillo-Manceilla, Jose R., M.D. "The Changing HIV Epidemic in Mexico," *ibid*, p. 2484.

36. Strathdee, S.A., and Magis-Rodriguez, C. "Mexico's Evolving HIV Epidemic," JAMA 300(5):571-573, 2008.

37. Stephenson, Joan, Ph.D. "HIV in Asia," JAMA 302(11):1161, 2009.

38. Abrams, D., M.D., et al. "Interleukin-2 Therapy in Patients with HIV Infection," the INSIGHT-ESPRIT Study Group and SILCAAT Scientific Committee," New England Journal of Medicine 361:1548-1559, 2009.

39. Tobian, Aaron A.R., M.D., Ph.D., et al. "Male Circumcision for the Prevention of HSV-2 and HPV Infections and Syphilis," New England Journal of Medicine 360:1298-1309, 2009.

40. Ridzon, Renee, M.D., and Singh, Kanwarjit, M.D. "Male Circumcision for the Prevention of HSV-2 and HPV Infections," New England Journal of Medicine 361:307, 2009.

41. Storms, Michelle R., M.D., *ibid*.

42. Stephenson, Joan, Ph.D. "AIDS in South Africa," JAMA 302(3):246, 2009.

43. Tohill, Beth C., M.D. "Nutritional Biomarkers Associated with Gynecological Conditions Among U.S. Women with or At Risk for HIV Infections," American Journal of Clinical Nutrition 85:1327-1334, 2007.
44. Belec, L., et al. "Vitamin A Deficiency and Genital Tract Infection in Women Living in Central Africa," Journal of Acquired Immunity Deficiency Syndrome 29:203-204, 2002.
45. Fawzi, Wafie W., et al. "Multivitamin Supplementation Improves Hematologic Status of HIV-Infected Women and Their Children in Tanzania," American Journal of Clinical Nutrition 85:1335-1343, 2007.
46. Mehta, Saurabh, et al. "Nutritional Indicators of Adverse Pregnancy Outcomes and Mother-to-Child Transmission of HIV Among HIV-Infected Women," American Journal of Clinical Nutrition 87:1639-1649, 2008.
47. Villamor, E., et al. "Pattern and Predictors of Weight Gain During Pregnancy Among HIV-Infected Women from Tanzania," Journal of Acquired Immune Deficiency Syndrome 32:560-569, 2003.
48. Koyangi, Ai, et al. "Effect of Early Exclusive Breastfeeding on Morbidity Among Infants Born to HIV-Negative Mothers in Zimbabwe," American Journal of Clinical Nutrition 89:1375-1382, 2009.
49. Jones, G., et al. "Bellagio Child Survival Study Group. How Many Deaths Can We Prevent This Year?" Lancet 362:65-71, 2003.
50. Black, R.E., et al. "Maternal and Child Under Nutrition: Global and Regional Exposures and Health Consequences," Lancet 371:243-260, 2008.
51. World Health Organization. "The Optimal Duration of Exclusive Breastfeeding: A Systematic Review," World Health Organization, Geneva, Switzerland, 2001.
52. McNeil, Donald G., Jr. "H.I.V. Spreads in China, Affecting New Populations and All Provinces," New York Times, October 7, 2008, p. D6.
53. Bartlett, John G., M.D., et al. "Opt-Out Testing for Human Immunodeficiency Virus in the United States," JAMA 300 (8): 945-951, 2008.
54. Hammer, Scott M., M.D., et al. "Antiretroviral Treatment of Adult HIV Infection—2008. Recommendations of the International AIDS Society-USA Panel," JAMA 300(5):555-570, 2008.
55. Hammer, Scott M., M.D., et al. "Treatment for Adult HIV Infection: 2006 Recommendations of the International AIDS Society-USA Panel," JAMA 296(7):827-843, 2006.

56. Zuccotti, Gianna, M.D., and Smith, Jeanette M., M.D. "HIV/AIDS—Still a Force to Be Reckoned with," JAMA 302 (20):2259, 2009.

57. Celum, C., et al. "Acyclovir and Transmission of HIV-1 from Persons Infected with HIV-1 and HSV-2," New England Journal of Medicine 362:427-439, 2010.

58. Severe, Patrice, M.D., et al. "Early Versus Standard Antiretroviral Therapy for HIV-Infected Adults in Haiti," New England Journal of Medicine 363:257-265, 2010.

59. "Study Confirms Importance of Nutrition in Southern Indian State of Tamil Nadu Shows That Good Nutrition Dramatically Increases the CD4 Count and Reduces Opportunistic Infections in HIV/AIDS Patients," HIV/AIDS Information Gateway, November 4, 2010.

4

MEASLES

Measles is a distressing viral illness that results in a characteristic rash and fever, according to the American Medical Association Home Medical Encyclopedia. Although it mainly affects children, it can occur at any age. An attack usually confers lifetime immunity.[1]

Highly infective, the measles virus is spread primarily by airborne droplets of nasal secretions. There is an incubation period of 9 to 11 days before symptoms appear. Infected children can transmit the virus from shortly after the attack up to 1 week following the development of symptoms. Infants under 8 months old are rarely affected because they have acquired some immunity from their mothers.

"Prevention of the illness is important since it can have rare but serious complications," the publication said. "It may also be serious or fatal in children with impaired immunity, such as those being treated for leukemia."

In developing countries, measles is very common, especially in malnourished children whose defenses against the infection are seriously impaired.

The illness begins with fever, runny nose, sore eyes, and cough, and the victim is very sick, the publication added. After 3 or 4 days, a rash appears, usually starting on the head and neck and spreading downward to cover the entire body. The spots sometimes join to produce large and blotchy areas, and the lymph glands may be enlarged. After 3 days the rash may fade and symptoms subside.

"The most common complications are ear and chest infections, which usually occur with a return of fever 2 to 3 days after the appearance of the rash," the publication continued. "Diarrhea, vomiting, and abdominal pain may occur. A more serious complication, occurring in about one in 1,000 cases, is encephalitis, an inflammation of the brain. It results in headache, drowsiness and vomiting, starting 7 to 10 days after the rash appears. Seizures and coma may follow, sometimes leading to mental retardation or death."

In rare cases, a progressive disorder—subacute sclerosing panencephalitis— can develop years after the acute illness.

"Measles during pregnancy results in death of the fetus in about one-fifth of the cases," the publication added. "However, there is no evidence that measles causes birth defects."

In the United States, children are routinely immunized early in the second year of life. Given by injection, the vaccine is usually combined with mumps and rubella vaccine, which produces immunity in about 97% of the people. Side effects of the vaccine are generally mild, although there may be a low fever, slight cold, and a rash 1 week after the vaccination.

The vaccine should not be given to children under the age of 1, or children with any of the usual risk factors for vaccination. For example, the vaccine may cause a seizure in those who have had a shot before, and if there is a history of epilepsy in the family. In those cases, simultaneous injection of measles-specific immunoglobulin—which contains antibodies against the virus—should be given, the publication continued.

If a pregnant woman comes in contact with anyone with measles, she should be passively immunized against measles with immunoglobulin within 5 days.

As a result of successful U.S. vaccination programs, measles elimination, that is interruption of endemic measles transmission, was declared in the United States in 2000, reported the June 11, 2008 issue of the Journal of the American Medical Association.[2,3]

In fact, the number of reported measles cases has declined from 763,094 in 1958 to fewer than 150 cases reported annually since 1997.

During 2000-2007, 29,116 measles cases were reported annually, however, during January 1-April 25, 2008, 64 confirmed cases were reported by the Centers for Disease Control and Prevention in Atlanta, Georgia.

The 64 confirmed cases were reported in New York City (22), Arizona (15), California (12), Michigan and Wiaconsin (4 each), Hawaii (3), and Illinos, New York state, Pennsylvania, and Virginia (1 each).

Patients ranged in age from 5 months to 71 years. Fourteen of the patients were hospitalized, but no deaths were reported. Sixty-three of the 64 patients had not been vaccinated, while the remaining patient had received 2 doses of the measles, mumps, and rubella vaccine.

"Although ongoing measles transmissions declared eliminated in the U.S. in 2000, and in the World Health Organization region of the Americas in 2002, many cases of measles occur annually worldwide," the publication said.

The 2008 upsurge in measles cases serves a reminder that measles is still imported into the U.S., and can result in outbreaks unless population immunity remains high through vaccination, the publication added.

"Before the introduction of measles vaccination in 1963, about 3 to 4 million people had measles annually in the U.S., and 400 to 500 died, 48,000 were hospitalized, and 1,000 developed chronic disability from measles encephalitis," the publication continued. "Even after elimination of endemic transmission in 2000, imported measles has continued to create a substantial U.S. public health burden. Of the 501 measles cases reported during 2000-2007, 1 in 4 patients were hospitalized, and 1 in 250 died."

Many of the measles cases in children in the U.S. in 2008 have occurred among children whose parents claimed exemption from vaccination because of religious or personal beliefs, and in infants too young to be vaccinated.

"Forty-eight states currently allow religious exemptions to school vaccination requirements, and 21 states allow exemptions based on personal belief," the publication said.

It went on to say that increases in the proportion of people declining vaccinations for themselves and their children might lead to large-scale outbreaks in the United States, such as those that have occurred in other countries, such as the United Kingdom and the Netherlands.

Sporadic importations of measles into the United States have been recorded since the disease was declared eliminated in the U.S. in 2000, but, during January-July, 2008, 131 measles cases were reported by the CDC, compared with an average of 63 cases annually during 2000-2007, reported the Journal of the American Medical Association on November 12, 2008. At that time, 2 recent outbreaks had been reported among unvaccinated schoolchildren in Washington and Illinois.[4]

"Among the measles cases reported during the first 7 months of 2008, 78% were in those less than 20 years of age, and 91% were in those who were unvaccinated or of unknown vaccination status," the publication continued.

Of the 131 measles cases, 89% were imported from or associated with importations from other countries, especially countries in Europe, where several outbreaks were then ongoing. The cases originated in Italy (3), Switzerland (3), Belgium (2), India (2), Israel (2), China (1), Germany (1), Pakistan (1), the Philippines (1), and Russia (1).

"The findings demonstrate that measles outbreaks can occur in communities with a high number of unvaccinated persons, and that maintaining high overall measles, mumps, and rubella (MMR) vaccination coverage rates in the United States is needed to continue to limit the spread of measles," the publication said.

In the United States, recommendations for MMR vaccination include a single dose at age 12-15 months, and a second dose at the time of school entry. Vaccination as early as age 6 months is recommended for U.S. children traveling abroad, and it is sometimes recommended within U,S. communities during outbreaks of measles.

Of the 131 measles cases reported to the CDC, the patients were in Illinois (32), New York (27), Washington (19), Arizona (14), California (14), Wisconsin (7), Hawaii (5), Michigan (4), Arkansas (2), and D.C., Georgia, Lousiana, Missouri, New Mexico, Pennsylvania, and Virginia, 1 each.

Before the measles vaccine became available in the U.S. in the 1960s, the disease caused 450 reported deaths and 4,000 cases of encephalitis annually.

"Measles is one of the first diseases to reappear when vaccination coverage rates fall," the publication continued. "Ongoing outbreaks are occurring in European countries where rates of vaccination coverage are lower than those in the U.S., including Austria, Italy, and Switzerland."

In June 2008, the United Kingdom's Health Protection Agency declared that, because of a drop in vaccination coverage levels (to 80 to 85% among children aged 2 years), measles was again endemic in the country, 14 years after the disease had been declared eliminated.

Since April 2008, 2 measles-related deaths have been reported in Europe, both in children ineligible to receive MMR vaccine because of congenital immunologic compromise.

"Such children depend on herd immunity for protection from the disease, as do children aged less than 12 months, who normally are too young to receive the vaccine," the publication added. "Otherwise healthy children with measles also are at risk for severe complications, including encephalitis and pneumonia, which can lead to permanent disability or death."

Adults without evidence of measles immunity should receive at least 1 dose of MMR vaccine. All those who travel internationally also should be up-to-date on their measles vaccination and other vaccination recommended for countries they might visit, the publication said.

The February 26, 2003 issue of the Journal of the American Medical Association reported that at that time Cambodia was recovering from almost 30 years of civil war that resulted in a breakdown of the country's public health infrastructure.[5,6]

In 1999, the Ministry of Health initiated a measles-control program with a goal of reducing the annual incidence of measles to less than 10,000 cases by 2003. This would be accomplished by strengthening measles surveillance, improving routine vaccination coverage, implementing supplementary measles immunization activities (SIAs), and providing vitamin A during outbreak investigations and SIAs.

From December 2000 to May 2001, authorities targeted 191, 327 children less than 5 years of age living in remote areas, who were given multiple vaccines (measles, polio vaccine, diphtheria-tetanus-pertussis vaccine), vitamin A, and mebendazole for helminth (an intestinal worm) control.

Phase II conducted during October 2001-April 2002 targeted 2,489,763 children aged 9 months to 14 years living in 8 provinces in densly populated central areas. The children were given measles vaccine, oral polio vaccine (OPV), vitamin A, and mebendazole.

Phase III, which began in October 2002 and was to last until April 2003, targeted about 2,300,000 children aged 9 months to 14 years living in the remaining 7 provinces. They received measles vaccine, OPV, vitamin A, and mebendazole (a drug against pinworms, hookworm, whipworm, and Ascaris (a parasitic roundworm).

In 1999, the World Health Organization assisted the Cambodian National Immunization Program (NIP) in conducting 30 measles outbreak investigations, in which they recorded 1,423 cases, including 14 deaths. In addition, 80 people showed signs of vitamin A deficiency, and six had encephalitis.

"On receiving a report of a measles outbreak from an outreach team, an investigation is conducted about 1 to 4 weeks later by provincial, district, and health center staff," the publication added. "In each village, treatment with vitamin A at the WHO recommended dosage is provided to all people with measles to prevent complications and as a prophylaxis in all children under the age of 12."

During January 2000-October 2002, a total of 94 to 99% of reported measles cases occurred among those less than 15 years of age. The proportion of cases among children less than 5 years of age decreased from 47% in 2000 to 36% in 2001, and 35% in 2002.

Among those less than 10 years of age, the proportion with a history of previous measles vaccination has remained steady, ranging from 23% in 2010 to 27% in 2002.

"Lessons learned in Cambodia might be useful in planning measles-control strategies in other postconflict settings, especially in areas with a few trained health staff and limited transportation and cold chain facilities," the publication added.

A measles outbreak in Gibraltar has infected about 1% of the territory's 28,000 people in just 3 months, according to the November 11, 2008 issue of the New York Times.[7]

The outbreak, most in school children, shocked authorities, since they had thought that 90% of the children had measles shots.

"Gibraltar is a British territory, and resistance to the MMR vaccine has been high in Britain since a 1998 report in The Lancet speculated that it could cause autism," the publication said.

Although that report was widely circulated, a number of other studies revealed no link between vaccines and autism. However, as a consequence of dropping vaccine rates, Britain has had several measles outbreaks.

From August to October 2008, there were 276 cases of measles in Gibraltar, whereas there were none in the previous 10 years, according to Vijay Kumar, M.D. The patients ranged in age from 4 months to 58 years, and most of the cases were mild.

The outbreak was said to have originated in the nearby Spanish town of Algeciras. Gibraltar is less than 10 miles from Algeciras, across the Bay of Gibraltar. Residents live in modern but unusually crowded conditions by Western Europe standards, the newspaper said.

The World Health Organization (WHO) and the United Nations Children's Fund (UNICEF) comprehensive strategy for measles mortality reduction is focused on 47 priority countries, according to the January 30, 2008 issue of the Journal of the American Medical Association.[8,9,10,11,12]

Components of the strategy include:

1. Achieving and maintaining high coverage (over 90%) with the first dose of measles vaccine by age 12 months in every district of each priority country through routine immunization services.
2. Ensuring that all children receive a second opportunity for measles vaccination.
3. Maintaining effective case-based surveillance and monitoring of vaccination coverage.

4. Providing appropriate clinical management, including vitamin A supplementation.

"Measles vaccination campaigns are an opportunity to provide other interventions aimed at improving child survival, such as distribution of vitamin A supplements, delivery of insecticide-treated bednets to prevent malaria, and delivery of deworming medication," the publication added.

The majority of measles supplementary immunization activities (SIAs) conducted in priority countries in 2006 were integrated with other child-survival interventions.

"Experience with combining essential health interventions with measles vaccination campaigns increases high-level political support, allows for resources to be pooled, and increases community participation," the publication continued. "However, these interventions should be integrated in such a way as not to cause delays or reduce the quality of the SIAs."

WHO/UNICEF reported that implementation of measles mortality reduction strategies had reduced measles mortality by 60%, from an estimated 873,00 deaths in 1999 to 345,000 in 2005.

The report concluded by saying that, "measles case management, including appropriate vitamin A supplementation for all children with diagnosed measles cases, should be strengthened."

In January 2007, the American Red Cross, U.S. Centers for Disease Control and Prevention, the United Nations, UNICEF, and the World Health Organization announced that, due to new data from the WHO, global deaths from measles fell from an estimated 873,000 deaths in 1999 to 345,000 in 2005.[13]

In Africa, measles deaths fell by 75% from an estimated 560,000 to 126,000.

Measles has long been a leading cause of death among young children globally, which still kills 500 children daily, reported USA Today on December 4, 2008. However, estimates indicate that millions of deaths have been avoided through interventions in recent years.[14]

The most dramatic improvements have been in Africa, Afghanistan, and Pakistan, where measles deaths have dropped by about 90%.

The least progress has been recorded in South-East Asia, where most of the world's measles deaths now occur. India alone accounted for about two-thirds of the world's deaths from measles.

Most children in India get only 1 dose of vaccine, whereas 2 doses are standard in other nations, the newspaper said.

Measles has resurged in the United States, where cases in 2008—135—reached their highest level in more than a decade.

A cross-sectional study was carried out during an outbreak of measles in Shivpuki, India, according to Ashok Mishra, and colleagues at the Gajara Medical College in Gwalior, and the Ghandi Medical College in Bhopal, India.[15]

The population of 193,000 was covered in house-to-house visits, where the caregivers found 1,204 cases of measles, including 214 patients with complications.

The coverage with routine measles vaccine and vitamin A supplements was 18.3% and 28.9%, respectively.

Both complications and case fatality rates were higher among the children who had not had vitamin A supplements during the previous 6 months.

Measles vaccine was also found to have a protective effect on the development of complications.

The researchers concluded that routine vitamin A supplements and measles vaccination reduce the chances of complications from the disease. The role of vitamin A supplements becomes more important when management of the cases is poor, the researchers added.

"While measles is frequently associated with complications in an Indian setting, there is a need for enhancing the efforts to improve the delivery of vitamin A supplements and measles vaccine to the children in rural areas," the research team said.

The researchers added that measles is one of the biggest causes of childhood illness and death among vaccine preventable diseases in India.

While recent reports suggest a decline in measles related deaths worldwide, evidence of the reduction in illness is still awaited from countries like India, where outbreaks are a common occurrence.

The administration of vitamin A at 100,000 IU at the time of measles immunization is recommended for infants in developing countries, according to Richard D. Semba, M.D., and colleagues, at the Johns Hopkins University School of Medicine in Baltimore, Maryland.[16]

He and his colleagues conducted a randomized, double-blind, placebo-controlled trial which evaluated the simultaneous supplementation of 100,000 IU of vitamin A or a look-alike pill in 336 infants immunized with the standard-titre Schwarz measles vaccine.

It was found that 82% of the infants seroconverted to measles. Seroconversion is the development of antibodies in the blood as a result of infection or immunization.

Vitamin A supplementation was associated with a lower likelihood of seroconversion to measles, and girls were less likely to seroconvert than boys. Simultaneous high vitamin A may interferes with seroconversion to the live measles vaccine in infants with maternal antibodies.

The researchers added that the immune enhancement by vitamin A may limit the ability of the live vaccine to result in a subclinical infection, thereby rendering the measles vaccine less effective and contributing to primary vaccine failure.

Existing data suggests that vitamin A may limit measles infection irresponsive of whether it is due to a wild type or the vaccine-strain measles virus, the researchers added. Infants who received vitamin A were less likely to develop a generalized rash after immunization, which suggests that the vitamin may be limiting the replication of the vaccine-strain measles virus. However, reasons for the sex difference in the seroconversion to the measles vaccine is not known.

The high seroconversion rates of measles in 6-month-old infants with standard titre-Schwarz measles vaccine support the potential of efficacy of vaccinating infants earlier than 9 months of age in this population, the researchers continued.

Vitamin A has an important impact on childhood mortality in infants and young children, and the WHO and UNICEF recommend that oral vitamin A at 100,000 IU be given at the time of the measles immunization at 6 and 9 months of age, depending on the vaccine schedules in developing countries, the researchers said.

The existing data suggests that simultaneous doses of vitamin A increase the risk of failure to seroconvert, and failure to reach protective levels of antibodies to measles. The finding that the mean titres against measles were reduced in infants who received vitamin A may have consequences for long-term immunity against measles. Titre (titer) refers to the strength of a solution.

The benefits of improving vitamin A status needs to be weighed against the potential risk of reduced seroconversion of measles, the researchers continued. Their data suggest that vitamin A is unlikely to interfere with seroconversion among infants with no detectable maternal antibodies to measles.

The 9-month-old infants who would be expected to have lower levels of maternal antibodies to measles, the impact of vitamin A supplementation with measles is known. For example, the oral polio virus vaccine depends on replication by live attenuated (weakened) vaccine-strain virus to be effective.

The researchers added that further study is needed to measure the risk and benefits of delivering vitamin A supplements along with live viral vaccines.

As reported in the Journal of Pediatrics, Antonio Arrieta, M.D., and colleagues, at Children's Hospital of Orange County in California, evaluated 20 children with measles from Long Beach, California, and found that 50% were deficient in vitamin A. This frequency of deficiency was surprising, since these were presumed to be well-nourished American children.[17]

The authors estimate that the number of U.S. children with measles who are vitamin A deficient exceeds 28%, and it is larger than expected in the population that was studied.

They added that it has been recorded in other studies that vitamin A has been given to children at 200,000 IU by mouth for 2 consecutive days, and it was found that there was a quicker recovery from measles. If the children are under 1 year of age, they usually get 100,000 IU of the vitamin.

According to the Centers for Disease Control and Prevention in Atlanta, Georgia, research of vitamin A supplements may result in preventing complications of severe measles in young children, and, therefore, save lives, reported Medical Tribune.[18]

It was discovered in 89 children in New York City, under 2 years of age with measles, that those with lower vitamin A levels were more likely to be hospitalized and to have higher fevers. Children with low levels of vitamin A had lower levels of antibodies against the measles virus.

Researchers at CDC said that vitamin A therapy could reduce deaths caused by measles. They recommended using a single or split dose of 100,000 to 400,000 IU, depending on the child's weight. However, higher doses may cause neurologic problems.

Researchers at the Children's Hospital in Milwaukee, Wisconsin, found that children with low vitamin A levels were more likely to become seriously ill when they contracted measles.

In a double-blind study of 60 African children with measles, 29 of whom were treated with 100,000 IU of retinyl palmitate (Arovite drops from Roache) if under 12 years of age, and 200,000 IU if 12 months and over, reported the Pediatric and Infectious Disease Journal. A control group received the equivalent amount of placebo.[19]

The vitamin A or look-alike medication was administered by the same person on admission and at days 2 and 8. It was found that the supplemented group had significant reductions in morbidity during the acute and chronic phases of the illness.

In the treated group, there was an increase in total number of lymphocytes and measles IgG antibody concentrations, both of which have consistently been shown to correlate more closely with outcome in measles than other immunologic, clinical, and radiologic factors.

Also, Interlukin II and plasma complement values were unaffected by vitamin A supplementation. These findings reinforce data from animal studies that show that vitamin A activity can decrease illness and death by selective immunopotentation," said Anna Coutsoudis, BsC., and colleagues, at the University of Natal, South Africa. Interleukin

II results in the proliferation of T lymphocytes or white blood cells.

The authors added that vitamin A supplementation had an effect on immune function, as shown by a more rapid reversal of measles-induced lymphopenia, and improvement of measles IgG antibody responses during the acute phase. Lymphopenia refers to a reduction of lymphocytes in circulating blood.

A heightened antibody response could lead to a reduction in the number of vaccine failures that occur in developing countries, the authors added.

Writing in the South African Medical Journal, C.B. Ijsselmuiden and colleagues of the Medical Association of South Africa in Pinelands, reported that vitamin A supplementation reduced illness and death from measles infection 30 to 50%, respectively, in a Cape Town study.[20]

Other studies from Indonesia, India, and Nepal have also shown marked reductions in childhood mortality in children with measles who were supplemented with vitamin A.

At Elim Hospital, an understaffed rural hospital, they introduced a therapeutic and prophylatic regimen of vitamin A almost a decade before its major beneficial effects could be demonstrated conclusively.

As early as 1968, low vitamin A levels were shown to occur in malnourished children without measles in Cape Town. Since then, vitamin A levels have been shown to be low in a variety of deprived populations in South Africa, the researchers said.

At the Harvard School of Public Health in Boston, Massachusetts, Wafaie W. Fawzi, MD., and colleagues, evaluated 12 vitamin A-controlled trials for the relationship between vitamin A and childhood deaths, reported the Journal of the American Medical Association.[21]

Vitamin A in hospitalized measles patients was highly protective against mortality. Supplementation was also protective in its overall mortality in community-based studies.

These results suggest that vitamin A supplementation is associated with a significant reduction in deaths when given in a periodic fashion to children at the community level.

The researchers suggest that vitamin A supplements should be given to all measles patients in developing countries, whether they have signs and symptoms of a vitamin A deficiency or not.

They added that large doses of vitamin A are life-saving in children with measles. Additional studies are needed to confirm that the vitamin is useful in treating diarrhea and lower respiratory tract infections.

As reported by Caroline Hall, M.D., in Pediatrics, a consensus statement by the Committee of Infectious Diseases of the American Pediatric Society regarding vitamin A and measles, the recommendations are:[22]

1. Patients 6 months to 2 years of age, who are hospitalized with measles or measles complications, should be considered for vitamin A supplementation.
2. Patients older than 6 months of age with measles, who have any of the following risk factors, who are not already receiving vitamin A, should be considered. The risk factors are immunodeficiency, ophthalmologic (eye) evidence of a vitamin A deficiency, impaired intestinal absorption, moderate to severe malnutrition, and recent immigrants from high mortality areas for measles. A vitamin A solution at 50,000 IU per milliliter is available for oral administration.

The World Health Organization and UNICEF's recommended daily dosage is 1 single dose of 200,000 IU by mouth for children 1 year of age and older or 100,000 IU of vitamin A for children 6 months to 1 year of age.

The higher dosage may be associated with vomiting and headaches within a few hours. The dose should be repeated the following day, and at 4 weeks for children with ophthalmologic evidence of a vitamin A deficiency, Hall added.

Since vitamin A was discovered in 1913, it has been reported that deficiencies of the vitamin result in stunting of growth, infection, and xerophthalmia, which results in blindness, according to Alfred Sommer, M.D., of Johns Hopkins University in Baltimore, Maryland.[23]

Although the correlation with vitamin A deficiency in ocular changes was most popular during the 1980s, a longitudinal prospective study found that a vitamin A deficiency had a dose-response relationship between the severity of mild pre-existing vitamin A deficiency, and the incidence of respiratory and diarrheal infections and death.

Community-based prophylactic trials using vitamin A retinyl palmitate, at doses of 200,000 IU every 6 months has shown significant reductions in childhood mortality by an average of 35%.

When children with measles in hospital-based trials were given vitamin A in dosages of 200,000 IU on 2 subsequent days, there was significant reductions in mortality of at least 50%, Sommer said.

He added that, in an article in the Journal of Infectious Diseases in 1993, improving vitamin A status of children worldwide would prevent 1 to 3 million childhood deaths annually.

As reported in Pediatrics, Jay C. Butler, M.D., and colleagues at the Centers for Disease Control and Prevention in Atlanta, Georgia, evaluated 114 patients with measles, who were less than 5 years of age. They were examined for vitamin A status within 4 days following the onset of a rash.[24]

Retinal concentrations ranged from 0.25 to 1.18 micromol/l. It was found that 72% of the children had low retinol (vitamin A) concentrations. Median retinol levels were lower among hospitalized patients and those with pneumonia. However, these levels of retinol were higher in the children with otitis media, an inflammation of the middle ear.

In addition, higher modified pediatric risk of mortality scores were associated with lower vitamin A levels. In this group of urban children with measles, serum retinol concentrations were depressed, and the degree of depression was associated with the severity of the illness. Serum means the same as blood.

The authors added that vitamin A therapy may be considered for children with measles in the United States who require hospitalization. Dose ranges recommended are 100,000 IU orally for children younger than 12 months, and 200,000 IU for children 12 months or older.

Vitamin A deficiency increases the severity of, as well as death from, measles and diarrhea, reported the British Medical Journal. Deficiency also increases infections and mortality even before the appearance of xerophthalmia, according to Alfred Sommer, M.D.[25]

Improving the vitamin A status of deficient children aged 6 months to 6 years can significantly reduce the illness and death from infection, Dr. Sommer added. Large doses of vitamin A given to children with moderate or severe measles, especially if children are vitamin A deficient, can reduce mortality 59%, and or attenuate the severity of complications. Doses used for measles have been 200,000 IU on 2 consecutive days.

Vitamin A supplementation has been used to restore normal vitamin A status, which increases resistance to several infections by restoring the normally differentiated epithelia, by providing a more effective barrier to infection, and by upgrading the immune system, Sommer added.

Children with measles are hyporetinemic with serum vitamin A levels less than 20 mcg/dl, according to Greg Hussey, M.D., and Max Klein, M.D., of the University of Cape Town, South Africa.[26]

This low blood level suggests a vitamin A deficiency at a tissue level. Even these children from communities that are not nutritionally vitamin-deficient are still at high risk of hyporetinemia during measles.

The researchers added that a high dose of vitamin A at 400,000 IU has shown a remarkable reduction in illness and death. There have been similar reductions in hospital stays, intensive care admissions, and death rates with vitamin A supplementation during measles outbreaks under conditions of routine hospital care in Cape Town.

Intervention studies have shown that there is a relationship between vitamin A status and severe measles, they added. The exact mechanism is unknown, but it is hypothesized that vitamin A deficiency in measles affects the same cell systems.

As reported in the American Journal of Diseases in Children, a research team headed by Thomas R. Frieden, M.D., of the New York City Department of Health, evaluated vitamin A levels in

89 children with measles, who were younger than 2 years of age.[27]

Vitamin A levels in the children with measles ranged from 0.42 to 3.0 micromol/l, and 20 of the children, or 22%, had low vitamin A stores.

Children with low levels of the vitamin were more likely to have fever at a temperature of 40 degrees C. or higher (68 vs 44%), to have fever for 7 days or more (54 vs 23%), and to be hospitalized (55 to 30%). Children with low vitamin A levels had lower measles-specific antibody levels.

The authors added that clinicians may consider vitamin A therapy for children under 2 years of age with severe measles. The vitamin is very inexpensive, and a single or split dose of 100,000 to 400,000 IU, depending on the weight of the child, is relatively safe.

Multiple or higher doses may cause a rash or severe neurological (nervous system) symptoms, and should not be given, the authors added.

Vitamin A supplementation substantially reduced mortality from severe measles, as well as reduced the severity of diarrhea, according to researchers at Royal Children's Hospital in Parkville, Victoria, Australia, in The Lancet.[28]

At Pennsylvania State University in University Park, Francisco J. Rossales, M.D., and colleagues, evaluated, in a double-blind study, vitamin A in oil at 200,000 IU in 90 non-xerophthalmic measles patients versus 110 controls.[29]

They reported that evidence for the efficacy of 1 dose of vitamin A in oil to prevent measles is not as strong as previously shown with 200,000 IU doses in water-miscible vitamin A.

In an article in the Bulletin of the World Health Organization in 1992, researchers estimated that 124 million children worldwide were vitamin A deficient. Improved vitamin A nutriture would be expected to prevent about 1 to 2 million deaths annually among children between 1 and 4 years of age.[30]

The researchers added that an additional 250,000 to 500,000 deaths could possibly be prevented if improved vitamin A nutriture could be achieved during the latter half of infancy.

In the highest-risk developing countries, improved vitamin A nutriture alone could prevent 1.3 to 2.5 million of the nearly 8 million late infancy and preschool deaths that occur each year, they said.

It is believed that improved vitamin A status would help to reduce the incidence of infection, diarrhea, respiratory diseases, and measles, added the research team at Johns Hopkins University. The vitamin may also be of benefit in enhancing immunization programs, they continued.

At the All India Institute of Medical Science in New Delhi, S.K. Kabra, M.D., and colleagues, evaluated 177 children with post-measles complications. They were divided into 2 groups. In the study, 89 children were given vitamin A in doses of 200,000 IU on 2 consecutive days, in addition to antibacterial and other supportive care. The controls consisted of 88 children who were not given the vitamin.[31]

The case fatality rate was 16% in those who were given vitamin A, compared with 32% not given the vitamin. However, there were no statistical differences in the mortality rate among the 2 groups when the children were suffering from severe malnutrition or encephalopathy (any disorder of the brain).

The researchers added that there is considerable evidence that vitamin A deficiency occurs during measles. It is possible that the beneficial effect of vitamin A is mediated by an effect on epithelial cell maturation.

While vitamin A therapy did not show any beneficial effect in severely malnourished children in the study, it is possible that there was a defect in utilizing the vitamin in those children, the researchers added.

At the University of Queensland in Australia, researchers evaluated 20 controlled trials dealing with vitamin A supplementation and a variety of infections. Twelve of the studies were randomized, six were community based in developing countries, 3 were in children admitted to the hospital with measles, and 3 were in very low-birth weight infants.[32]

The results from the community study suggests a 30% reduction in all case mortality with vitamin A supplementation.

There was a reduction in deaths from diarrheal disease (community studies) by 39%, from respiratory disease (measles study) by 70%, and from other causes of death in the community studies by 34%.

The authors concluded that an adequate supply of vitamin A, either by appropriate dietary means, or through supplementation, has a major role in preventing illness and death in children in developing countries. It was also noted that children in developed countries may receive benefit from vitamin A supplementation during life-threatening infections, such as measles, and for relative deficiencies such as premature infants, they reported in the British Medical Journal.

In spite of a safe and effective vaccine since 1963, measles has been a major killer of children in developing countries, causing an estimated 750,000 deaths as recently as 2000, primarily because of underutilization of the vaccine, reported the April 8, 2009 issue of the Journal of the American Medical Association.[33]

At the World Health Assembly in 2008, all World Health Organizations (WHO) member states reaffirmed their commitment to achieve a 90% reduction in measles mortality by 2010, compared with 2000, a goal that was promulgated in 2005 as part of the Global Immunization Vision and Strategy.

The WHO-UNICEF comprehensive strategy for measles mortality reduction focuses on 47 priority countries.

Of 23.3 million infants in 2007 who missed receiving their first dose of measles vaccine through routine immunization services by the age of 1 year, 15.2% (65%) resided in 8 highly populated countries:

India (8.5 million children); Nigeria (2.0 million); China (1.0 million); Ethiopia (1.0 million); Indonesia (0.9 million); Pakistan (0.8 million); the Democratic Republic of the Congo (0.6 million); and Bangladesh (0.5 million).

During 2000-2007, an opportunity for measles immunization was provided in the 47 priority countries to almost 576 million children aged 9 months to 14 years through supplementary immunization activities (SIAs)," the publication reported.

In 2007, 20 (43%) of these 47 countries conducted SIAs, reaching about 91 million children. Sixteen (80%) of these SIAs integrated at least 1 other child-survival intervention—insecticide-treated bed nets, vitamin A supplements, and deworming medications.

Countries with high measles disease were urged to adopt a strategy to reduce measles cases by 90% by 2010. These include:

1. Accelerated measles mortality reduction activities, e.g., SIAs coupled with efforts to improve routine measles-containing vaccine (MCVI) coverage, especially in the South-East Asian Region, notably India.
2. Vaccination system need to be improved to ensure that over 50% of infants are given their MCVI on schedule.
3. Countries need to monitor accumulation of susceptible children, and conduct follow-up SIAs when the number of susceptible children approaches the size of a birth cohort.
4. Disease surveillance systems need to be strengthened at all levels.
5. Measles case management should be improved, for example, by including the use of vitamin A.
6. Additional efforts are needed to ensure sustainability of measles control activities.

Children with severe measles should be given vitamin A supplements, according to a placebo-controlled trial of vitamin A in 189 Cape Town, South African children with severe measles, reported the South African Medical Journal.[34]

This therapy reduced the death rate by more than 50%, and the duration of pneumonia, diarrhea, and hospital stays by 33%.

The researchers also found that vitamin A also reduced the incidence of croup and herpes stomatitis (inflammatory disease of the mouth). The children were given 400,000 IU (120 mg) of water-soluble vitamin A (retinyl palmitate/Arovite drops/Roche) or a placebo. Half of the doses were given initially on admission, and the other 200,000 IU was given a day later.

The researchers added that hyporetinemia is present in severe measles. Also, all children hospitalized for measles should receive the just-named dosages of vitamin A. Children under 2 years of age should be given preference where resources are limited, the researchers added.

An editorial in the New England Journal of Medicine commented positively on the use of vitamin A as an adjunct to disease prevention, along with combined efforts at sanitation, hygiene, good quality health care, immunizations, and adequate water supplies.[35]

Vitamin A's benefit for decreasing the incidence of diarrhea, respiratory diseases, illness and death, and measles progression, may be due to the activity to mediate maturation of epithelial cell integrity, explained Gerald T. Keusch, M.D., of the New England Medical Center in Boston, Massachusetts.

While the ultimate mechanism is not yet known, the previous study (NEJM 323: 160-164, 1990), using vitamin A administration in measles, utilized a much larger dose, compared to the lower weekly dose reported in NEMJ 323:929, 1990.

The potential benefit against menigococcal meningitis needs to be assessed and is intriguing, the researchers added. The annual costs of such prevention measures may be $1.64 to $2.20 per recipient (1990), which may significantly stress the resources of developing nations. It was suggested that the international community help out.

Measles remains a public health problem in Europe, and there are serious doubts that it can be eliminated by 2010 as health officials had predicted, reported Donald G. McNeil, Jr., in the January 13, 2009 issue of the New York Times.[36]

As originally tabulated in The Lancet, for 2006 and 2007, there were 12,132 cases in measles in Europe, mainly in Britain, Germany, Italy, Romania, and Switzerland. Seven deaths were reported.

While most European cases were in the general population, there were outbreaks among Roma and Sinti—sometimes called gypsies—in Italy and Romania, travelers in Britain and Norway, and Orthodox Jews in Belgium and Britain, McNeil continued.

The Swiss cases were mostly in Lucerne, the German patients in Bavaria and Hesse, where vaccination rates are reportedly lower, and families rated "hard to reach" by authorities, and the medical philosophy of the 19th and early 20th century theorist Rudolf Steiner (1861-1925).

Countries Where Measles is Most Prominent

Afghanistan, Angola, Bangladesh, Benin, Burkina Faso, Burundi, Cambodia, Cameroon, Central African Republic, Chad, Congo, Cote e'Ivoire.

Democratic Republic of the Congo, Djibouti, Equatorial Guinea, Eritrea, Ethiopia, Gabon, Ghana, Guinea, Guinea-Bisseau.

India, Indonesia, Kenya, Lao People's Democratic Republic, Liberia, Madagascar, Mali, Mozambique, Myanmar.

Nepal, Niger, Nigeria, Pakistan, Papua New Guinea, Rwanda, Senegal, Sierre Leone, Somalia, Sudan, Timor-Leste, Togo, Uganda, United Republic of Tanzania, Vietnam, Yemen, and Zambia.

Source: JAMA 299(4):402, January 30, 2008.

References

1. Clayman, Charles B., M.D., medical editor. The American Medical Association Home Medical Encyclopedia. New York: Random House, 1989, pp. 668-669.
2. "Measles—United States, January 1-April 25, 2008," JAMA 299(22)2621-2623, 2008.
3. Orenstein, W.A., et al. "Measles Elimination in the United States," Journal of Infectious Diseases 189:5138, 2004.
4. Update: "Measles—United States, January-July, 2008," JAMA 300(18):2111-2112, 2008.
5. "Accelerated Measles Control—Cambodia, 1999-2002," JAMA 289(8): 977-978, 2003.
6. "Expanded Programs on Immunization. Joint WHO/UNICEF Statement on Vitamin A for Measles," Weekly Epidemiological Record 62:133-134, 1987.
7. McNeil, Donald G., Jr. "Fast-Spreading Outbreak Reveals Lower Immunization Rate in Gibraltar," New York Times, November 11, 2008, p. D8.
8. "Progress in Global Measles Control and Mortality Reduction, 2000-2006," JAMA 299(4): 400-402, 2008.

9. World Health Organization, United Nations Children's Fund Measles Mortality Reduction and Regional Elimination Strategic Plan—2001-2005. Geneva, Switzerland, World Health Organization, 2001.

10. World Health Organization, United Nations Children's Fund. Global Immunization Visition and Strategy—2006-2015. Geneva, Switzerland: World Health Organization, 2005.

11. Wolfson, L.J., et al. "Has the 2005 Measles Mortality Reduction Goal Been Achieved: A Natural History Modelling Study," Lancet 369(9557): 191-200, 2007.

12. Hussey, G.D., and Klein, M. "A Randomized Controlled Trial of Vitamin A in Children with Severe Measles," New England Journal of Medicine 323:160-164, 1990.

13. "Global Goal to Reduce Measles Deaths in Children Surpassed," World Health Organization, Geneva, Switzerland, January 19, 2007.

14. "WHO, CDC Report Drop in Measles Deaths Worldwide," USA Today, December 4, 2008.

15. Mishra, Ashok, et al. "Measles Related Complications and the Role of Vitamin A Supplements," Indian Journal of Pediatrics 75(9): 887-890, 2008.

16. Semba, Richard D., M.D., et al. "Reduced MM Seroconversion of Measles in Infants Given Vitamin A with Measles Vaccination," The Lancet 345:1330-1332, May 1995.

17. Arrieta, Antonio, M.D., et al. "Vitamin A Levels with Measles in Long Beach, California," Journal of Pediatrics 121(1): 75-78, July 1992.

18. Slom, Celia. "Vitamin A May Ease Severity of Measles in Children" Medical Tribune, March 12, 1992, p. 7.

19. Coutsoudis, Anna, Bs.C., et al. "Vitamin A Supplementation Enhances Specific IgG Antibody Levels and Total Lymphocyte Numbers While Improving Morbidity in Measles," The Pediatric Infections Disease Journal 11(3): 203-209, March 1992.

20. Ijsselmuiden, C.B., et al. "Vitamin A, Childhood Mortality, Foresight and Epidemiology," South African Medical Journal 81(4):182-183, February 15, 1992.

21. Fawzi, Wafaie, M.D., et al. "Vitamin A Supplementation and Child Mortality: A Meta-Analysis," JAMA 269(7): 893-903, 1993.

22. Hall, Caroline, M.D. "Vitamin A Treatment for Measles," Pediatrics 91(5):1014-1015, May 1993.

23. Sommer, Alfred, M.D. "Vitamin A, Infectious Disease, in Childhood Mortality: A 2-Cent Solution," Journal of Infectious Diseases 167:1003-1007, May 1993.

24. Butler, Jay C., M.D., et al. "Measles Severity and Serum Retinol (Vitamin A) Concentrations Among Children in the United States," Pediatrics 91(6): 1176-1181, June 1993.
25. Sommer, Alfred, M.D. "Vitamin A Prophylaxis," British Medical Journal, 1997, pp. 191-194.
26. Hussey, Greg, M.D., and Klein, Max, M.D. "The Interaction Between Vitamin A Status and Measles Infection, Beyond Deficiency: New Views on the Function and Health of Vitamins," New York Academy of Sciences, February 9-12, 1992; Abstract 17.
27. Frieden, Thomas R., M.D., et al. "Vitamin A Levels and the Severity of Measles: New York City," American Journal of Diseases of Children 146:182-186, February 1992.
28. Shann, Frank, M.D., and Duke, Trevor, "Micronutrients, Measles, Malaria, and Mortality," The Lancet, December 23-30, 1995, p. 16.
29. Rossales, Francisco J., M.D., et al. "Efficiency of a Single Oral Dose of 200,000 IU of Oil-Soluble Vitamin A in Measles-Associated Morbidity," American Journal of Epidemiology 143:413-422, 1996.
30. Humphrey, J.H., et al. "Vitamin A Deficiency and Attributable Mortality Among Under-Five-Year Olds," Bulletin of the World Health Organization, Geneva, Switzerland 70(2): 225-232, 1992.
31. Kabra, S.K., M.D., et al. "Vitamin A Supplementation in Post-Measles Complications," Journal of Tropical Pediatrics 40:305-307, October 1994.
32. Glasziou, P.P., and Mackerras, D., et al. "Vitamin A Supplementation in Infectious Diseases: A Meta-Analysis," British Medical Journal 306:366-370, February 6, 1993.
33. "Progress in Global Measles Control and Mortality Reduction, 2000-2007," JAMA 301(14): 1430-1431, 2009.
34. Klein, Max, and Hussey, Gregory D. "Vitamin A Reduces Morbidity and Mortality in Measles," South African Medical Journal 78: 56-57, July 21, 1990.
35. Keusch, Gerald T., M.D. "Vitamin A Supplements—Too Good Not to Be True," New England Journal of Medicine 323: 985-987, 1990.
36. McNeil, Donald G., Jr. "With Measles Still a Threat in Europe, Eradication Goal Is Unlikely, Report Says," New York Times, January 13, 2009, p. D6.

5

CANCER

Although the word cancer has no precise medical meaning, it is a term used and understood by both the laymen and the medical profession, according to Foods and Nutrition Encyclopedia. Neoplasia—new growth—is a more precise term.[1]

The ancient Greeks called it karkinos, meaning crab, because of the clawlike spread of the new growth. The Romans adopted the idea from the Greeks and gave it the Latin name for crab—cancer.

"Cancer is a word that stands for a large group of diseases—malignant tumor (malignant neoplasia, carcinoma, sarcoma, melanoma, lymphoma, and others)—that afflict man and animals," the encyclopedia said.

The characteristic of cancer is wild, uncontrolled growth of cells which can arise in any organ or tissue of the body. Cancer cells have a rather primitive appearance when compared to normal cells, since they are rather irregular in shape and have large irregular nuclei.

"All cells have the capacity to divide," the encyclopedia continued. "This process is called mitosis—one cell becomes two, two cells become four, four cells become eight, etc. When a cell divides, it goes through a cell cycle and the cell receives some sort of signal that averts and stops the process."

Out of 100 cancer cells, 10 or 20 will continuously be going through division, and many cells will pile up. The cancer cell then has an apparent autonomy due to some abnormality in the chromosomes. It will continue to grow regardless of the size of the mass it creates.

"As cancers continue to grow, they interfere with body function by crowding normal organs and outstripping the food supply available to the patient, eventually killing the patient," the encyclopedia added.

Tumor cells are either benign (harmless) or malignant. Benign tumors are the ones that cannot invade the surrounding tissues, but remain as strictly local growths. Malignant tumors spread from their site of origin, and, therefore, can reach the bloodstream and lymphatic system. These cancers are divided into three groups:

1. Carcinomas, which arise in the epithelial tissues, that is, the sheets of cells covering the surface of the body and lining the various glands.
2. Sarcomas arise in supporting structures such as fibrous tissue or connective tissue and blood vessels.
3. Leukemias and lymphomas arise in blood-forming cells of the bone marrow and lymph nodes.

"Cancers are further classified by the organ in which they originate—lung, colon and rectum, breast, prostate, uterus, skin, oral, etc.—and by the kind of cell involved," the encyclopedia said. "In this way, there are 100 or more distinct varieties of cancer, however, most of these are rare."

A number of clinical studies have linked nutrient deficiencies in the development of cancer. Deficiencies of vitamins A, C, E, and the B Complex have been associated with the increased susceptibility of chemically-induced tumors, as have protein, iodine, iron, magnesium, and selenium deficiencies, the encyclopedia added. Some studies have shown that those with a higher vitamin A (carotene) intake or blood levels are less susceptible to cancer. Nontoxic vitamin A analogs have been successfully used to prevent cancer.

Although there are many theories regarding the causes of cancer, the fundamental idea underlying these theories is that the genetic material, the DNA of the cell, has been changed, and the various theories attempt to explain how this change was brought about, explained Mukti H. Sarma, Ph.D.[2]

"The DNA of a cancer cell is slightly different from that of a normal cell," Sarma said. "This means that the sequence of their bases—adenine (A), guanine (G), thymine (T), and scytosine (C)—in a given strand of DNA is not the same. These sequences dictate the sequence of the transcribed messenger RNA, which in turn, specifies the kinds of proteins to be synthesized in a cell. The change in the DNA sequence in the cancer cells results in abnormal proteins. These new proteins influence the mechanism of growth control in such a way that cell division continues indefinitely."

Sarma goes on to say that one of the important characteristics of a cancer cell is its lack of "contact inhibition." Normal cells reproduce by dividing, but they stop dividing when the number of cells reaches a certain point. Precise control of cell division is a basic function of all multicultural organisms. The growth-control signal is transmitted by various proteins that interact with the cell-surface protein receptors.

"The basic change in the DNA, known as mutation, can be caused by a number of factors, such as ultra-violet and ionizing radiation, chemicals, so-called free radicals, and viruses, Sarma added.

"However, mutation does not necessarily cause cancer. This happens only when proteins that result from mutation affect cellular growth-control mechanisms."

In multicultural organisms, interaction between cells is crucial in maintaining the structural and functional integrity of the organism. The interaction between cells depends on two types of signals—growth stimulating and growth inhibiting. Recent research has shown that tumor suppression genes can inhibit cell growth in three possible ways: (1) cells may not enter the DNA synthesis phase, and, thus, cell division does not occur; (2) cells may divide but at the end of division will differentiate and will not divide again (called terminal differentiation); or (3) the most dramatic, the cell goes through apoptosis or programmed cell death.

On December 23, 1971, the United States declared war on cancer, when President Richard H. Nixon, urged on by members of Congress and lobbyists, proposed that the same concentrated effort that resulted in the splitting of the atom, and put a man on the Moon, to go forward in conquering the disease, reported William J. Cromie.[3]

At that time, Congress passed the National Cancer Act of 1971, unmindful of the differences in solving problems in space and knowing engineering principles. In the following decades, $22 billion was spent on research and development concerning cancer. While vaccines were won against cancers of the stomach, cervix, rectum, testis, thyroid, mouth, larynx, and some childhood malignancies, incidences of the major killers such as lung, prostate, breast, colon, and skin cancers rose.

"Much, but not all, of that rise came from better methods of detection," Cromie added. "Finding cancer early significantly increases the chances of successfully containing or curing it with the most effective treatments that have become available."

The battle against breast cancer reflects lack of progress in the war in general, Cromie said. Over $1 billion was spent on this part of the struggle from 1971 to 1991, and, while treatment has improved and survival has increased—the 5-year rate having reached 77%— the death rate has not been reduced.

"Much of this increase resulted from the timely discovery of localized lumps by self-examination and X-ray mammography, but there remains an unexplained portion of the rise that has been linked to hormonal changes, diet, breast-feeding, breast implants, and radiation," Cromie continued.

Long-term use of estrogen replacement therapy produces about a 10% increase of breast cancer for every five years of therapy, he added. Rise of breast cancer is apparently lowered 10 to 20% for each year if menarche—the onset of menstruation—is delayed. Women who stop menstruating before age 45 experience half the rise of those who continue to menstruate at age 55 and beyond.

"Progestin, taken to counteract estrogen's tendency to cause uterine cancer, has been shown in trials to increase the risk of breast cancer rather than reduce it, as had been originally assumed," Cromie said.

Attempts to link breast cancer with animal or vegetable fats have been inconsistent, he continued. A better case can be made for the claim that women who nurse their babies reduce their risk of this malignancy. And some women with silicone breast implants have tested positive for a substance suspected of causing cancer, but the risk is not clear enough to warrant removal of this procedure.

"In 1991, researchers reported that women who carry a single copy of the gene responsible for ataxia-telanglectasia might be especially sensitive to damage from low-dose X-rays," Cromie continued. "Some physicians recommend that such women avoid mammography when possible in favor of periodic physical examinations by an expert who feels for lumps."

A slowly progressive multisystem disorder, ataxia-telanglectasia—also called Louis-Bar Syndrome—results in the onset of walking problems, dilation of conjunctiva and skin of the face, neck, and ears; recurring infections of the respiratory system; involuntary movemens; etc.

About 70% of the patients have an IgA deficiency consistent with decreased T-helper cell function. There may also be many chromosome breaks.[4]

Approximately 35% of all cancers may be preventable through dietary modification, according to Charles H. Hennekens, M.D., of the Harvard Medical School and Brigham and Women's Hospital in Boston, Massachusetts.[5]

As an example, beta-carotene is one of the most efficient quenchers of singlet oxygen molecules, and it can prevent tissue damage by trapping organic free radicals.

In evaluating a large number of studies, results suggest that those with the highest dietary intakes or blood levels of beta-carotene tend to have a 20 to 40% lower risk of cancer than those with the lowest intakes or blood levels. It could be that other constituents of beta-carotene-rich foods, or some dietary or non-dietary lifestyle factors, are responsible, he added.

Four large-scale trials of beta-carotene supplementation in cancer prevention have been completed, Hennekens said. The Chinese Cancer Prevention Trial involved some 29,000 poorly nourished residents in Linxian, China. The participants were given 15 mg of beta-carotene, 30 mg of vitamin E, and 50 mcg of selenium daily for 5.25 years. There was a significant 9% decrease in total mortality, which was largely due to the 21% decrease in gastric cancer deaths.

While other studies with beta-carotene have not always been supportive, in a 12-year study of 12,000 male physicians, it is possible that 12 years of treatment was inadequate to provide benefit on cancer, a disease that may take as long as 15 to 20 years to show symptoms, Hennekens added. The anticancer benefit of beta-carotene may also be confined to poorly nourished people.

Vitamin supplementation should be an adjunct, not alternative, to lifestyle practices, which reduce cancer risk, such as smoking avoidance or cessation, and increased consumption of carotene-rich fruits and vegetables, Hennekens added.

A precancerous state of squamous metaplasia from tissue vitamin A deficiency can occur without systemic deficiency, reported researchers at the University of Missouri at Columbia.[6]

A deficiency may occur through direct epithelial exposure to the carcinogen stimulating vitamin A metabolism locally. Enhancement of beta-carotene cleavage could explain the cancer protective effect of dietary beta-carotene over the active form of vitamin A.

They added that beta-carotene can prevent carcinogenic-induced vitamin A tissue deficiency that can occur from exposure to carcinogens such as benzopyrene.

In one study, researchers found that the number of T-helper cells in male volunteers jumped 30% after they took 180 mg—almost 299,000 IU of beta-carotene—daily for two weeks, according to Prevention's Healing with Vitamins.[7]

In a study at the University of Arizona at Tucson, men and women were given daily doses of 15 mg (about 25,000 IU); 30 mg (about 50,000 IU); 45 mg (about 75,000 IU); or 60 mg (almost 100,000 IU) of beta-carotene for two months, reported Ronald R. Watson, Ph.D.

It was found that an enhanced immune response was noticeable at 30 mg and above, with increased numbers of both natural killer cells and activated lymphocytes, which are important immune system components.

While some physicians believe that antioxidants interfere with chemotherapy, others argue that they might actually enhance the effects of chemotherapy.[8]

Researchers reviewing the evidence, reported in Gynecologic Oncology on the anti-cancer properties of vitamin A, vitamin C, vitamin E, and mixed carotenoids.

They reported that, "while it is accepted that antioxidants are useful in the reduction of adverse effects of chemotherapy, the prevailing opinion is that antioxidants reduce the effectiveness of chemotherapy and radiation therapy's neoplastic toxicity. However, there is evidence that antioxidants may also be a choice for therapeutic intervention alongside chemotherapy with demonstrated benefit in tumor size reduction and/or increased longevity."

Considerable research has shown that antioxidant supplements prevent free-radical damage to DNA, an early step in the development of cancer. While simple DNA damage can often be repaired, chromosome damage is far more serious and difficult to repair, according to Mutagenesis.[9]

In the study, researchers asked 57 healthy men from rural areas, and 28 men who had survived a heart attack, to take either placebos or a daily supplement containing vitamin E (100 mg); vitamin C (100 mg); beta-carotene (6 mg); and selenium (50 mcg) for 12 weeks.

Lymphocytes, a type of immune cell, were studied from blood samples at the beginning and end of the study. The researchers were especially interested in the number of lymphocytes with chromosome damage.

It was reported that antioxidant supplements significantly decreased the number of cells with chromosome damage in the healthy men. The percentage of cells with chromosome aberrations decreased by 57% with supplementation.

The most significant effect was in smokers, who had only 0.12% chromosome damage, compared with 0.81% in smokers taking placebos. The supplements did not alter chromosome damage in the men who had had a heart attack.

An extensive review of the role of vitamins A, C, E, beta-carotene, selenium, and zinc was reported by the Food and Drug Administration in Washington, D.C., in Nutrition Cancer Prevention and Treatment.[10]

The authors stated that the protective effects of supplemented antioxidants have been observed in clinical trials, the reduction in cancer risk strongly relates to diets containing high amounts of carotene-rich fruits and vegetables.

We know from large population studies, low intakes of beta-carotene are associated with higher incidence of cancer, according to Sheldon Saul Hendler, M.D., Ph.D. It also appears likely that beta-carotene exerts a protective effect through its unique antioxidant properties.[11]

The nutrient is especially good at attacking a very toxic form of di-oxygen—singlet oxygen—that contributes to the malignant processes in tissues. Researchers studying this antioxidant effect have called beta-carotene "the most efficient quencher of singlet oxygen thus far discovered," he said.

Equally exciting is vitamin A's role in immunity, a role which almost certainly contributes to its anti-cancer properties," Hendler added. "It appears that many of the hopes that were related for vitamin A as the 'anti-infective vitamin' more than 50 years ago are now being realized. Studies in third-world populations have demonstrated the enormous power of this vitamin in boosting resistance to infection and reducing the related mortality."

He went on to say that vitamin A, even in the wake of all its "miracles," continues to be the most feared vitamin.

"It is surprising," he continued," how many physicians still warn patients to stay away from vitamin A, neglecting to mention that beta-carotene has the same benefits as preformed vitamin A and almost none of its adverse side effects."

Increases in cellular immunity have been reported among lung cancer patients given very high doses of vitamin A for three weeks, Hendler continued. And depression of immune function has been blocked in surgical patients given high doses of the vitamin.

Supplementation was given just before surgery and for a few days afterward. In the case of cancer patients, 1.5 million IU were given daily, and in the case of the surgical patients the daily dose was 300,000 to 450,000 IU. These doses require medical supervision and cannot be tolerated for long periods.

"Some especially exciting research has shown that supplemental beta-carotene in high, but still non-toxic doses of 180 mg/day, can increase the number of very important immune cells—T-lymphocyte helper cells. In healthy males, after only two weeks of supplementation, there was a 30% increase in T-helper cell numbers" he continued.

There are hundreds of papers demonstrating that vitamin A, primarily in the preformed variety, can suppress the malignant behavior of cultured cells adversely transformed by radiation, chemicals, or viruses, can delay the development of transplanted tumors, and can even completely prevent malignancy in animals exposed to various potent cancer-causing sustenances, Hendler said.

The drug derivatives of vitamin A are also showing promise in the fight against cancer, he continued. Accutane has been shown to be of benefit in the treatment of cutaneous T-cell lymphoma, a blood cancer that affects the skin. The drug may also be useful in the treatment of myelodysplastic syndrome, a premalignant condition with leukemia-like characteristics. Accutane has also been able to shrink dramatically, and, in some cases, completely eradicate oral leukoplakia, the precancerous lesions found on the lips and inside the mouth.

"Both preformed vitamin A (liver, fish oils, eggs, etc.), and beta-carotene, either in combination or alone, are capable of shrinking and sometimes eradicating these leukoplakias, especially common among smokers," Hendler continued. "They are particularly good at preventing the development of new leukoplakias, which resemble white spots and patches."

Breast Cancer

A number of factors are associated with the risk of breast cancer, including age, smoking, alcohol consumption, and diet. A number of studies have demonstrated that eating foods rich in antioxidant carotenoids may reduce the risk of breast cancer and other types of cancer also, according to the American Journal of Clinical Nutrition.[12]

In the study, a research team evaluated the dietary habits of 414 women with breast cancer and 429 healthy women to evaluate the influence of carotenoids and essential fatty acids on breast cancer risk. The women were French Canadians, a relatively genetically and culturally related group.

In women who had never used hormone replacement therapy, high intakes of beta-carotene was associated with a 43% lower risk of breast cancer. In contrast, in premenopausal women who smoked, the highest intakes of alpha-carotene was associated with a 140% increased risk of breast cancer.

Breast cancer risk was also related to an interaction among intakes of carotenoids and essential fatty acids. As an example, in postmenopausal women, who combined high intakes of carotenoids and omega-3 fatty acids (fish oils) was associated with a 48% lower risk of breast cancer.

The researchers concluded that a high intake of total carotenoids and omega-3 fatty acids—specifically docosahexaenoic acid or DHA—may reduce the risk of breast cancer in postmenopausal women. Other studies have also suggested that diets rich in carotenoids and omega-3 fatty acids may reduce the risk of breast cancer, they added.

According to an article in Epidemiology, researchers analyzed the diets of 273 women with breast cancer, and 371 healthy women at various stages of their lives.[13]

The researchers reported that postmenopausal women who had been consuming diets rich in beta-carotene for 20 to 45 years had a decreased risk of breast cancer when compared to women with low intakes of the vitamin.

In 12 women who were given 150,000 IU/day of vitamin A, after three months there was complete or partial responses in five patients, and a marked pain reduction in nine, according to Preventive Medicine.[14]

Side effects were minimal. The dosage of one patient was reduced due to side effects, however, no hepatoxicity was observed.

In 3,543 cancer patients, compared with 9,406 controls, eating carrots and spinach—rich sources of vitamin A—more than twice weekly, compared to no intake, was associated with an odds ratio of 0.56 in developing breast cancer.[15]

These data, reported in Cancer, Epidemiology, Biomarkers

and Prevention, are consistent with a diet rich in vegetables having a modest protective effect against breast cancer.

Free radicals are known to damage DNA, cause mutations, and give rise to cancerous cells, reported the Journal of Nutrition. Since antioxidants neutralize free radicals, they have the potential for reducing a person's long-term risk of cancer.[16]

In the study, researchers analyzed blood levels of antioxidants, nutrients, and other substances in the blood of 153 women recently diagnosed with breast cancer, and 151 healthy controls.

Women with the highest blood levels of total antioxidants, retinol (vitamin A), bilirubin, or beta-carotene, were about one-half less likely to be diagnosed with breast cancer. Therefore, vitamin A and beta-carotene may offer some protection against breast cancer, the researchers said. Bilirubin is a red bile pigment found in gallstones.

It is estimated that about 55% of breast cancer can be explained by recognized risk factors, according to Louise A. Brinton, Ph.D., in the Journal of the National Cancer Institute. Risk factors include familial susceptibility, menstrual characteristics, reproductive behavior, and socioeconomic status.[17]

She added that evidence suggests that breast cancer risk can be reduced by vitamin A, vitamin C, vitamin D, vitamin E, carotenoids, and fiber intake. Physical activity may also reduce the risk, since it has been shown that women who were athletes during college had a reduced risk of the disease.

There appears to be growing evidence that long-term use of oral contraceptives increase the risk of early-onset breast cancer. Whether this extends to older women is unclear. However, extended or recent use of menopausal estrogens is associated with approximately 50 to 80% elevation in the risk of this cancer, Brinton said.

There is a distinct north-south Latitudinal trend in breast cancer deaths, as well as a correlation with levels of solar radiation, which is where vitamin D may be protective, she added.

Numerous studies have shown that diets high in vegetables and fruits are associated with a low risk of breast cancer and other types of cancer. The theory is that the antioxidants in the foods can prevent cellular damage and mutations in genes, according to Nutrition Research.[18]

In the study, researchers compared blood levels of vitamin E, beta-carotene, a combination of lutein and zeaxanthin, cryptoxanthin, lycopene, alpha-carotene, and vitamin A in 160 breast cancer patients and 229 healthy controls.

High blood levels of several antioxidants were strongly associated with a low risk of breast cancer. In premenopausal women, high levels of vitamin E, beta-carotene, lutein/ zeaxanthin, and vitamin A were associated with 59, 67, 87, and 85% reduction in breast cancer, respectively.

In postmenopausal women, high levels of vitamin E, vitamin A, beta-carotene, alpha-carotene, lycopene, and lutein/ zeaxanthin were associated with 87, 92, 72, 75, and 88% reduction in adjusted breast cancer risk, respectively.

Patients with advanced cancer typically have low blood levels of antioxidants, generally thought to be the result of poor dietary intake. However, a high systemic (body-wide) inflammatory response, which is known to occur in cancer, may lower antioxidant levels, according to Clinical Nutrition.[19]

A research team evaluated blood levels of several antioxidants and C-reactive protein, a marker and promoter of inflammation in 15 patients with breast cancer; 15 with prostate cancer; and 11 with colorectal cancer, along with 30 healthy controls.

It was reported that cancer patients had significantly higher levels of C-reactive protein and lower levels of antioxidants when compared with the healthy controls.

In the cancer patients and normal controls, C-reactive protein levels were inversely related to blood levels of vitamin A, vitamin E, lutein, lycopene, alpha-carotene, and beta-carotene.

The research team added that low levels of antioxidants in patients may be due to the high levels of inflammation associated with cancer. Since antioxidant levels are known to be low in cancer patients because of inadequate dietary intake, the study hints at a possibility that anti-inflammatory treatment may offer an alternative manner in which to restore antioxidant concentrations in these patients.

Breast cancer is the second leading cause of cancer-related deaths in women in most industrialized countries, explained researchers at Centre Hospitalier de l' Universite de Montreal-Hotel-Dieu in Canada.[20]

In fact, the disease is about five times that in women in developing countries and Japan.[21]

In Canada, breast cancer is the most common type of cancer in women, with an age-standardized incidence rate of 103 per 100,000, or 30% of all cancers in women. In 2002, some 20,700 new cases and 5,400 deaths were attributed to breast cancer.[22]

Their study involved 414 cases and 429 controls, which involved a French Canadian population in Montreal. Dietary intake was estimated with the use of a validated food-frequency questionnaire in face-to-face interviews.

"Carotenoids include a large array of substances with different properties," the researchers reported in the American Journal of Clinical Nutrition. "Besides their overall influence on enhancement of immune function, cellular protection against DNA damage, stimulation of gap junctions intercellular communication, induction of detoxifying enzymes, and inhibition of cellular proliferation."

For example, alpha-carotene may decrease the activity of a cytochrome substance, which is an activator of procarcinogens. Beta-carotene is effective in protecting lipid membranes from damage by free radicals and reactive species. Lycopene is the most efficient quencher of singlet oxygen species, while lutein and zeaxanthin are scavengers of radical oxygen species, the researchers added. (These are all carotenoids).

The research team concluded by saying that, "we found a high intake of total carotenoids in combination with a high intake of DHA is associated with a reduced risk of breast cancer in postmenopausal women. As a whole, our data suggest a diet high in fruit, carotenoid-rich vegetables, and DHA-rich fish may reduce the risk of breast cancer."

While all forms of cancer involve mutations in genes that regulate cell growth and proliferation, most of these changes occur over the course of a lifetime, according to Beverly Merz. A few such mutations are inherited, however, and therefore the gene defect is present at birth.[23]

In 1993, she added, investigators came closer to identifying two such genes, one responsible for breast cancer, and the other one believed to predispose those who inherit it to colon and possibly other cancers.

"Inherited mutations in three genes, a tumor suppressor, ER, the estrogen receptor, and BRCAI—the function of which is yet to be identified—have been associated with breast cancer," Merz added. "Of these, the gene called BRCAI, which has been traced to chromosome 17, seems to be responsible for the disease in families at high risk for the disease, and in families in which both breast and overian cancers are highly prevalent."

In April 1993, a research team from the University of Michigan at Ann Arbor, and the Dana-Farber Cancer Institute in Boston, Massachusetts, reported that they had used molecular markers on chromosome 17 to identify those women in families with high rates of breast cancer, overian cancer, or both, who have inherited the abnormal form of the BRCAI gene.

"Cancer specialists believe that inherited gene defects are responsible for 5 to 10% of all cases of breast and overian cancer, and are carried by one women in 200 to 400," Merz continued. "Women who inherit a defective copy of the BRCAI gene are estimated to have an 85% chance of developing breast cancer over their lifetime. On the other hand, women in the same family who have not inherited the defect are likely to have only 10 to 11% lifetime risk—the same as the general population."

At the Aviano Cancer Center in Italy, Silvia Franceschi, M.D., and colleagues evaluated 2,000 women with breast cancer and an equal number of controls, ranging in age from 20 to 74 years of age. The women came from six different Italian areas, including two from the north.[24]

The researchers reported that the risk of breast cancer increased with increasing intake of starch, chiefly from refined bread and pasta. Conversely, high intake of unsaturated fatty acids was associated with a decreased risk.

In the study, refined white flour products accounted for about 90% of the starch, and 75% of carbohydrate intake.

"One-fifth of our women derived more than 60% of their total calories from carbohydrates," Franceschi said. "White flour products end up being, in Italy, a source of empty calories, which can lead to reduced intake of some beneficial micro nutrients."

In addition to olive oil and seed oils, high intakes of raw vegetables and fish conferred a significant protection against breast cancer—about 30% decreased risk in the highest intake quintile. In addition, a variety of vegetable types consumed weekly seemed to have a beneficial effect. Among vitamins, beta-carotene and vitamin E seemed to be beneficial, Franceschi continued.

"In our studies, high vegetable intake conferred 30 to 50% protection against virtually all cancer sites and types," she added. "The mechanisms are unclear, but vegetables are essential in order to curb energy intake and provide vitamins and fiber. In the so far useless waiting for chemopreventive agents, carrots, tomatoes, and lettuce should be taken far more seriously by the medical community."

Colon Cancer

Since the mid-1980s, numerous studies have investigated the relation between colorectal cancer and consumption of fruits and vegetables, reported Amy. E. Millen of the University of Buffalo in New York, and colleagues at various facilities.[25,26,27]

The hypothesis as to how fruit and vegetable intake may reduce the risk of colon or rectal cancer are numerous and involve independently or additively the many potential anti-carcinogenic compounds found in fruits and vegetables—fiber, carotenoids, vitamin C, folic acid (a B vitamin), glucinolates and allium (garlic) compounds.

In the study, 3,057 men and women, 55 to 74 years of age, were screened for colorectal cancer in the Prostate, Lung, Colorectal, and Ovarian Cancer Screening Trial (PLCO) from 1993 to 2001. The controls consisted of 29,413 people.

"Overall, this study showed that diets high in fruit, dark green vegetables, deep-yellow vegetables, onions, and garlic are associated with decreased risk of colorectal adenomas," the researchers said.

As a result of their study, the research team concluded that to reduce the risk of development of colorectal adenoma—a precursor of colorectal cancer—people should continue to consume diets rich in fruits and vegetables, which contain many potential anti-carcinogenic compounds.

In two human colon cancer cell lines, carotenoids, including alpha, and beta-carotene, and canthaxanthin, significantly suppressed cell viability, DNA synthesis, and cell proliferation, thus slowing growth-inhibitory effects on both cancer cell lines, according to Nutrition and Cancer.[28]

The effective dose of retinoic acid was considerably higher than that of alpha- and beta-carotene. Like canthaxanthin, alpha- and beta-carotene might exert their tumor-suppressing effects without being converted to retinoids.

The researchers added that their results suggest that a certain antitumor activity of carotenoids may not necessarily require their provitamin A activity.

At the Institute de Patologia Medica in Moderna, Italy, a research team evaluated 225 patients following polypectomy (excision of a polyp), who were divided into two groups, reported Diseases of the Colon and Rectum.[29]

Group 1 received 30,000 IU/day of vitamin A; 1 g/day of vitamin C; and 70 mg/day of vitamin E. Group 2 was given lactulose at 20 g/day. Group 3 received no treatment. Lactulose is a synthetic disaccharide used to treat chronic constipation.

Of the 209 people who remained in the study, the recurrence rate for Group 1 was 5.7%; 14.7% in Group 2; and 35.9% in Group 3.

The antioxidant vitamins, and, to a lesser extent lactulose, lowered the recurrence rate of adenomas of the large bowel, and can be suggested as chemopreventive agents in high-risk individuals, reported Luca Roncucci, M.D., and colleagues.

In evaluating 18 people, of whom four were healthy, seven had adenomatous polyps, and seven suffered from colon cancer. Blood and colonic biopsy samples were taken before and after beta-carotene supplementation at 30 mg/day for 43 days, except in the colon cancer patients, in which the supplement was terminated usually within 15 days, according to the European Journal of Clinical Nutrition.[30]

Tissue and blood concentrations of carotenoids, retinol (vitamin A), and vitamin E were evaluated. Tissue concentrations of each carotenoid were similar in all intestinal sites.

Only beta-carotene made significant increases after supplementation. The people with cancer showed tissue levels for each carotenoid lower than those of the healthy controls or those with polyps.

While the blood levels of vitamin E did not change after supplementation, significant increases were noted for retinol, alpha-carotene, and beta-carotene.

The researchers noted that those with colon cancer have a significant reduction in their antioxidant reserves compared with normal people and those with polyps. Oral beta-carotene supplementation at 30 mg/day resulted in an increase in blood levels of alpha-carotene in all groups.

A research team at the University of Bologna in Italy, reported that vitamins A, C, and E effectively reduced abnormalities in cell kinetics that otherwise might be associated with precancerous lesions, according to the Journal of the American Cancer Institute.[31]

Patients with colorectal adenomas were supplemented with vitamins A, C, and E for six months after surgical removal of polyps. Another 21 patients with adenomas were given a placebo. Six biopsy specimens were lifted from each patient prior to supplementation, and after 3- and 6-month treatment periods.

Biopsies taken from the vitamin-supplemented group showed reduced numbers of abnormal cell kinetics associated with precancerous conditions, while no significant changes were noted in cell kinetics in the controls.

Prostate Cancer

Writing in the September 2007 issue of the American Journal of Clinical Nutrition, a large number of researchers, headed by Timothy J. Key, of the University of Oxford, United Kingdom, and colleagues from various facilities in Europe, reiterated that previous studies indicated that dietary carotenoids, vitamin A, and vitamin E may affect the development of prostate cancer.[32,33,34]

However, they added, "overall, this research was inconclusive, but it suggested that any associations may be more marked for advanced than for localized prostate cancer, and there was particular interest in the possibility that high concentrations of lycopene (from tomatoes) may be associated with a reduced risk."

They added that, "further research on the effects of lycopene and other carotenoids on the prostate would be valuable. Although this is the largest prospective study of plasma carotenoids, vitamin A, vitamin E, and prostate cancer risk published so far, more data are needed to clarify to differentiate the associations of lycopene and total carotenoids with localized and advanced disease, to examine whether these associations vary according to the time between blood collection and diagnosis, and to examine whether these associations are confounded or modified by other potential risk factors for prostate cancer."

As reported in Cancer Epidemiology, Biomarkers and Prevention, consumption of foods rich in beta-carotene and lycopene may reduce the risk of prostate cancer. In the study, researchers tracked the diets, blood carotenoid levels, and health of over 51,000 men participating in the Health Professionals Follow-up Study.[35]

When the study began in 1986, the men ranged in age from 60 to 75. During follow-up from 1993 to 1998, 450 of the men were diagnosed with prostate cancer. They were compared with 450 controls without the disease.

It was reported that men who were under age 65 when blood samples were taken were 64% less likely to develop prostate cancer if they had high blood levels of beta-carotene. Also, men over 65 without a family history of the disease were 57% less likely to develop prostate cancer if they had high levels of lycopene in their blood. However, in the total population, there was no significant inverse association between carotenoid levels and the risk of prostate cancer.

The research team added that tomato products may exhibit more potent protection against specific prostate cancer, rather than those with a stronger familial or hereditary component.

In the 12-year Physicians' Health Study, which involved 22,000 male doctors, half were given beta-carotene supplements every other day, and the other half received placebos.[36]

Those with low beta-carotene levels were one-third more likely to develop prostate cancer, according to Nutrition Week.

It was also reported that beta-carotene deficient participants who took the supplements were 36% less likely to develop prostate cancer than those lacking beta-carotene who did not.

As reported in Cancer, researchers evaluated almost 15,000 men who participated in the Physicians' Health Study. Some of the men were given 50 mg of beta-carotene supplements every other day, while the controls received a placebo.[37]

It was found that the men with low blood levels of beta-carotene when the study began, suggesting that they ate few fruits and vegetables, had a 45% increased risk of developing prostate cancer. However, men in this study who took beta-carotene supplements had a 32% lower risk of that cancer. There was additional evidence that beta-carotene supplements lowered the overall risk of cancer among the men.

The research team concluded by saying that, among men who do not eat many fruits and vegetables, beta-carotene supplements appear to bridge the dietary gap and reduce the risk of prostate cancer.

In evaluating 800 new cases of prostate cancer out of over 47,800 men, a combined intake of tomatoes, tomato sauce, tomato juice, and pizza, were inversely associated with the risk of prostate cancer, according to Edward Giovannucci, M.D., in the Journal of the National Cancer Institute.[38]

Lycopene or other compounds in tomatoes may reduce prostate cancer risk, he added.

Lung Cancer

While the protective value of carotenoids has been debated, it is believed that carotenoids may work against cancer through a number of mechanisms, quenching dangerous free radicals, improving cell-to-cell communications, increasing production of detoxifying enzymes, and inhibiting proliferation of cancer cells, according to the American Journal of Epidemiology.[39]

In their study, researchers evaluated the diets, as well as blood levels of some nutrients, of about 27,000 male smokers, ranging in age from 50 to 69. The researchers tracked correlations between specific carotenoids and the risk of developing lung cancer.

It was reported that men with high intakes of fruits and vegetables, and foods containing lycopene, lutein/zeaxanthin, beta-carotene, or cryptoxanthin, and total carotenoids, were less likely to develop lung cancer after 14 years of follow-up.

The researchers added that men with high blood levels of vitamin A and beta-carotene also had a lower risk of developing lung cancer. Men consuming large amounts of lycopene were the least likely to develop lung cancer.

As often reported, diets high in fruits and vegetables reduce the risk of many types of cancer. That is because of the antioxidants they contain.[40]

In Nutrition and Cancer, researchers compared the diets of 541 patients with lung cancer, and 540 other patients hospitalized with other health conditions.

The researchers found that those who ate the largest quantities of fruits and vegetables had about one-half the risk of lung cancer, compared with those who ate few or none of these foods. Beta-carotene, alpha-carotene, lutein, vitamin E, and glutathione were associated with a reduced risk of this cancer.

At the National Cancer Institute, Niguarda Hospital, and the San Carlo Hospital in Milan, Italy, researchers conducted a randomized clinical trial on the effectiveness of retinol/vitamin A supplementation in preventing post-surgery recurrences of lung cancer.[41]

In the study, 181 patients were enrolled, and 87 patients received 30,000 IU of vitamin A as retinol palmitate daily for three years. The controls were 94 patients not receiving the vitamin.

Prior to the study, the participants had undergone resection of Stage la non-small-cell lung cancer. Signs of toxicity from vitamin A were evaluated at approximately 14 months.

Occurrences of mestatases and new cancers were evaluated for the 3-year period.

A majority of the patients developed skin and mucous membrane desquamation (shedding of the cuticle in scales or the outer layer of any surface) and dryness, and symptoms of vitamin A toxicity, but the symptoms were mild, and the therapy was continued. A few patients experienced headache, hair loss, dyspepsia (upset stomach), or itching, and treatment was discontinued in three patients who experienced more severe toxicity symptoms.

In the final analysis, however, only 18% of the patients who were given vitamin A had a recurrence of cancer during the study, compared with 28% of the controls.

The greatest differences between the two groups were found for bone metastases, brain metastases, and squamous histology. Two of the controls developed new primary cancers, whereas none of the treated patients did. Metastasis means the moving of cancer cells around the body.

The research team added that high-dose oral retinol palmitate was a well tolerated treatment, with only limited toxicity. While the number of patients was small and the follow-up period short, the results are promising in terms of both tolerance and efficacy of treatment, they reported in Acta Oncologia.

A research team reported in Cancer Letters that beta-carotene may help to prevent lung cancer.[42]

In the study, the researchers deposed laboratory mice to a tobacco carcinogen, then provided them with 1 of 4 chemopreventive nutrients, either through diet or by injection.

The nutrients were fumaric acid, N-acetylcysteine—a form of the amino acid cysteine—a synthetic form of vitamin A, and beta-carotene.

Although none of the nutrients lowered the total number of tumors, injections of beta-carotene and dietary supplementation with N-acetylcysteine retarded the progression of lung adenomas—a type of cancer—to adenocarcinomas, a more lethal form of lung cancer.

A research team from Louisiana State University, the National Cancer Institute, and the Illinois Cancer Institute reported in Cancer that retinol, beta-carotene, and vitamin C reduce lung cancer risk.[43]

"In the study, dietary levels of the three nutrients were assessed between 1979 and 1982 in 1,253 lung cancer patients and 1,274 controls.

Beta-carotene was found to have a protective effect for squamous and small-cell carcinoma, while vitamin A showed a protective effect for adenocarcinoma, especially among African-Americans. Vitamin C intake was more protective than beta-carotene for squamous small-cell carcinoma, the researchers added.

In evaluating blood levels of vitamin A, beta-carotene, and vitamin E in 58 patients with lung cancer, and 22 patients with stomach cancer, compared with 63 controls in China, it was found that the lung cancer patients had significantly lower blood levels of vitamin A, beta-carotene, and vitamin E than controls, reported Cancer Letters.[44]

Lower blood levels of the three vitamins were associated with an increased risk of lung cancer, and lower levels of vitamin A and beta-carotene increase the risk of stomach cancer. Lower levels of vitamin A and vitamin E were more evident in lung cancer with heavy smokers than non-smokers.

In a randomized study of 307 surgically-cured lung cancer patients given 300,000 IU of vitamin A daily for 12 months, or no supplements, it was found that 37% of the supplemented group and 48% of the controls developed new primary tumors.[45]

However, the tumor-free interval was significantly longer in the patients given vitamin A. Second primary tumors developed in 18 supplemented patients, compared with 29 in the controls.

The researchers reported in the Journal of Clinical Oncology that their study confirms that high doses and prolonged administration of vitamin A can effectively reduce the incidence of new primary tumors and increase the tumor-free interval in heavy-smoking people cured of lung cancer.

As reported in Medical Tribune, Richard Shekelle, M.D., of the University of Texas Health Center in Houston, analyzed 24 years of data and found that, in 1960, middle-aged men who rarely or never ate foods rich in beta-carotene had up to a 48% increased risk of developing lung cancer. Men with the lowest risk of lung cancer consumed at least 5,000 IU/day of beta-carotene.[46]

Beta-carotene is transported through the bloodstream by LDL-cholesterol, and Shekelle and colleagues theorized that too little LDL-cholesterol would not allow enough beta-carotene to be available to inhibit tumor cells.

A high intake of fruits and vegetables, rich in beta-carotene, or high blood concentrations of the vitamin, are associated with reduced risks of cancers of the lung and stomach, according to Geeri van Poppel and Alexandra Goldbohm of the TNO Nutrition and Food Research Institute in Zeist, Netherlands.[47]

For colorectal cancer, there is a modest reduction, and for breast and prostate cancer there was no consistency, the researchers said.

Low blood levels of beta-carotene are associated with increased risk for lung, stomach, and colon cancers, according to a research team at the University of Basel and the University of Berne in Switzerland.[48]

As reported in the American Journal of Clinical Nutrition, the Basel Study began in 1959 as a prospective study on major causes of disease and death. Blood levels and antioxidant nutrients were measured in 2,974 men at the third examination of this study in 1971 and 1973.

A subsample and their families were assessed in 1977 and 1979. During that time, over 500 men died, involving 204 from cancer (68 from lung cancer; 20 from stomach cancer; and 17 from colon cancer). During the 12-year study, 99 men died from other malignancies.

It was found that those who developed lung cancer had low blood levels of beta-carotene (less than 0.23 micromol/l) prior to the detection of cancer. Higher risks for developing cancer were noted for all cancers when both blood levels of vitamin A (retinol) and beta-carotene were low.

Bladder Cancer

As reported in the International Journal of Cancer, researchers assessed dietary habits and blood antioxidant levels of 771 men and women diagnosed with bladder cancer in Los Angeles, California. Similar data was obtained from 775 controls.[49]

The research team found that those consuming the largest amount of vitamin C and carotenoid-rich fruits and vegetables had about a 25% lower risk of developing bladder cancer.

Those who consumed the most fruits and vegetables had about one-half the risk of bladder cancer, compared with smokers who ate few of these foods. The research benefit also applies to those who smoke, former smokers, and those with a genetic predisposition to cancer, the researchers added.

In a study at the University of Toronto in Canada, Michael Jewett, M.D., and colleagues observed 40% of 35 patients with Stage Ta or T1 traditional cell carcinoma, who were given intravesical bacillus Calmette-Guerin (BCG), plus high doses of vitamin A (40,000 IU); vitamin B6 (100 mg); vitamin C (2,000 mg); and vitamin E (400 IU). They developed new tumors compared with 80% of 30 patients given BCG alone.[50]

While patient survival in those with and without bladder cancer was roughly 75% in both groups, the mean time of death was 18.8 months in the BCG-only group, compared with 33 months in the vitamin group.

There were no side effects with these mega-doses of vitamins, and researchers believe that high doses of vitamins may provide protection against high recurrence rates observed with bladder cancer.

At West Virginia University in Morgantown, Donald L. Lamm, M.D., and colleagues evaluated high doses of vitamins A, B6, C, and E in 65 patients with biopsy confirmed bladder cancer, who were randomized to intravesical (within the urinary bladder) using the TB vaccine BCG, with or without additional precutaneous admiñistration.[51]

"My interest in bladder cancer research began in 1973, during my research year of residence at the University of California at San Diego, which involved immunotherapy of bladder cancer using BCG," Lamm said. "That very controversial approach has now become the treatment of choice for superficial bladder cancer."

In the study, reported in the Journal of Urology, the dose of vitamins studied were 40,000 IU of vitamin A; 100 mg of vitamin B6; 2,000 mg of vitamin C; 400 IU of vitamin E; 90 mg of zinc daily; plus the daily recommended allowances of the remaining multiple vitamins. Controls were given the RDA of multiple vitamins.

"Similar to the previous control trial, we found no evidence in reduction of tumor recurrence during the first year of vitamin administration," Lamm continued. "However, beyond one year there was a dramatic reduction in the recurrence of cancer in patients given high doses of vitamins. Specifically, with an average follow-up of over 4 years, tumor recurrence was reduced by 40% in those given high-dose vitamins."

He went on to say that their work has been confirmed by two European studies. Statistically, significant reductions in tumor recurrence was seen in two controlled trials using the vitamin A derivative Etretinate. Although he did not mention it, this retinoid is also used in the treatment of severe recalcitrant psoriasis.

Skin Cancer

A research team at the University of Texas M.D. Anderson Cancer Center in Houston, evaluated 131 patients with confirmed basal cell cancer, and 200 cancer-free controls with nonmalignant skin disorders.[52]

The use of vitamins, especially vitamins A, C, and E, was associated with reduced risk of basal cell cancer. After controlling for variables, which included age, sex, use of tobacco, lifetime number of severe sunburns, and skin actinic lesions, regular vitamin supplementation was associated with significantly reduced risk of basal cell cancer. Actinic relates to the chemically active rays of the electromagnetic spectrum.

The researchers added that the odds ratio decreased as the regular use and daily dosage of the supplements increased. This was especially noted with vitamin A and vitamin E.

In a study in Melbourne, Australia, 88 consecutive men admitted for the surgical removal of nonmelanocytic skin cancer, and 88 male controls admitted for small elective surgeries.[53] Melanocyte is a pigment-producing cell located in the basal layer of the epidermis.

Gabriel A. Kune, M.D., reported in Nutrition and Cancer a statistically significant inverse relationship was found between the risk of skin cancer and high intakes of fish, vegetables, especially cruciferous vegetables, beta-carotene, and vitamin C-containing foods.

In addition, those who developed skin cancer had lower beta-carotene and vitamin A levels than the controls. The incidence of skin cancer was inversely related to the blood levels of beta-carotene. Smoking and alcohol consumption had no significant association with this cancer, Kune added.

Head and Neck Cancer

Vitamin A, into which beta-carotene is transformed, may protect against cancer by neutralizing unstable oxygen molecules known as free radicals that can kill and injure cells, reported William J. Cromie.[54]

In addition to this antioxidant effect, vitamin A initiates the rapid proliferation of cells so characteristic of cancerous growth. This capacity provides a rationale for testing both natural vitamin A and synthetic substances called retinoids.

He reported that, in 1990, researchers at the M.B. Anderson Cancer Center in Houston, found that treatment with a retinoid compound prevented patients with head and neck cancers from developing more primary tumors. However, the compound failed to halt the spread of the original tumor.

Stomach Cancer

Studies of various populations have found that high intakes of fruits and vegetables are associated with a low risk of gastric (stomach) cancer, at least in this Japanese study reported in Nutrition and Cancer.[55]

Gastric cancer is the leading cause of cancer deaths in Japan, even though the prevalence of the disease varies between regions. The researchers studied the relationship between antioxidant levels and stomach cancer in five regions of Japan.

Regions in which people had the highest levels of alpha-carotene, lycopene, and total (mixed) carotenoids, and vitamin E, had the lowest incidence of stomach cancer. By contrast, the highest incidence of gastric cancer was in the area in which people had the lowest blood levels of beta-carotene, alpha-carotene, lutein, lycopene, and mixed carotenoids. In general, beta-carotene and vitamin E appeared to be the most protective nutrients against gastric cancer.

Worldwide, gastric cancer is the fourth most common malignancy and the second leading cause of death due to cancer, according to researchers at the National Institute of Environmental Medicine, Karolinska Institute, in Stockholm, Sweden, reported the American Journal of Clinical Nutrition in 2007.[56,57]

While infection with the bacterium Helicobacter pylori has been recognized as a major risk factor for noncardia gastric cancer, it probably accounts for less than half the causes in Western populations.[58]

It is thought that dietary factors play a significant role in the development of gastric cancer (59), however, the specific dietary components have yet to be identified.

"Vitamin A may influence gastric gastrogenesis through its essential role in controlling cell proliferation and differentiation," the researchers said.

In the study, the research team evaluated 82,002 Swedish adults, ranging in age from 45 to 83, who completed food-frequency questionnaires in 1997. The volunteers were studied through June 2005.

During 7.2 years of follow-up, 139 cases of gastric cancer were diagnosed, and high intakes of vitamin A and retinol from foods only (dietary intake) and from foods and supplements combined (total intake) and of dietary alpha-carotene and beta-carotene were associated with a lower risk of stomach cancer.

As we know, vitamin A is a generic term referring to both preformed vitamin A (retinol and its esters), and some of the carotenoids. Retinol is found only in foods from animal origin, such as liver, kidney, dairy products, and eggs, whereas fruits and vegetables are major sources of provitamin A carotenoids (mostly beta-carotene, alpha-carotene, and beta-cryptoxanthin.

"Retinoic acid, the primary active metabolite of vitamin A, exerts most of its function via interaction with retinoic acid receptors and retinoid X receptors, both of which are expressed in human gastric epithelium," the researchers added.

Besides their ability to be converted into vitamin A, carotenoids have antioxidant properties and may reduce gastric cancer risk by neutralizing DNA-damaging free radicals generated by various factors, including chronic H. pylori infection, the researchers added.

Endometrial Cancer

In evaluating 368 patients with histologic confirmed endometrial cancer, compared to 713 controls, the relative risk of this cancer in the highest quintile of intake compared to the lowest was 1.2 for retinol; 0.5 for beta-carotene; 0.6 for vitamin C; 1.8 for vitamin D; 0.9 for vitamin E; 2.9 for methionine; 0.7 for folic acid, the B vitamin; and 1.5 for calcium, according to Eva Negri, Sc.D., and colleagues at Institut di Richerche Farmacologiche Mario Negri in Milan, Italy.[60]

Total energy intake and beta-carotene are related to the development of endometrial carcinoma, Negri added in Cancer.

Cervical Cancer

According to researchers at the Albert Einstein College of Medicine in New York, blood levels of beta-carotene and vitamin E, both effective antioxidants, are inversely associated with cervical dysplasia and cancer. The cervix is the narrow outer end of the uterus.[61]

The researchers reported in Nutrition and Cancer that blood levels of beta-carotene and vitamin E were measured in a cross-sectional sample of 116 women. Data found that women with cervical dysplasia and cancer had low levels of both nutrients. Dysplasia is abnormal tissue development.

The research team added that the cervical cells exhibited increasingly greater degrees of cancer-like abnormalities when blood levels of the two antioxidants dropped.

Also, women with advanced dysplasia were most likely to be smokers, perhaps because of the strong inverse association noted between smoking and plasma beta-carotene levels.

The researchers concluded that the two antioxidant nutrients play significant and independent roles in the development of cervical lesions and cervical cancer.

As reported in Clinical Cancer Research, researchers, in a cross-sectional sample of 235 women who were not pregnant, and who were attending a family planning clinic, found that mean plasma levels of carotenoids—beta-carotene, lycopene, and canthaxanthin—and vitamin E, were significantly lower in women with cervical intraepithelial neoplasia (CIN) and cervical cancer.[62]

The mean plasma levels of gamma-tocopherol (vitamin E) was higher among patients with CIN, while mean plasma levels of retinol were considerable among the participants.

Plasma beta-carotene concentrations in smokers were significantly lower, regardless of cervical pathology, and blood levels of lycopene and canthaxanthin were significantly lower in smokers with CIN.

The reduction in all plasma antioxidant nutrient levels, except for vitamin E, in women with CIN and cancer indicate a role for antioxidant deficiency in the pathogenesis of CIN and cancer of the cervix, the research team added.

According to an article in the British Journal of Cancer, in 156 women with cervical dysplasia, higher serum levels of alpha-carotene were significantly associated with a reduced risk of cervical dysplasia after controlling for human papillomavirus infection and smoking status.[63]

A reduced risk for the highest tertile of serum lycopene was marginally significant, the researchers said.

In studying 257 cases of cervical dysplasia and 133 controls, vitamin A intake showed a significantly increased risk at the lowest quartile when compared with the highest quartile of intake, according to Cancer Epidemiology, Biomarkers and Prevention.[64]

There was a significant trend of increasing risk also observed with lower intake of vitamin A. And there was an increased risk at the two lower quartiles of vitamin B2 (riboflavin) intake.

It was also reported that there was an increased risk with lower intakes of vitamin C, folic acid, and the calcium-phosphorus ratio, the research team added.

Two large trials have shown benefit with folic acid in regression of cervical intraepithelial neoplasia (CIN I and II), according to Frank I. Meyskins, Jr., and Alberto Manetta of the University of California at Irvine in Orange, California, in the American Journal of Clinical Nutrition.[65]

However, cervical caps with sponges containing 1.0 ml of 0.372% of beta-trans retinoic acid or placebo showed a histologic regression rate of CIN II from 27% in the placebo group to 43% in the retinoic acid group. No benefit was recorded with severe dysplasia.

In 30 patients given 30 mg of beta-carotene orally for 6 months showed a greater than 70% response rate in patients with CIN I and II by six months, which was not related to the severity of the diseases but to the extent it had progressed.

Lower vitamin A and beta-carotene intake and a deficiency of intracellular retinal binding protein (the protein that transports vitamin A/retinol) are significantly associated with higher-grade severe dysplasia and in situ cervical carcinoma, reported Seymour L. Romney, M.D., and colleagues at the Albert Einstein College of Medicine in Bronx, New York.[66]

Smokers have lower levels of beta-carotene, vitamin A, and vitamin C, and smoker's effect on dysplasia is mediated in part to deficient levels of vitamin C. Smoking is known to generate free radicals.

Cervical cancer risk has been consistently shown to increase with lower dietary intake of carotenoids as well as antioxidants. Decreased levels of beta-carotene, vitamin E, and vitamin C have been documented in cervical cancer patients, the researchers added.

They added that pharmacologic antioxidant intervention may be a valuable chemopreventive addition to clinical management. It is estimated that 35 to 40% of cancer deaths are related to diet, and there are very serious nutritional consequences in advanced malignant disease.

As reported in the International Journal of Cancer, researchers reported that dietary beta-carotene or some related compound of a vegetable-rich diet is protective against cervical cancer.[67]

In comparing the risk for women consuming a monthly intake of 150,000 IU or more of beta-carotene, the estimated reduced risk for those with 100,000 to 149,000 IU, and those with less than 100,000 IU per month, were 2.8 and 6.1, respectively.

In evaluating 30 patients who had cervical intraepithelial neoplasia Stage I and II, who were treated with 30 mg of beta-carotene daily for 6 months, the response rates were 60, 70, and 33% at 3, 6, and 12 months, according to a research team at the University of California at Irvine.[68]

There were significant increases noted in the beta-carotene levels of the vaginal mucosa, compared to those at the beginning of the study, and a significant correlation was noted between serum and vaginal beta-carotene levels.

The research team reported that there is a positive relationship between serum and tissue levels of beta-carotene, which suggest that blood levels can be used for monitoring responses.

In evaluating 116 women, significantly reduced plasma levels of beta-carotene and vitamin E were seen in women with histopathologically diagnosed cervical dysplasia and cancer, reported Nutrition and Cancer.[69]

Also, there was an inverse association between the plasma levels of both beta-carotene and vitamin E, and increasingly severe graded cervical histopathology.

In women with advanced dysplasia, the percentage of smokers was markedly increased, and the women were comparatively older. It was also found that there was a strong association between smoking status and blood beta-carotene levels. This was not evident with respect to vitamin E, the researchers added.

In 82 women with abnormal cervical cytology, compared with 82 controls, it was reported that retinol binding protein was absent or in very minute amounts, and inversely related to the severity of cervical dysplasia, according to Seymour L. Romney and colleagues in the American Journal of Obstetrics and Gynecology.[70]

In 44% of the controls, compared with 68% of the patients, with severe dysplasia or carcinoma in situ, dietary intake of total vitamin A was below the pooled median of 3,450 IU/day. And in 41% of the controls, compared with 68% of the women with severe dysplasia and carcinoma in situ, dietary intake of beta-carotene was low (below 2,048 IU/day). Also, in 38% of the controls, compared with 73% of the women with severe dysplasia and carcinoma in situ, dietary intake of vitamin C was found to be low.

In this in vivo study, a research team at Gifu University School of Medicine in Japan, the authors suggest that the prevention of cervical cancer by beta-carotene is due to the induction of apoptosis (cell death) in cervical dysplasia cells, which are premalignant cells in a cervical multi-step carcinogenesis process through down-regulation of epidermal growth factor (EGF) receptor-protein.[71]

In 187 women with cervical dysplasia or carcinoma in situ in the original place, compared with 82 controls, the cases of severe cervical dysplasia or carcinoma in situ were more likely to have a total dietary vitamin A intake below the median of 3,450 IU and/or a beta-carotene intake below the median of 2,072 IU than were the controls.[72]

The research team found that there was a 3-fold risk for severe dysplasia or carcinoma in women with lowered vitamin A or beta-carotene intake.

Retinal binding protein was either absent or undetectable in 78.8% of the dysplasia tissue samples, compared with 23.5% of the normal tissue samples.

Cervical intraepithelial neoplasia, or cancer of the cervix, is the most common lethal cancer in the developing countries, especially Asia, Africa, and parts of Latin America, reported Alberto Manetta, M.D., and Carlos Cuchtner, M.D., of the University of California at Irvine. The disease also affects many American women.[73]

A number of epidemiological studies report an association between the incidence of cervical intra-epithelial neoplasia (CIN) and dietary levels of vitamin A, the researchers added. For example, the use of retinoic acid in CIN has shown the extent of the lesion being decreased by 50% or more in 80% of the patients. In addition, histologic severity improved in 32% of the women.

A retinal acetate gel applied intravaginally in women with mild or moderate cervical dysplasia showed no intolerable side effects at any dosage between 3 and 10 mg/day for 7 days in 3 consecutive months.

Local symptoms were mild in the 3 and 9 mg range, but severe at 18 mg. In a study using vaginal-B-trans-retinoic acid and in women with CIN II and III, patients were treated for four consecutive days and the response rate was assessed by colposcopy, which is examination of the vagina and cervix using an endoscope.

The researchers reported that 33 of the patients had a minimum 25% regression in the side of the lesions, and post treatment conization revealed complete resolution of CIN in two patients. Conization is the excision of a cone of tissue for examination.

Oral Cancer

It was initially reported that 13-CIS-retinoic acid had benefit in treating leukoplakia, which is a precancerous condition presenting as white patches of the skin and mouth that can turn malignant, reported K.A. Fackelmann in Science News.[74]

However, once the patient stopped taking the nutrient, the precancerous conditions returned.

In one preventive trial, 53 people with leukoplakia received a very large dose of 13-CIS-retinoic acid for three months. Then the patients, for 9 months, were given a maintenance therapy with either low-dose 13-CIS-retinoic acid or beta-carotene.

The researchers reported that the premalignant changes progressed only in 2 of 24 patients given 13-CIS-retinoic acid, when compared to 16 of 29 patients given beta-carotene, a difference of 8 and 55%.

It is estimated that 8% of Americans will develop leukoplakia, mostly in smokers and heavy drinkers. The standard treatment is surgery, but this does not work for the premalignant patches that have spread all over the areas of the mouth, Fackelmann said.

Oral cancers rank sixth in overall cancer incidence worldwide, and they are the most often-found malignancies in India, Southeast Asia, and parts of Latin America, according to Harlinder S. Garewal, M.D., Ph.D., of the University of Arizona Health Sciences Clinic in Tucson.[75]

The main causative agents are tobacco and alcohol. Nutritional epidemiology suggests a strong protective role for carotenoids as preventive agents for oral cancer, since low intakes of fruits and vegetables are associated with increased cancer rates, Garewal continued.

He went on to say that, since the 1960s, it has been known that retinoids, both natural and synthetic, can reverse oral leukoplakia.

In 1986, the researcher and colleagues showed that beta-carotene resulted in a 70% response rate in 24 people treated over a 3- to 6-month period with the vitamin. However, lesions tend to return when treatment is stopped.

In a study in India and Southeast Asia, beta-carotene, alone or in combination with vitamin A, reversed leukoplakia. In a trial in Canada, there was a 67% response rate with beta-carotene in 18 people. In other studies, beta-carotene, and vitamins C and E have reversed leukoplakia, he said.

At the Isituto Nazionale per la Ricerca Sul Can Sancro in Genoa, Italy, Prof. S. Toma and colleagues evaluated 23 patients, 17 to 85 years of age, who were included in a study using beta-carotene at 90 mg/day in those with oral leukoplakia.[76]

Eighteen patients completed the study, and 44% had positive responses to the therapy, of which 6 were complete and 2 were partial. In 4 complete responders and one partial responder, leukoplakia appeared unexpectedly between 2 to 7 months after the therapy ended.

When lesions were evaluated at the beginning of the study, 2 types of alterations were found: atypical hyperplasia in 16 patients and dysplasia in 2 patients. No toxicity was recorded. Hyperplasia denotes an increase in the number of cells in a tissue or organ. Dysplasia is abnormal tissue development.

The study demonstrates that there is fair efficiency of beta-carotene against oral leukoplakia, and further confirmation is needed. Perhaps higher doses would bring better results, Toma added.

Epidemiologic studies have suggested that blood levels of nutrients, including vitamin A, vitamin B2, and beta-carotene are deficient in inhabitants of regions with a high incidence of oral cancers, reported John P. Richie, Ph.D., of the American Health Foundation in Valhalla, New York.[77]

In one study, vitamin A at 32,000 IU was administered to tobacco/betal quid chewers with oral leukoplakia for 6 months. The results showed a reduction in the formation of new lesions, and complete remission of existing lesions in over 50% of the patients.

In several epidemiologic studies, low intakes of vitamin E and carotenoids have been associated with increased oral cancer risk, according to the American Journal of Clinical Nutrition. Smoking lowers beta-carotene levels in blood and oral mucosa cells.[78]

Also, beta-carotene and vitamin E can result in clinical regression of oral leukoplakia, a premalignant form of oral cancer, reported Harlinder Garewal.

In the study, 30 mg/day of beta-carotene for 3 to 6 months in 24 patients showed a response rate of 71%. Beta-carotene at 40 mg/day, retinol at 100,000 IU/week, and vitamin E at 80 mg/week for 6 months showed a significant reduction in oral leukoplakia, Garewal added.

Alcohol and tobacco use generate the increased production of reactive free radicals, as well as eliciting immunosuppression, according to researchers at the University of Maryland at Baltimore.[79]

The most widely used chemotherapeutic agents against oral cancer are antioxidant/free radical scavengers such as vitamins A, E, C, and beta-carotene, the researchers added. These antioxidants neutralize the reactive oxygen species, interfere with the activation of procarcinogens, prevent binding of carcinogens to DNA, inhibit chromosome alterations, inhibit the replication of transformed cells, suppress the action of cancer promoters, and may even cause regression of precancerous oral lesions such as leukoplakia or erythroplakia, which are red velvety plaque-like lesion of mucous membranes.

Alcohol, tobacco and/or malnutrition-immunosuppression impairs parasalivary gland function and oral mucosal immunity, a reduction of the number of helper CD4 cells, with less changes in the number of suppressor T-cells, and depresses natural killer cell activity, the researchers continued.

Daily consumption of fruits and vegetables is encouraged, and vitamin and mineral supplementation in high-risk groups may be useful adjuncts, the researchers added.

Researchers at the British Columbia Cancer Research Center in Vancouver, Canada, reported that vitamin A and beta-carotene supplementation reduced the incidence of oral precancerous lesions in those who chew tobacco, according to Cancer Detection and Prevention.[80]

Chewing mixtures and their link to oral cancer rates were studied in Guam, Taiwan, the Philippines, India, Peru, and Canada.

The research team studied the response of micronucleated mucosal cells and oral leukoplakia of tobacco chewers to twice weekly dosages of beta-carotene (180 mg/week); vitamin A (100,000 IU), or 200,000 IU/week; or beta-carotene (180 mg/week); and vitamin A at 100,000 IU/week.

The researchers reported that both beta-carotene and vitamin A produced substantial reduction in frequency of micronucleated mucosal cells, and remission of leukoplakia within 3 to 6 months of treatment. Micronucleus refers to a small nucleus in a large cell.

In addition, supplementation also reduced the frequency of new leukoplakias. When the supplements were discontinued, micronucleated cells and leukoplakia returned in the oral cavity.

Vitamin A in doses of 50,000 IU/week maintained the protective effect for the 12-month post-treatment period. However, beta-carotene at 60 mg/week was less effective, suggesting larger doses might be necessary to produce long-term benefits, the researchers added.

An extensive review in Oral Oncology, European Journal of Cancer, reported on the role of oral chemopreventive agents and cancer. In the study, beta-carotene (30 mg/day); vitamin C (1,000 mg/day); and vitamin E (800 IU/day); given for 9 months, produced a 55.7% clinical improvement in 79 patients with histologically confirmed oral leukoplakia, or dysplasia, and this improvement was most likely to occur in those with reduced alcohol and tobacco use.[81]

Added Takuji Tanaka, M.D., even if these natural substances are half-active, they are more likely to be usable as chemopreventive agents than the other toxic compounds.

As reported in Archives of Otolarygology-Head and Neck Surgery, a research team gave 60 mg/day of beta-carotene supplements to 50 patients with oral leukoplakia. Six months into the study, patients responding to beta-carotene therapy were given either beta-carotene or a placebo for 12 more months.[82]

At 6 months, 26 of the volunteers improved, as evidenced by thinning of their leukoplakia lesions. Three of the patients didn't stop taking the supplement since their condition was improving. Of the 23 people randomized to take beta-carotene or placebo for 12 more months, 19 had no further progression of their disease.

The study suggests that beta-carotene supplements can reverse oral leukoplakia, and benefits can remain for another year, even if the patients decide not to continue with the supplements, the researchers said.

At the National Institute of Nutrition in Hyderabad, India, a research team supplemented 150 patients with vitamin A (25,000 IU/day); vitamin B2 (50 mg/day); zinc (12.5 mg/day); and selenium (100 mcg/day); for 1 to 4 months. Participants were evaluated for precancerous lesions.[83]

The dosages were reduced between 5 and 8 months, except for zinc, which was increased to 25 mg/day. Between 9 and 12 months, the dosages were 25,000 IU/day for vitamin A; 25 mg/day for B2; and 50 mcg/day for selenium. A placebo was given to 148 volunteers.

The supplements improved the vitamin A, riboflavin, and selenium nutriture in the supplemented group with a concomitant regression of precancerous lesions present on the palate.

It was also found that clinical remission of white, red, and combination lesions were seen in 57% of the people on the supplements, whereas 8% of the placebo group showed a positive response.

An additional progression of the lesions was seen in 10% of the treated people, compared to 47% in the placebo group. In the nonlesion group, lesions appeared in 12% on supplements, but over 38% in the controls, the researchers added.

Of the 34,000 volunteers from the Women's Health Study, 59 developed cancers of the upper digestive tract over a 6-year period, according to Wei Zheng, M.D., and colleagues at the University of Minnesota at Minneapolis.[84]

After adjusting for variables, higher intakes of carotene and vitamins C and E were related to lower risks of oral/pharyngeal/esophagus and gastric cancers.

Glioblastomas

As reported in Acta Nuerochir, two human glioblastoma cell lines were exposed to 25-dihydroxyvitamin D3, and its metabolite 1-alpha, 25-dihydroxyvitamin D3. Both substances had the ability to induce a significant reduction, which was greater than 50%, in growth of the two glioblastoma cell lines at dosages over 5 micromolar. Glioblastomas are malignant tumors of the central nervous system.[85]

The combination of vitamin D3 and 1 micromolar of all-trans-retinoic acid (vitamin A) resulted in a significant inhibition, the researchers said.

The reduction of growth was due to cell death. The data gives evidence in vitro that vitamin D metabolites alone or in combination with retinoids may be potential therapies in human malignant gliomas, according to a research team from the University of Pavia in Matteo, Italy.

Leukemia

Researchers have reported that children diagnosed with cancer may not be malnourished, however, this study found that children undergoing chemotherapy for newly diagnosed leukemia ate only 66% of the dietary recommendations for vitamin E; 30% of total carotenoids; 59% for beta-carotene; and 29% of vitamin A.[86]

The research team added in the American Journal of Clinical Nutrition that children with the lowest intake of antioxidants were most likely to experience adverse side effects of chemotherapy. Conversely, those with higher antioxidant intake had fewer side effects. Higher intakes of vitamin E were associated with a lower incidence of infection, and those with a higher intake of beta-carotene were less likely to experience toxic reactions to chemotherapy. Higher intakes of vitamin C were associated with less toxicity, fewer delays in chemotherapy, and fewer days in the hospital.

A research team at Sammelweis University School and the John F. Hospital in Budapest, Hungary, have found that vitamin A therapy restores the depressed cellular immunity seen in patients with chronic lymphocytic leukemia (CLL).[87]

The patients were given 100,000 IU/day of vitamin A for two weeks. Changes in immunity seen at the end of the supplementation period included enhanced antibody-dependent cell-mediated cytotoxicity, enhanced natural killer cell activity, as well as enhanced blastogenic responses to plant mitogens. Blastogenesis is the reproduction of unicellular organisms by budding/gemmation in which the parent cell does not divide.

The decreased cell-mediated immune responses often lead to secondary viral infections, such as herpes zoster (shingles), the researchers added.

The researchers said that vitamin A supplementation may be necessary in restoring immune competence in CLL and other conditions that lead to secondary immune deficiencies.

In a study reported in the New England Journal of Medicine, 346 patients with previously untreated acute promyeloctic leukemia were randomly assigned to be given either all-trans-retinoic acid or daunorubicin, an antibiotic used in treating leukemia. It is obtained from Streptomyces peucetius, a bacteria. Promyelocyte is a large uninuclear cell occurring in the blood of those with myeloctic leukemia.[88]

All-trans-retinoic acid was given orally in 2 divided doses of 45 mg per square meter per day, by intravenous bolus on days 1 through 3, plus 100 mg of cytarabine per square meter per day by continuous intravenous infusion on days 1 through 7. Cytarabine, also called arabinosylcytosine, is a chemotherapeutic agent.

Patients less than 3 years of age received lower doses of each of the medications. It was found that all-trans-retinoic acid treatment improved disease-free and overall survival as compared with chemotherapy alone, and should be included in the treatment of acute promyelocytic leukemia, according to Martin S. Tallman, M.D., and colleagues.

A number of studies have found that people who consume large amounts of carotenoids have a decreased risk of cancer, cardiovascular disease, and other age-related degenerative diseases, reported Free Radical Research.[89]

In a study using human leukemia cells, researchers grew cells with levels of several carotenoids much higher than would normally be found in the blood, except through supplementation. They were specifically interested in the ability of carotenoids to induce cancer cell death (apoptosis), and investigated the mechanisms by which carotenoids exert their effects on human health.

The research team reported that beta-carotene was the most effective in destroying leukemia cells, with the effect related to dosage and the length of exposure.

They added that carotenoids have numerous effects, including enhancement of immune-cell activity, improved cell-to-cell communication, and the inhibition of cancer cell growth. Beta-carotene can induce apoptosis in different types of cancer cells.

As reported in Annals of Internal Medicine, a research team evaluated 56 patients, 34 of which were newly diagnosed leukemia patients, and 22 had relapse from previous treatment.[90]

The patients were given all-trans-retinoic acid in 2 divided doses of 45 mg/m2 per day, rounded out to the nearest 10 mg after meals.

The 13 patients given all-trans-retinoic acid as a maintenance therapy had a median duration of remission of only 3.5 months. Only 3 of the 19 patients who relapsed from a remission induced by all-trans-retinoic acid could be brought into remission again using the nutrient.

At the time of the article, the mean survival time of all newly-diagnosed patients exceeded 31 months. No decrease in early mortality rate was observed compared with a historical control group comprised of 80 consecutive, newly-diagnosed patients treated only with chemotherapy.

The researchers said that overall survival was superior. The results suggest that all-trans-retinoic acid is an effective agent to induce remission in patients with a molecular diagnosis of acute promyeloctic leukemia, but remissions are short and resistance develops rapidly.

While the incidence of early death was not reduced, the use of all-trans-retinoic acid to induce remission, followed by cytotoxic chemotherapy for "consolidation," was associated with longer survival times when compared with historical controls treated with only chemotherapy, reported Stanley R. Frankel, M.D., and colleagues, at Memorial Sloan-Kettering Cancer Center in New York.

How Antioxidants Might Prevent Cancer?

Antioxidants—vitamins A, C, and E, beta-carotene, lycopene, etc.—neutralize free radicals as the natural by-product of normal cell processes. Free radicals are molecules with incomplete electron shells, which make them more chemically reactive than those with complete electron shells.

Exposure to various environmental factors, including tobacco smoke and radiation, can also lead to free radical formation.

In humans, the most common form of free radicals is oxygen. When an oxygen molecule (O_2) becomes electrically charged or "radicalized," it tries to steal electrons from other molecules, causing damage to DNA and other molecules.

Over time, such damage may become irreversible and lead to disease, including cancer. Antioxidants are often described as "mopping up" free radicals, meaning they neutralize the electrical charge and prevent the free radical from taking electrons from other molecules.

Source: "Antioxidants and Cancer Prevention," National Cancer Institute, Bethesda, Maryland, November 12, 2008.

Cancer Deaths in India

In India, in 2010, 1 million people were expected to die from tobacco smoking, and smoking already accounts for 900,000 deaths annually, according to the BBC News.

A study predicts that smoking could soon account for 20% of male deaths in India, and 5% of female deaths for those between the ages of 30 and 69.

Researchers have calculated that men who smoke bidi—small, hand-rolled cigarettes in India—lose about 6 years of their lives, compared to those who smoke full-size cigarettes, who shorten their lives by 10 years. Women who smoke bidi reduce their lives by 8 years.

Among the men who died between the ages of 30 and 69, smoking caused about 38% of the deaths from TB, 32% from cancer, and 20% of the deaths from vascular diseases.

"It is truly remarkable that 1 single factor—smoking—which is entirely preventable, accounts for nearly 1 in 10 of all deaths in India," said Amartya Sen, M.D., of Harvard University in Boston, Massachusetts.

Added Anbumani Ramadoss, M.D., India's health minister, "I am alarmed by the results of this study."

Source: "India Facing Smoking Death Crisis," BBC News, February 13, 2008.

Worldwide Cancer Deaths

The World Health Organization has reported that cancer has become the leading cause of death worldwide, and the number of cases is influenced in part by the aging population, reported The Times of India.

The number of cancer deaths globally is projected to increase by 45% from 2007 to 2030, from 7.9 million to 11.5 million.

Experts suggest that 46% of cancer deaths can be prevented by curbing tobacco sales. This alone will avoid 1.8 million cancer deaths annually. Sadly, 60% of those deaths occur in low- and middle-income countries.

"Having an active lifestyle can reduce cancer deaths by 274,000, which are otherwise caused by obesity and physical inactivity," the newspaper said. "Alcohol is responsible for 350,000 cancer deaths annually, while the sexually transmitted human papilloma virus (HVP) infection accounts for 235,000 deaths each year."

Source: "Cancer Deaths will go up by 45% by 2030," *The Times of India,* February 9, 2010.

References

1. Ensminger, A., et al. Foods and Nutrition Encyclopedia. Clovis, CA: Pegus Press, 1983, pp. 316-317, 322, 327.
2. Sarma, Mukti H., Ph.D. "Cancer." Medical and Health Annual. Chicago, IL: Encyclopaedia Britannica, Inc., 1994, pp. 250ff.
3. Cromie, William J. "Cancer." Medical and Health Annual. Chicago, IL. Encyclopaedia Britannica, Inc., 1993, pp. 257 ff.
4. Spraycar, Majory, editor. Stedman's Medical Dictionary, 26th Edition. Baltimore, MD: Williams & Wilkins, 1995, p. 161.
5. Hennekens, Charles H., M.D. "Beta-Carotene Supplementation and Cancer Prevention," Nutrition 13(7/8): 697-699, 1997.
6. Edes, Thomas E., and Gysbers, Daniel S. "Carcinogen-Induced Tissue Vitamin A Depletion: Potential Protective Advantages of Beta-Carotene," Annals of the New York Academy of Sciences 686:203-212, May 28, 1993.
7. Feinstein, Alice, editor. Prevention's Healing with Vitamins. Emmaus, PA: Rodale Press, Inc., 1996, pp. 323-324.
8. Drisko, J.A., et al. "The Use of Antioxidant Therapies During Chemotherapy," Gynecologic Oncology 88:434-439, 2003.
9. Dusinska, M., et al. "Nutritional Supplements with Antioxidants Decrease Chromosomal Damage in Humans," Mutagenesis 18:371-376, 2003.
10. Kornhauser, Andrija, et al. "Antioxidants and Cancer Prevention: In Vivo and In Vitro," Nutrition in Cancer Prevention and Treatment 83-100, 1995.
11. Hendler, Sheldon Saul, M.D., Ph.D. The Doctors' Vitamin and Mineral Encyclopedia. New York: Simon & Schuster, 1990, pp. 39ff.
12. Nkondjock, Andre, et al. "Intake of Specific Carotenoids and Essential Fatty Acids and Breast Cancer Risk in Montreal, Canada." American Journal of Clinical Nutrition 79:857-864, 2004.
13. Jumaan, A.C., et al. "Beta-Carotene Intake and the Risk of Postmenopausal Breast Cancer," Epidemiology 10:49-53, 1999.
14. Band, P.R., et al. "Treatment of Benign Breast Disease with Vitamin A," Preventive Medicine 13:549-554, 1984.
15. Longnecker, Matthew P., et al. "Intake of Carrots, Spinach, and Supplements Containing Vitamin A in Relation to Risk of Breast Cancer," Cancer, Epidemiology, Biomarkers and Prevention 6:887-892, 1997.
16. Ching, S., et al. "Serum Levels of Micronutrients, Antioxidants, and Total Antioxidant Status Predict Risk of Breast Cancer in a Case-Control Study," Journal of Nutrition 132:303-306, 2002.

17. Brinton, Louise A., Ph.D. "Ways That Women May Possibly Reduce Their Risk of Breast Cancer," Journal of the National Cancer Institute 86(18): 1371-1372, 1994.
18. Kim, M.K., et al. "Relationship of Serum Alpha-Tocopherol, Carotenoids, and Retinol with the Risk of Breast Cancer," Nutrition Research 21:797-809, 2001.
19. McMillan, D.C., et al. "The Relationship Between Reduced Vitamin Antioxidant Concentrations and the Systemic Inflammatory Response in Patients with Common Solid Tumors," Clinical Nutrition 21:161-164, 2002.
20. Nkondjock, Andre, and Ghadirian, Parvis. "Intake of Specific Carotenoids and Essential Fatty Acids and Breast Cancer Risk in Montreal, Canada, *ibid.*
21. International Agency for Research on Cancer, Globocan, Internet, May 29, 2003.
22. Canadian Cancer Society. Canadian Cancer Statistics, 2002. Toronto: National Cancer Institute of Canada, 2002.
23. Merz, Beverly. "Genetics." Medical and Health Annual. Chicago, IL: Encyclopaedia Britannica, Inc., 1994, pp. 300 ff.
24. Hamilton, Kirk. The Experts Speak. Sacramento, CA: I.T. Services, 1997, pp. 29-30. Also Franceschi, Silvia, M.D., "Intake of Macronutrients and Risk of Breast Cancer," The Lancet, May 18, 1996.
25. Millen, Amy E., et al. "Fruit and Vegetable Intake and Prevalence of Colorectal Adenomas in a Cancer Screening Trial," American Journal of Clinical Nutrition 86:1754-1764, 2007.
26. Papas, M.A., et al. "Fiber from Fruit and Colorectal Neoplasia," Cancer Epidemiology, Biomarkers and Prevention 13:1267-1270, 2004.
27. Steinmetz, K.A., and Potter, J.D. "Vegetables, Fruit and Cancer," II. Mechanisms, Cancer Causes and Control 2:427-442, 1991.
28. Onogi, N., et al. "Antiproliferation Effect of Carotenoids on Human Colon Cancer Cells without Conversion to Retinoic Acid," Nutrition and Cancer 32(1):20-24, 1998.
29. Roncucci, Luca, M.D., et al. "Antioxidant Vitamins or Lactolose for the Prevention of the Recurrence of Colorectal Adenomas," Diseases of the Colon and Rectum 36(3):227-233, March 1993.
`30. Pappalardo, G., et al. "Plasma (Carotenoids, Retinol, Alpha-Tocopherol) and Tissue (Carotenoids) Levels After Supplementation with Beta-Carotene in Subjects with Precancerous and Cancerous Lesions of Sigmoid Colon," European Journal of Clinical Nutrition 51:661-666, 1997.

31. Paganelli, G., et al. "Effect of Vitamins A, C, and E Supplementation on Rectal Cell Proliferation in Patients with Colorectal Adenomas," Journal of the American Cancer Institute 84:47-51, 1992.

32. Key, Timothy J., et al. "Plasma Carotenoids, Retinol, and Tocopherols and the Risk of Prostate Cancer in the European Prospective Investigation into Cancer and Nutrition Study," American Journal of Clinical Nutrition 86:672-681, 2007.

33. International Agency for Research on Cancer. IARC Handbooks of Cancer Prevention. Carotenoids. Vol. 2. Lyon, France, International Agency for Research on Cancer, 1998.

34. Chan, J.M., et al. "Role of Diet in Prostate Cancer Development and Progression," Journal of Clinical Oncology 23:8152-8160, 2005.

35. Wu, K., et al. "Plasma and Dietary Carotenoids, and the Risk of Prostate Cancer: A Nested Case-Control Study," Cancer Epidemiology, Biomarkers and Prevention 13:260-269, 2004.

36. "Prostate Cancer and Beta-Carotene," Nutrition Week 27(23):7, June 13, 1997.

37. Cook, N.R., et al. "Beta-Carotene Supplementation for Patients with Low Baseline Levels and Decreased Risks of Total and Prostate Carcinoma," Cancer 86:1783-1792, 1999.

38. Giovannucci, Edward, M.D. "Intake of Carotenoids and Retinol in Relation to the Risk of Prostate Cancer," Journal of the National Cancer Institute 87(23):1767-1776, December 6, 1995.

39. Holick, C.N., et al. "Dietary Carotenoids, Serum Beta-Carotene, and Retinol and Risk of Lung Cancer in the Alpha-Tocopherol, Beta-Carotene Cohort Study," American Journal of Epidemiology 156:536-547, 2002.

40. De Stefani, E., et al. "Dietary Antioxidants and Lung Cancer Risk: A Case-Control Study in Uruguay," Nutrition and Cancer 34:100-110, 1999.

41. Pastorino, U., et al. "Lung Cancer Chemoprevention with Retinol Palmitate: Preliminary Data from a Randomized Trial on Stage Ia Non Small-Cell Lung Cancer," Acta Oncologia 27:773-782, 1988.

42. Conaway, C.C., et al. "Chemopreventive Potential of Fumaric Acid, N-Acetylcysteine, N-(4-Hydroxyphenyl) retinamide and Beta-Carotene for Tobacco Nitrosamine-Induced Lung Tumors in A/J Mice," Cancer Letters 124: 85-93, 1998.

43. Fontham, E., et al. "Dietary Vitamin A and C and Lung Cancer Risk in Louisiana," Cancer 62:2267-2273, 1988.

44. Kumugai, Y., et al. "Serum Antioxidant Vitamins and Risk of Lung and Stomach Cancer in Shenyang, China," Cancer Letters 129:145-149, 1998.

45. Pastorino, U., et al. "Adjuvant Treatment of Stage 1 Lung Cancer with High-Dose Vitamin A," Journal of Clinical Oncology 11:1216-1222, 1993.

46. "Low LDL May Prevent Beta-Carotene Transport," Medical Tribune, August 6, 1992, p. 25.

47. van Poppel, Geeri, and Goldbohm, Alexandra. "Epidemiologic Evidence for Beta-Carotene and Cancer Prevention," American Journal of Clinical Nutrition 62:1393S-1402S, 1995.

48. Stahelin, H., et al. "Beta-Carotene and Cancer Prevention: The Basel Study," American Journal of Clinical Nutrition 53:265S-269S, 1991.

49. Castaleo, J.E., et al. "Carotenoids/Vitamin C and Smoking Related Bladder Cancer," International Journal of Cancer 110:417-423, 2004.

50. Laino, Charlene "Vitamins Boost Bladder Cancer Survival Rates," Medical Tribune, June 10, 1993, p. 3.

51. Hamilton, Kirk. The Experts Speak. Sacramento, CA: I.T. Services, 1997, pp. 24-25. Also Lamm, Donald L., M.D., et al. "Magadose Vitamins in Bladder Cancer: A Double-Blind Clinical Trial," The Journal of Urology 151:21-26, January 1994.

52. Wei, Qingyi, M.D., Ph.D., et al. "Vitamin Supplementation and Reduced Risk of Basal Cell Carcinoma," Journal of Clinical Epidemiology 47(8) : 829-836, 1994.

53. Kune, Gabriel A., M.D. "Diet, Alcohol, Smoking, Serum Beta-Carotene, and Vitamin A in Male Nonmelanocytic Skin Cancer Patients and Controls," Nutrition and Cancer 18: 237-244, 1992.

54. Cromie, William J. "Cancer." Medical and Health Annual. Chicago, IL: Encyclopaedia Britannica, 1993, p. 264.

55. Tsubono, X., et al. "Plasma Antioxidant Vitamins and Carotenoids in Five Japanese Populations with Varied Mortality from Gastric Cancer," Nutrition and Cancer 34: 56-61, 1999.

56. Larsson, Susanna C., et al. "Vitamin A, Retinol, and Carotenoids and the Risk of Gastric Cancer: A Prospective Cohort Study," American Journal of Clinical Nutrition 85: 497-503, 2007.

57. Parkin, D.M., et al. "Global Cancer Statistics, 2002," CA Cancer Journal of Clinology 55: 74-108, 2005.

58. Kelly, J.R., and Duggan, J.M. "Gastric Cancer Epidemiology and Risk Factors," Journal of Clinical Epidemiology 56 :1-9, 2003.

59. World Cancer Research Fund and American Institute for Cancer Research. Food, Nutrition and the Prevalence of Cancer: A Global Perspective, Washington, D.C. American Institute for Cancer Research, 1997.

60. Negri, Eva, Sc.D., et al. "The Risk of Endometrial Carcinoma," Cancer 77(5): 917-923, March 1, 1996.

61. Palan, P., et al. "Plasma Levels of Antioxidant Beta-Carotene and Alpha-tocopherol in Uterine Cervix Dysplasia and Cancer," Nutrition and Cancer 15: 13-20, 1991.

62. Prabhudas, P.R., et al. "Plasma Levels of Beta-Carotene, Lycopene, Canthaxanthin, Retinol and Vitamin E in Cervical Intraepithelial Neoplasia and Cancer," Clinical Cancer Research 2: 181-185, January 1996.

63. Nagata, C., et al. "Serum Carotenoids and Vitamins and Risk of Cervical Dysplasia from a Case-Control Study in Japan," British Journal of Cancer 81(7): 1234-1237, 1999.

64. Liu, T., et al. "A Case-Control Study of Nutritional Factors and Servical Dysplasia," Cancer Epidemiology, Biomarkers and Prevention 2(6): 525-530, 1993.

65. Meyskins, Frank I., Jr., and Manetta, Alberto. "Prevention of Cervical Intraepithelial Neoplasia and Cervical Cancer," American Journal of Clinical Nutrition 62:1417S-1419S, 1995.

66. Romney, Seymour L., M.D., et al "Nutrient Antioxidants in the Pathogenesis and Prevention of Cervical Dysplasia and Cancer," Journal of Cellular Biochemistry 23:96S-103S, 1995.

67. La Vecchia, C., et al "Dietary Vitamin A and the Risk of Invasive Cervical Cancer," International Journal of Cancer 34:319-322, 1984.

68. Manetta, Alberto, et al. "Beta-Carotene Treatment of Cervical Intraepithelial Neoplasia: A Phase II Study," Cancer Epidemiology, Biomarkers and Prevention 5:929-932, November 1996.

69. Palan, P.R., et al. "Plasma Levels of Antioxidant Beta-Carotene and Alpha-Tocopherol in Uterine Cervix Dysplasia and Cancer," Nutrition and Cancer 15(1): 13-20, 1991.

70. Romney, Seymour L., et al. "Retinoids and the Prevention of Cervical Dysplasia," American Journal of Obstetrics and Gynecology 141: 890-894, 1981.

71. Muto, Yasutoshi, et al. "Growth Retardation in Human Cervical Dysplasia-Derived Cell Lines by Beta-Carotene Through Down-Regulation of Epithelial Growth Factor Receptor," American Journal of Clinical Nutrition 62: 1535S-1540S, 1995.

72. Wylie-Rosett, J.A., et al. "Influence of Vitamin A on Cervical Dysplasia and Carcinoma in Situ," Nutrition and Cancer 6(1): 49-56, 1984.

73. Manetta, Alberto, M.D., and Cuchtner, Carlos, M.D. "The Role of Beta-Carotene in Cancer Chemoprevention," Drug Therapy, July 1992, pp. 55-60.

74. Fackelmann, K.A. "Vitamin-Like Drug May Ward Off Cancers," Science News 141:358, May 30, 1992.

75. Garewal, Harlinder S., M.D., Ph.D. "Beta-Carotene and Antioxidants in Oral Cancer Prevention," The Nutrition Report 10(2): 89, 96, December 1992.

76. Toma, S., et al. "Treatment of Oral Leukoplakia with Beta-Carotene," Oncology 49: 77-81, 1992.

77. Richie, John P., Ph.D. "Role of Nutrition in Cancer of the Oral Cavity," Journal of Applied Nutrition 43(1) :49-57, 1991.

78. Garewal, Harlinder S., M.D., Ph.D. "Antioxidants in Oral Cancer Prevention," American Journal of Clinical Nutrition 62: 1410S-1416S, 1995.

79. Enwonwu, C.E., and Meeks, V.I. "Bionutrition and Oral Cancer in Humans," Clinical Reviews in Oral Biology and Medicine 6(1): 5-17, 1995.

80. Stich, H., et al. "Remission of Oral Precancerous Lesions of Tobacco/ Areca Nut Chewers Following Administration of Beta-Carotene and Vitamin A and Maintenance of the Protective Effect," Cancer Detection and Prevention 15: 93-98, 1991.

81. Tanaka, Takuji, M.D., "Chemoprevention of Oral Carcinogenesis," Oral Oncology-European Journal of Cancer 31B(1): 3-15, 1995.

82. Garewal, Harlinder S., M.D., Ph.D., et al. "Beta-Carotene Produces Sustained Remissions in Patients with Oral Leukoplakia," Archives of Otolaryngology-Head and Neck Surgery 124:1305-1310, 1999.

83. Krishnaswamy, K., et al. "Case Study of Nutrient Intervention of Oral Precancerous Lesions in India," Oral Oncology-European Journal of Cancer 31B(1): 41-48, 1995.

84. Zheng, Wei, M.D., et al. "Retinol, Antioxidant Vitamins, and Cancers of the Upper Digestive Tract in a Prospective Cohort Study of Postmenopausal Women," American Journal of Epidemiology 142(9): 955-960, 1995.

85. Magrassi, I., et al. "Effects of Vitamin D and Retinoic Acid on Human Glioblastoma Cell Lines," Acta Neurochir 133: 184-190, 1995.

86. Kennedy, D.D., et al. "Low Antioxidant Vitamin Intakes Are Associated with Increases in Adverse Effects of Chemotherapy in Children with Acute Lymphoblastic Leukemia," American Journal of Clinical Nutrition 79: 1029-1036, 2004.

87. Gergeley, P., et al. "Effects of Vitamin A Treatment of Cellular Immune Reactivity in Patients with CLL," Acta Medica Hu 45:307-311, 1988.

88. Tallman, Martin S., M.D., et al. "All-Trans-Retinoic Acid in Acute Promyeloctic Leukemia," New England Journal of Medicine 337(15): 1021-1028, 1997.

89. Muller, K., et al. "Carotenoids Induce Apoptosis in the T-Lymphoblast Cell Line Jurkat E6.1," Free Radical Research 36: 791-802, 2002.

90. Frankel, Stanley R., M.D., et al. "All-Trans-Retinoic Acid for Acute Promyeloctic Leukemia: Results of the New York Study," Annals of Internal Medicine 120(4):278-286, February 15, 1994.

6
WOMEN'S HEALTH

Oxidative stress has been implicated in the pathogenesis of chronic disease related to aging, such as cancer and cardiovascular disease, according to Xianfeng Zhao and colleagues at Tufts University in Boston, Massachusetts, and colleagues in the United States, Italy, Germany, and Denmark.[1]

They added that it is possible that carotenoids found in fruit and vegetables act as a major group of antioxidants, thereby preventing damage from harmful reactive oxygen species, which are continuously produced in the body from normal cellular functions.

In the study, 37 healthy, nonsmoking women, ranging in age from 50 to 70, were assigned to 1 of 5 groups, who were instructed to consume a daily dose of mixed carotenoids (beta-carotene, lutein, and lycopene, 4 mg each; 12 mg of a single carotenoid (beta-carotene, lutein, or lycopene); or placebo for 56 days.

At day 57, all carotenoid groups showed significantly lower endogenous DNA damage than at the beginning of the study, whereas the placebos (controls) did not show any significant change. In fact, less endogenous DNA damage was found as early as day 15 in the mixed carotenoid and beta-carotene groups.

"Our results indicate that carotenoid supplementation decreases DNA damage and that a combination of 4 mg/day of lutein, beta-carotene, and lycopene—an intake that can be achieved by diet—or a larger dose—12 mg—of individual carotenoids exert protection against DNA damage."

Pregnancy : As reported in Journal of Nutrition, in evaluating 15,832 Nepali women in a placebo-controlled, double-blind trial, who were between 12 and 45 years of age, they were given 7,000 mcg retinol equivalents of vitamin A as retinyl palmitate, 42 mg of beta-carotene, or a placebo.[2]

All treatments were given in identical gelatin capsules containing peanut oil, and 5 mg of synthetic vitamin E as an antioxidant. There was no effect of either supplement on morbidity rates reported up to 28 weeks of gestation.

However, in the late pregnancy, over 28 weeks, symptoms of nausea, faintness, and night blindness were reduced with vitamin A but not with beta-carotene. Vitamin A supplementation reduced the length of labor by 1.5 hours among 11 muliparous women, and by 50 minutes among multiparous women. Multiparous means having other children.

It was also found that vitamin A and beta-carotene reduced the postpartum prevalence of at least 4 loose stools and night blindness. Beta-carotene supplementation reduced the symptoms of high fever postpartum.

In the women who were given vitamin A, the total number of days of illness symptoms that occurred over the last 12 weeks of pregnancy was lower by 5 days when compared with placebo.

In addition, maternal vitamin A or beta-carotene supplementation reduced the prevalence of selected illness symptoms during late pregnancy, at the time of birth, and during 6 months postpartum, the researchers said.

Researchers at Queen Elizabeth Hospital for Children in London, England, evaluated concentrations of vitamins A and E, copper, magnesium, and zinc in cord blood from pregnant women in Hackney, an inner city of London.[3]

Esters of vitamin A were not detected in any samples which indicated there was no biochemical evidence of toxicity. Vitamin A intake correlated significantly with birthweight, head circumference, length, and gestation.

The data suggested that most of the mothers evaluated may have been marginal with respects to vitamins A and E and zinc. Higher levels of these nutrients may have benefited low birthweight infants, the researchers added.

For low-income mothers, liver and liver products are the cheapest and best sources of vitamins A, E, heme iron, B vitamins, and other essential nutrients. However, pregnant women who consume large amounts of liver need to be monitored so as not to intake too much vitamin A. It does not harm the mother but could harm the fetus.

The improvement of vitamin A status may help to control anemia in pregnant women, reported a research team at Wageningen Agricultural University in The Netherlands.[4]

The study involved 251 Indonesian women, 17 to 35 years of age, with varying weeks of gestation. Hemoglobin levels between 80 and 109 g/l were evaluated for the role of vitamin A and iron supplementation in nutritionally anemic pregnancies.

The women were assigned to 1 of 4 treatment groups: (1) vitamin A at 2.4 mg of retinol and placebo iron tablets; (2) iron at 60 mg of elemental iron and a placebo vitamin A; (3) vitamin A and iron; or (4) both placebos daily for 8 weeks.

Maximum hemoglobin was achieved with both vitamin A and iron supplementation, with one-third of the response attributable to vitamin A and two-thirds to the iron.

Following supplementation, the proportion of women who became nonanemic was 35% in the vitamin A-supplemented group, 68% in the iron supplemented group; 97% in the women who supplemented with both supplements; and 16% in the controls.

As reported in the British Medical Journal, researchers evaluated 44,646 married women, of whom 20,119 became pregnant 22,189 times in a double-blind placebo-controlled trial. Participants who came from 270 wards were randomized into 3 groups of 90 women, each who received a weekly single oral supplement of placebo, vitamin A at 7,000 mcg retinol equivalents, or beta-carotene at 42 mcg (7,000 RE) over 3 ½ years.[5]

All-cause mortality was measured in the women during pregnancy and up to 12 weeks postpartum, and mortality during pregnancy to 6 weeks postpartum.

Mortality related to pregnancy in the placebo, vitamin A, and beta-carotene groups were 704, 426, and 361 deaths per 100,000 pregnancies, respectively, holding relative risks of 0.60 and 0.51.

This represented reductions of 40 and 49 among those getting vitamin A, and beta-carotene, respectively. Combined vitamin A and beta-carotene lowered mortality by 44%, and reduced the maternal mortality ratio from 645 deaths to 385 deaths per 100,000 live births, or by 40%.

Supplementation levels of vitamin A or beta-carotene in these women were the recommended dietary amounts, the researchers said.

In evaluating 57 healthy, lactating women, 18 to 35, it was found that, during the third trimester, 33% of the women had vitamin A intakes from diet and supplements of less than 800 mcg/day, which is the recommended value, reported the American Journal of Clinical Nutrition.[6]

The study reported that vitamin A and serum vitamin A concentrations during pregnancy influenced the composition of breast milk. Less than 1.4 micromol of vitamin A/1 was found in mature breast milk in 12.3% of the women.

Vitamin A status should be monitored and improved during pregnancy and lactation. Dietary counseling is warranted to insure vitamin A adequacy during pregnancy and lactation, reported Rosa M. Ortega and colleagues.

At the University of New Mexico in Albuquerque, a research team evaluated 7 eclampic, 9 preeclampic, and 56 normal pregnancies, whose blood levels of vitamin A were significantly reduced in the preeclampic and eclampic women, when compared to healthy women in the third trimester. Preeclampsia is the development of high blood pressure or edema, or both, usually during the 20th week of gestation. However, it can develop earlier than that. Eclampsia is the occurrence of one or more convulsions, often in conjunction with preeclampsia.[7]

In addition, blood levels of vitamin E of preeclampic and eclampic women were 15 to 30% lower, respectively, than in the controls.

This data supports the hypothesis that preeclampic/eclampic conditions depletes natural lipid antioxidants. A pregnancy, if they happen to be infected with the HIV-1 virus, may place them at an increased risk for a mother/child transmission of the virus, the researchers said.

Vitamin A supplements are not generally needed by most pregnant women in western countries, who consume the RDA during their reproductive period, according to Barbara A. Underwood of the World Health Organization in Geneva, Switzerland. However, increasing the consumption of vitamin A-rich foods can meet increasing demands during lactation.[8]

However, women in developing countries, whose vitamin A intakes are near their basic needs, should receive an additional 100 mcg retinol equivalents (RE) during pregnancy, and 300 mcg RE during lactation.

Supplements not above 3,000 mcg RE (10,000 IU) daily are safe for fertile women where circumstances preclude obtaining the needed increment through diet, Underwood added.

The first postpartum month is the only safe period during which to provide deficient lactating women with a single, high-dose supplement of vitamin A to benefit the mother and breast-feeding infant for several months, she said.

Breast feeding : In a trial involving 48 infants, the children were given either 3,000 IU/day of vitamin A in the form of retinol acetate and 5 IU/day of vitamin E orally, or a placebo.[9]

Results showed that vitamin A and vitamin E levels increased with age in both groups of breast-fed infants. At 3 months, levels were higher in the supplemented group than in the controls.

In a randomized, double-blind trial in 153 Indonesian mothers, 1 to 3 weeks postpartum, researchers at Cornell University in Ithaca, New York, found that a daily dose of 312 micromol of vitamin A as retinol palmitate, or a placebo, can enhance the vitamin A status of the mother and infant significantly.[10]

The milk retinol concentrations of the vitamin A group was considerably higher than that of the placebo group, reported Rebecca Stoltzfuse and colleagues.

In children 6 years of age, the presence of low serum retinol concentrations less than 0.52 micromol/l were 36%, and in the placebo group 15%. It was also reported that the serum retinol concentrations in the vitamin A group were lower at baseline than the placebo group.

Fibrocystic disease : Referring to a promising pilot study of the effects of vitamin A on fibrocystic disease, as well as her own work with patients, Susan M. Lark, M.D., believes that vitamin A may be effective for soothing sore, lumpy, breasts.[11]

She referred to a study at the University of Montreal in Canada, in which 12 women with moderate to severe breast pain were given high doses of vitamin A for 3 months. Nine of the women reported significant pain relief, and 5 women experienced decreases in breast lumps. Fibrocystic disease involves cystic lesions in fibrous connective tissues.

Pierre R. Band. M.D., lead researcher of the Canadian study, said that, "from my experience, I believe that women who have substantial breast pain from benign breast disease are likely to get relief from vitamin A."

He went on to say, however, that, you are dealing with a potentially toxic substance (they used 150,000 IU/day), so you have to be careful. He added that researchers have used smaller doses with good results.

"My answer is to use beta-carotene instead," Lark said.

She recommends between 25,000 and 50,000 IU/day of beta-carotene for fibrocystic disease, since you don't have to worry about toxicity with this provitamin A.

Other doctors have recommended these daily amounts of nutrients for painful breasts: iodine (150 mcg); vitamin B6 (100 to 150 mg, taken in 2 or 3 divided doses; and vitamin E (600 IU).

Premenstrual syndrome (PMS) : In 30 women, who were between 17 and 47 years of age, with premenstrual tension and complaints of breast pain, tenderness to the abdomen, edema (swelling), and a variety of nervous symptoms, the patients were given 200,000 IU/day of vitamin A orally during the second half of the menstrual cycle, which was stopped at the onset of menstruation, and resumed 2 weeks later, reported the Journal of Clinical Endocrinology.[12]

During a 2- to 6- month period, results showed a disappearance of breast pain, a reduction in mammary nodules, a marked reduction in abdominal pain, disappearance of edema, and a great improvement in nervous symptom complaints in the majority of the women.

This improvement continued 1 year after the therapy began. However, the results were not as successful in patients given vitamin A irregularly, or for short periods of time, the researchers said.

Endometriosis : For women with endometriosis, Susan M. Lark, M.D., recommends 50 mg/day of B1, B2, B3, and pantothenic acid (a B vitamin), and 30 mg/day of B6; 50 mcg of B12; 400 mcg/day of folic acid (another B vitamin); and 200 mg/day of biotin, another B vitamin. She also recommends beta-carotene, vitamins C and E, and the mineral selenium.[13]

Antioxidants are best known for their ability to fight free radicals, the naturally occurring unstable molecules that cause tissue damage in the body by stealing electrons from healthy molecules to balance themselves. Doctors know that antioxidants can also build immunity, lessen cramping, and reduce excessive menstrual bleeding.

Endometriosis is the presence and growth of functioning endometrial tissue in places other than the uterus, which results in pain and infertility.

"While you can't just pop these supplements and expect instant relief from acute pain, I've found that doses of antioxidants, along with dietary changes, can treat the chronic problems of endometriosis," Lark added.

She recommends a daily regimen of 1,000 to 4,000 mg of vitamin C; 25,000 to 50,000 IU of beta-carotene; 400 to 2,000 IU of vitamin E; and 25 mcg of selenium, assuming this agrees with your doctor.

She added that antioxidants can have a dramatic effect on the regulation of bleeding as well as on the reduction of pain and cramps that may accompany endometriosis. Vitamin C controls excessive bleeding, vitamin A lessens profuse menstrual bleeding; and vitamin E helps in pain management, she continued.

Birth defects : As reported in the American Journal of Obstetrics and Gynecology, a study evaluated the relationship between vitamin A and pregnancies, which produced offspring with neural tube defects (548 participants), or major malformations other than neural tube defects (387 women), and 573 normal controls.[14]

The proportion of women consuming doses of vitamin A between 8,000 IU and 25,000 IU/day was no greater in the major malformation group, or the group with neural tube defects, than in the normal controls.

For exposure to vitamin A from supplements and fortified cereals combined, women consuming over 8,000 IU/day and greater than 10,000 IU/day had odds ratios for major malformation of 0.79 and 0.73, respectively, compared with women consuming less than 5,000 IU/day.

The study found no association between periconceptional vitamin A exposure at doses greater than 8,000 IU/day or doses greater than 10,000 IU/day and malformations in general or neural tube defects.

Compared with iron and folic acid supplementation, the administration of multimicronutrients to undernourished pregnant women may reduce the incidence of low birth weight and early neonatal morbidity, reported Archives of Pediatrics and Adolescent Medicine.[15]

The supplemented group were given a supplement containing 29 vitamins and minerals once daily, from enrollment until delivery, with a median duration of 58 days.

The women were also given supplements of iron, given in the form of ferrous sulfate—which contained 60 mg of elemental iron—at 60 mg/day, and folic acid, at 500 mcg/day.

Beta-carotene can only improve vitamin A status when zinc is also available, reported Marjoleine A. Dijkhuizen, and colleagues at Wageningen University in the Netherlands.[16]

Supplementation during pregnancy with beta-carotene and zinc—but not beta-carotene alone—is effective in improving the vitamin A status of both mothers and infants 6 months postpartum.

"Increased breast-milk vitamin A content is an important contributor to the improved vitamin A status of the infants," the researchers said. "In view of the high prevalence of vitamin A deficiency in infants and lactating mothers in developing countries and the direct relation between micronutrient deficiencies and increased morbidity and mortality, supplementing pregnant women with beta-carotene and zinc is clearly indicated."

They added that because iron supplementation of pregnant women is already widely implemented, the addition of beta-carotene and zinc to these supplements could be an efficient and cost-effective measure for improving the health of both infants and lactating mothers.

A Vitamin A Deficiency and Pregnancy

A study reported in an International Journal of Obstetrics and Gynecology evaluated 736 pregnant women in their third trimester of pregnancy, who belonged to low- and high-socio-economic groups.

The researchers found that 2.9% of the women suffered from night blindness, and 27% were found to have a subclinical vitamin A deficiency.

Moderate to severe anemia was reported in 41.2% of the volunteers, and 15.8% of the women developed pregnancy-induced high blood pressure.

The researchers suggested that subclinical vitamin A deficiency is a problem during the third trimester of pregnancy, and blood levels of retinol (vitamin A) less than 20 mcg/dl appears to indicate a deficient status, and this is associated with an increased risk of preterm delivery and maternal anemia.

Source: Radhika, M.S., et al. "Effects of Vitamin A Deficiency During Pregnancy on Maternal and Child Health," An International Journal of Obstetrics and Gynecology 109(6): 689-693, June 2002.

Vitamin A and Pregnancy

An excessive dietary intake of vitamin A has been associated with fetal abnormalities in humans in less than 20 reported cases over the past 30 years, according to Veronique Azais-Braesco, M.D., and Gerard Pascal, M.D., of the Vitamin Research Group in Paris and Clermont-Ferrand, France.

However, caution must be exercised to avoid unnecessary supplementation of women of child-bearing age.

Low levels of vitamin A affect millions of women and children worldwide, and a vitamin A deficiency is associated with a depressed immune system, and a high illness and death due to infectious diseases such as diarrhea, measles, and respiratory infections.

A vitamin A deficiency is often associated with an increased mother-to-child transmission of HIV-1.

Supplemental vitamin A should be carefully examined in each case according to risk-to-benefit ratio.

The final decision should take into account the estimated vitamin A status of the woman, the availability of vitamin A-rich foods in her diet, and whether supplementation can be supervised.

Source: Azais-Braesco, Veronique, M.D., and Pascal, Gerard, M.D. "Vitamin A in Pregnancy: Requirements and Safety Limits," American Journal of Clinical Nutrition 71(5): S1325-S1333, May 2000.

References

1. Zhao, Xianfeng, et al. "Modification of Lymphocyte DNA Damage by Carotenoid Supplementation in Postmenouausal Women," American Journal of Clinical Nutrition 83: 163-169, 2006.
2. Christian, P., et al. "Vitamin A and Beta-Carotene Supplementation Reduces Symptoms of Illness in Pregnant and Lactating Nepali Women," Journal of Nutrition 130: 2675-2682, 2000.
3. Ghabremeskel, K., et al. "Vitamin A and Related Essential Nutrients and Cord Blood Relationships with Anthropometric Measurements At Birth," Early Human Development 39: 177-188, 1994.
4. Suharno, Djoko, et al. "Supplementation with Vitamin A and Iron for Nutritional Anemia in Pregnant Women in West Java, Indonesia," The Lancet 342: 1325-1328, November 27, 1993.
5. West, K.P., Jr., et al. "Double-Blind, Cluster Randomized Trial of Low Dose Supplementation with Vitamin A or Beta-Carotene on Mortality Related to Pregnancy in Nepal," British Medical Journal 318: 570-575, February 27, 1999.
6. Ortega, Rasa M., et al. "Vitamin A Status During the Third Trimester of Pregnancy in Spanish Women: Influence on Concentrations of Vitamin A in Breast Milk," American Journal of Clinical Nutrition 66: 564-568, 1997.

7. Ziari, Shahed A., et al. "Serum Vitamin A, Vitamin E, and Beta-Carotene Levels in Preeclampic Women in Northern Nigeria," American Journal of Perinatology 13(5): 287-291, July 1996.

8. Underwood, Barbara A. "Meternal Vitamin A Status and Its Importance in Infancy and Early Childhood," American Journal of Clinical Nutrition 59: 517S-524S, 1994.

9. Delvin, E.E., et al. "Vitamin A and E Supplementation in Breast-Fed Newborns," Journal of Pediatric Gastroenterology and Nutrition 31(5): 562-565, November 2000.

10. Stoltzffuse, Rebecca, et al. "High Dose Vitamin A Supplementation of Breast-Feeding Indonesian Mothers: Effects on the Vitamin A Status of Mothers and Infants," Journal of Nutrition 123: 666-675, 1993.

11. Feinstein, Alice, editor. Prevention's Healing with Vitamins. Emmaus, PA: Rodale Press, Inc., 1996, pp. 251-253.

12. Argonz, J., and Abinxano, C. "Premenstrual Tension Treated with Vitamin A," Journal of Clinical Endocrinology 10: 1579-1590, 1950.

13. Feinstein, Alice, editor. *Ibid*, p. 235.

14. Mills, James L., M.D., et al. "Vitamin A and Birth Defects," American Journal of Obstetrics and Gynecology 177: 31-36, 1997.

15. Gupta P., et al. "Multimicronutrient Supplementation for Undernourished Pregnant Women and Birth Size of Their Offspring: A Double-Blind, Randomized, Placebo-Controlled Trial," Archives of Pediatrics and Adolescent Medicine 161: 58-64, 2007.

16. Dijkhuizen, Marjoleine A., et al. "Zinc Plus Beta-Carotene Supplementation of Pregnant Women is Superior to Beta-Carotene Supplementation Alone in Improving Vitamin A Status in Both Mothers and Infants," American Journal of Clinical Nutrition 80: 1299-1307, 2004.

7

CHILDREN'S HEALTH

Children with vitamin A deficieny have a greater risk of irreversible blindness, and dying of infectious disease than do children who are vitamin A replete, according to Rebecca L. Surles and Colleagues at the University of Wisconsin at Madison.[1, 2, 3, 4, 5, 6, 7]

Globally, over 250 million children under the age of 5 have vitamin A deficiency, and supplementation programs are commonly used to address the issue.

Studies found little or no improvement in infant vitamin A status after supplementation with either low-dose beta-carotene or 25,000 IU of vitamin A in the form of retinyl palmitate.

At about the same time, the recommendation was made to increase the dose to 50,000 IU, the researchers added. The World Health Organization currently recommends that infants receive 50,000 IU of vitamin A at immunization contacts at age 6, 10, and 14 weeks, and that children 6 to 11 months receive 100,000 IU of vitamin A, and those 12 to 59 months old be given 200,000 IU of vitamin A every 4 to 6 months.

Since studies have been inconsistent, the research team aimed to quantify liver vitamin A after the administration of vitamin A doses in piglets. The animals are good models in this regard because of their similar size to infants, gastrointestinal anatomy, and vitamin A requirements.

Male piglets born to sows who were fed a vitamin A-depleted diet were randomly assigned to receive 1 of 4 vitamin A doses: (1) 0, (2) 25,000 IU; (3) 50,000 IU; or (4) 100,000 IU; at weaning (9 to 14 days).

A vitamin A-depleted diet was fed until the piglets were 10 days old. Blood retinol was measured on days 1, 2, 4, 7 and 10.

The research team found that 25,000 IU did not result in a mean liver retinol reserve—over 0.07 micromol/g liver—the deficiency cutoff. The 50,000 IU dose increased mean reserves above 0.07 micromol/g only in parity (the condition of giving birth). Liver vitamin A reserves with the 100,000 IU treatment were only 5% above those with the 50,000 IU measurement.

"The piglet model suggests that, for supplementation to infants less than 6 months old, a 50,000 IU dose is likely to be more efficacious in mitigating deficiency than is a 25,000 IU dose," the researchers added.

They said that, as developing countries search for sustainable strategies to improve community vitamin A status, biofortification of staple crops and promotion of the consumption of vegetables are viable options that can be safely introduced alongside vitamin A supplementation programs.

Marginal vitamin A status is associated with an increased incidence in the severity of infections, poor growth, iron deficiency anemia, and excessive childhood mortality, according to researchers at the University of Stellenbosch in Tygerberg, South Africa.[8]

Improvement in vitamin A status in children results in improved growth and iron status, a decrease in infections morbidity, a 30% reduction in overall childhood mortality, they added.

The researchers added that clinical vitamin A deficiency is still one of the leading causes of childhood blindness in many developing countries, with over 500,000 children going blind annually.

Controlled trials of vitamin A in hospitalized children with measles have showed vitamin A supplementation can reduce mortality rates significantly, and, in some cases, by 50%.

The World Health Organization has recommended vitamin A supplements for children with severe measles. The recommended dose is 200,000 IU orally for two days, but in children one year of age, half that dose.

Vitamin A helps to maintain the integrity of epithelial tissues, and cellular and humoral immune function are affected by a vitamin A deficiency. Serum retinol concentrations in mcg/dl are used to assess vitamin A status per the WHO, the researchers added.

The following oriteria should be used: less than 10 mcg/dl, deficient; 10 to 19, low; 20 to 50, normal; over 50, high. If more than 5% of the population have levels below 10 mcg/dl, then vitamin A deficiency is a major public health problem.

The researchers added that intervention strategies using regular vitamin A supplementation include giving capsules every 4 to 6 months at a dose varying from 50,000 to 200,000 IU, food fortification, as well as dietary diversification and nutrition education with regard to the consumption of vitamin A-rich foods. Until policy is formulated, dietary diversification, and consumption of vitamin A-rich foods, should be encouraged in all individuals and communities.

Also, education of vitamin A should be part of a nutrition education program. If supplementation is deemed necessary on clinical grounds, children with measles, malnutrition, chronic diarrhea, and pneumonia should receive a dose of 200,000 IU for children older than 1, and 100,000 IU for those less than 1 year of age.

In children under 6 months of age, vitamin A supplements should be used with extreme caution, and no more than a single 50,000 IU dose should be given within a 6-month period, the researchers said.

While studying the effects of vitamin A in children, Ranjit Kumet Kumar Chandra, M.D., of Memorial University of Newfoundland in Canada, observed that even a moderate deficiency of vitamin A can weaken the immune defenses of a child's respiratory tract, according to Prevention's Healing with Vitamins.[9]

Vitamin A deficiency causes damage to the naturally protective mucous membrane barrier of the respiratory tract, and it is thought that bacteria and viruses take advantage of that damage, Chandra said.

As an example, after flu virus attacks, the lining of a normal throat will repair itself. But this is not the case in those who are vitamin A deficient.

"Instead, you might get that once-healthy cell replaced by an abnormal cell," added Charles B. Stephenson, Ph.D., of the

University of Alabama in Birmingham. "That may predispose you to having a more severe episode of an infection, or having another infection on top of the viral infection."

Many experts suggest that the immune-compromising vitamin A deficiencies are widespread among children in the United States, added Martha Rumore, Pharm. D., of the Arnold and Marie Schwartz College of Pharmacy and Health Sciences in Brooklyn, New York. She reported that vitamin A deficiency has been correlated with decreased resistance to pneumonia, tuberculosis, whooping cough, and infectious diarrhea.

Another study, which involved 20 U.S. children with measles, showed that half of them were vitamin A deficient. For one thing, measles depletes vitamin A stores, and many people, especially children, do not eat many vitamin A-rich foods.

Over one-third of the global population is affected either by a vitamin A or iodine deficiency, according to researchers at the Swiss Federal Institute of Technology in Zurich.[10]

These deficiencies often coexist, and 32 to 50% of school-age children in rural West and North Africa have both vitamin A deficiency and goiter, which is due to an iodine deficiency.

High-dose oral vitamin A supplementation is recommended strategy to control a vitamin A deficiency in the affected populations, many of whom are also iodine deficient.

Thyroid metabolism and the response of iodine prophylaxis (iodized salt) in areas of iodine deficiency are influenced by various nutritional factors, including vitamin A status.

A vitamin A deficiency has numerous effects on thyroid function in animals: (1) in the thyroid, vitamin A deficiency decreases thyroidal iodine uptake and iodine incorporation into the thyroglobulin and increases thyroid size; (2) in the periphery, vitamin A deficiency increases circulating thyroid hormone concentrations; and (3) in the pituitary, vitamin A status modulates thyrotropin (thyroid-stimulating hormone).

In the 6-month study, 404 South African children, ranging in age from 5 to 14 years, who had mild-to-moderate vitamin A and iodine deficiencies.

At the beginning of the study, and after 3 months, children were given: (1) iodine (191 mg as oral iodized oil or a placebo; (2) 200,000 IU of vitamin A as retinyl palmitate or a placebo; and (3) both vitamin A and iodine.

Serum vitamin A and retinol-binding protein increased significantly vitamin A supplementation. For urinary iodine, serum retinol/ vitamin A, and retinol-binding protein, there were no significant treatment interactions between the two nutrients.

"Our data indicate that iodine prophylaxis will be effective in controlling iodine deficiency, even in cases of poor vitamin A status, and high vitamin A supplementation is likely to be safe and effective in areas of mild iodine deficiency," the researchers said.

They added that their findings suggest that high-dose vitamin A supplementation can modify indicators of iodine deficiency, such as thyroglobulin and goiter, independent of change in iodine nutrition.

In areas of endemic goiter, through suppression of transcription of the primary TSH-beta gene, vitamin A supplementation may decrease excess thyroid-stimulating hormone (TSH), stimulation of the thyroid and thereby reduce the risk of goiter and its sequelae (a condition following as a consequence of a disease).

As reported in the American Journal of Clinical Nutrition, in 1,407 Indonesian children, between 6 and 47 months of age, were randomly assigned to receive either 214 micromol of vitamin A (206,000 IU/1), or 107 micromol of vitamin A/1 if the child was less than 12 months of age, or a placebo.[11]

Results revealed that high-dose vitamin A supplementation improved the linear growth of children with very low blood levels of retinol, and this effect was modified by age and by breastfeeding, the researchers added.

The World Health Organization recommends Bacille Calmette-Guerin (BCG) vaccination at birth in low-income countries. BCG is a strain of Mycobacterium bovis that is used in the preparation of a vaccine that is used for immunization against tuberculosis and in cancer chemotherapy.[12] Leon A. Calmette (1863-1933) was a French bacteriologist, and Camille Guerin (1872-1961), was also a French bacteriologist.

There are conflicting reports as to whether or not vitamin A supplementation should also be given at birth, added a research team from Copenhagen, Denmark, and other colleagues in Denmark, the Netherlands, and Sweden.

Vitamin A supplementation with BCG vaccination does not appear to interfere with the long-term immune response of BCG, the researchers reported in the American Journal of Clinical Nutrition.

However, the vitamin supplement temporarily altered the delayed-type hypersensitivity (DTH) reaction in Mycobacterium tuberculosis in boys at 2 months of age, suggesting sex differences in the immunological response to vitamin A supplementation when given with the vaccine.

In any event, 50,000 IU of vitamin A given at birth has been associated with decreased mortality in Asian countries. Previous studies have demonstrated that vitamin A therapy may influence immune response to vaccines, they added.

As reported in the International Journal of Vitamin and Nutrition Research, the study evaluated antioxidant capacity in malnourished Nigerian children, of which 15 were marasmic (wasting), 8 were severely marasmic, 12 had kwashiorkor, and 18 were normally nourished children. Kwashiorkor is often seen in children 1 to 3 years of age. It is caused by a dietary deficiency, especially protein, and it results in anemia, edema, pot belly, loss of hair, depigmentation of the skin, etc.[13]

Retinol levels were found to be reduced in severe marasmic, when compared to controls. There was a strong correlation between plasma retinol and retinol binding protein found in all groups. The vitamin E/lipid ration was lower in the kwashiorkor children. Retinol-binding protein transports vitamin A in the blood.

It was reported that alpha-carotene, beta-carotene, cryptoxanthin, and lycopene were below the detection limits in most of the malnourished children.

The authors conclude that there is a depletion of antioxidant vitamins present in malnourished Nigerian children, especially significant is the depletion in kwashiorkor syndrome.

A research team at the University of Queensland Medical School in Australia, reported in the British Medical Journal that vitamin A, either in foods or supplements, is essential in reducing the morbidity and mortality associated with infectious diseases in children.[14]

The researchers reviewed data from controlled trials on vitamin A. From 20 trials, 12 were identified that also were randomized, and it was found that adequate vitamin A intake reduced the incidence of mortality from all causes by 30%.

Death from diarrheal diseases were reduced by 39%, and a 70% reduction in deaths from respiratory diseases was found when vitamin A intake was adequate.

The research team added that adequate vitamin A status must be maintained either through diet or supplements to help prevent sickness and death in children, especially from infectious diseases such as measles, and improved survival rates of premature infants.

In 56 preschool-age children, who had recurrent acute respiratory infections, or recurrent diarrhea, compared with 35 healthy controls, blood levels of vitamin A were 51.66 mcg/dl, and beta-carotene levels were 82.88 mcg/dl in children with acute respiratory infections, according to the Journal of Tropical Pediatrics.[15]

This was considerably lower than in the control group of 58.14 mcg/dl and 131 mcg/dl, respectively.

Blood levels of vitamin A at 42.21 mcg/dl and beta-carotene levels at 81.63 mcg/dl in children with recurrent diarrhea were significantly lower than the controls, with 58.14 and 131.43 mcg/dl, respectively.

The researchers suggested that vitamin A supplementation during recurrent diarrhea and acute respiratory infections may be warranted.

Researchers at the Harvard School of Public Health in Boston, Massachusetts, evaluated the dietary intake of vitamin A and the incidence of diarrhea and respiratory infections in over 28,000 Sudanese children between 6 months and 6 years of age, reported the Journal of Nutrition.[16]

Total dietary vitamin A intake was strongly and inversely associated with the risk of diarrhea. There was also a strong inverse association with the risk of having a cough or fever.

The researchers added that there was a significant positive association with dietary vitamin A intake and the incidence of cough alone, which is a sign associated with a healthy respiratory epithelium. The study emphasized the importance of adequate vitamin A intake to protect the health of children in developing countries.

In 147 preschool children with a history of frequent respiratory illnesses who received either 450 mcg/day of vitamin A or a placebo, those children who were given the supplement over an 11-month period showed 19% fewer episodes of respiratory infections than their placebo counterparts, in spite of the fact that their plasma retinol levels did not change, reported the Australian Pediatrics Journal.[17]

Children who had a prior history of lower respiratory illness or of allergy benefitted the most from the supplementation, the researchers added.

Parasites that impair the utilization of certain nutrients or reduce food intake may be especially detrimental to young children during vulnerable stages of growth and development, according to M.C. Nesheim of Cornell University in New York.[18]

Parasites also depend on their hosts for their own nutrient supply, and diets of the host can influence growth and development of specific parasites.

The tapeworm—Diphyllobothrium latum—results in a high incidence of those with pernicious anemia due to a vitamin B12 deficiency, because of the interference with B12 absorption by the tapeworm. Hook worm, Trichuris (related to the trichina worm), and chistosomia infections may cause significant blood loss, which may elevate iron needs and contribute to anemia.

Ascaris lumbriooides (a large roundworm) infection may reduce fat absorption and interfere with the absorption of vitamin A precursors from food. When infection causes diarrhea, there may be serious nutrient loss, and nutrient deficiency can impair immune function.

As an example, populations of children with marginal vitamin A status have greater mortality and morbidity compared to populations given vitamin A supplements. Malaria parasites need a host with sufficient iron stores to grow and develop, reported Parasitology.

At Children's National Medical Center in Washington, D.C., 24 infants in 2 groups, with a mean birth weight of less than

1,000 grams, and a mean gestation of 27 weeks, were evaluated for vitamin A levels, and were given two different supplement regimens, according to the Journal of Parenteral and Enteral Nutrition.[19]

In Group 1, vitamin A levels were assessed after the first week of parenteral nutrition, and, if low, the infants were given a 2,000 IU supplement intramuscularly 3 times a week, beginning in the 10th and 14th day of life.

In Group 2, the same supplementation was begun on the 2nd and 4th day of life. In both groups, when enteral feeding reached 60 kcal/kg/day, 25,000 IU of vitamin A were given orally.

The incidence of oxygen support at 28 days was similar in both groups, although Group 2 had a trend towards less vigorous ventilatory support, reported Sandra T. Robbins, R.D., and Anne B. Fletcher, M.D.

They added that there was a significantly smaller proportion of infants in Group 2 who had bronchopulmonary dysplasia at 36 weeks gestation than in Group 1. The length of time in neonatal intensive care unit stay was significantly reduced from 81 to 60 days.

The researchers added that vitamin A supplementation should be given early tc small, premature infants who are at risk for bronchopulmonary dysplasia, and that monitoring of plasma levels of vitamin A are important to avoid toxicity.

As reported by the World Health Organization, their research reassures that 4-month interval between high-dose vitamin A supplementation using 100,000 IU for infants 0 to 11 months of age, and 200,000 IU for those 12 months of age or older, is an adequate public health measure in a population where disease rates are high and xerophthalmia (dryness of the conjunctiva and cornea) is low, according to the American Journal of Public Health.[20]

A vitamin A deficiency has been associated with compromised immune function in children, according to Richard D. Semba, M.D., and colleagues in the Journal of Nutrition.[21]

In this study in Indonesia, 236 children who received the diphtheria-pertussis-tetanus vaccine, and their responses to tetanus exposure, were evaluated after receiving either 60,000 mg of vitamin A or a placebo.

It was found that both the vitamin A-deficient and the healthy children who received the vitamin A supplement showed significantly greater IgG response to tetanus than the children who acted as controls.

Semba added that children who were marginally vitamin A deficient had suppressed immune function relative to those with optimal vitamin A status.

Very low birth weight in neonates, especially those who need mechanical ventilation and supplementary oxygen therapy in the early postnatal period, are susceptible to bronchopulmonary dysplasia, which affects the bronchial tubes and lungs, reported Jayant P. Shenai, M.D., and colleagues at the Vanderbilt University School of Medicine in Nashville, Tennessee.[22]

The healing of tissues in the lung and tracheobronchial tree involves nutrients, antioxidants, inflammatory cells, eicosanoids, growth factors, peptide hormones, and components of the extracellular matrix, the researchers reported in the Journal of Pediatrics.

They added that vitamin A is an essential nutrient in the promotion of growth and in the orderly differentation of regenerating epithelial cells, which make it important in the recovery of lung injury.

A number of clinical studies have reported on vitamin A and the relationship to bronchopulmonary dysplasia, showing that very low birth weight neonates are born with low blood concentrations of vitamin A and retinol-binding protein, and they also have low liver stores of the vitamin.

The authors have shown in a controlled trial that vitamin A supplementation from early potential life in very low birth weight neonates improves their vitamin status, and it also promotes normal regenerative healing from lung injury, as shown by a decreassed incidence of bronchopulmonary dysplasia and associated morbidity. Bronchopulmonary relates to the bronchi tubes and lungs.

At Osaka University Medical School in Japan, Yuichi Fukul, M.D., and colleagues, evaluated the vitamin A status of 19 patients with corrected biliary atresia, who were given 5,000 IU of oral vitamin A postoperatively. This is essentially neonatal hepatitis, which does not normally occur until several days after birth, they explained in the Journal of Pediatric Surgery.[23]

Plasma vitamin A levels in the jaundiced group were significantly low compared to the controls. In the severely-jaundiced group, blood levels of vitamin A increased from 13.5 to 30 mcg/dl following supplementation, compared to controls.

This data suggests that nutritional support to facilitate the synthesis of retinol-binding protein may be an important factor in addition to vitamin A supplementation. As previously reported retinol-binding protein carries vitamin A through the blood.

Branched-chain amino acids may also be useful in malnourished patients with liver cirrhosis, the researchers continued. Liver vitamin A levels are a good indicator of vitamin A status, since plasma vitamin A levels are homeostatistically controlled as long as liver storage is maintained at more than 20 mcg/g liver.

Nutritional management of very low birth weight infants often requires initial treatment with total parenteral nutrition before weaning to preteram formulas or breast milk with nutritional fortifiers, according to Peter J. Porcelli, M.D., and colleagues, at Wake Forest University in Winston-Salem, North Carolina.[24] Parenteral refers to providing nutrition via intravenous, subcutaneous, intramuscular, or intramedullary (within bone marrow) injection.

Very low birth weight infants are prone to deficiency of vitamin A and vitamin B2 (riboflavin), the researchers continued. Fetal hepatic vitamin A stores are negligible until 36 to 46 weeks of gestation.

Vitamin B2 deficiency has been described repeatedly in exclusively breast-fed infants who receive phototherapy for hyperbilirubinemia (large amounts of bilirubin in the blood, which may indicate jaundice).

The authors recommend that existing parenteral multivitamin preparations be reformulated specifically for low birth weight intants, and that the recommended daily dosage of vitamin A be increased to 500 mcg/day. Vitamin B2 administration at 0.15 mg/kg/day is also recommended for these infants.

Low vitamin A levels in the preteram infant may affect healthy respiratory epithelial development, the researchers added. One study using 2,000 IU (650 mg) intramuscularly given retinol palmitate every other day for 28 days, and another study using 4,000 IU of supplemental retinol palmitate on alternate days in 37 infants, reduced the incidence of bronchopulmonary dysplasia.

The therapeutical recommended amounts for very low birth weight infants by the researchers is: (1) 0.15 mg/kg/day of B2 parenterally; (2) 0.15 to 0.30 mg/kg/day of B2 enterally; (3) 500 mcg/kg/day of vitamin A parenterally; and (4) 500 to 750 mcg/kg/day of vitamin A enterally.

The Journal of Pediatrics reported on 2 very low birth weight infants who had inadequate blood levels of vitamins A and E. The infants had been given a parenteral multivitamin/mineral preparation at 1.5 ml/kg/day in a dextrose-amino acid solution.[25]

A different delivery system was tried, using 2 ml/kg/day and infused for 6 hours from the first day of life. This procedure offered significant improvement in vitamin A and E levels during the first 28 days of life in very low birth weight infants, the researchers said.

At Vanderbilt University School of Medicine in Nashville, Tennessee, Jayant P. Shenai, M.D., reviewed the beneficial effects of vitamin A supplementation in low birth weight infants, who were at risk of developing bronchopulmonary dysplasia.[26]

In one study, infants received intramuscular supplemental vitamin A (2,000 IU of retinyl palmitate) or a 0.9% saline solution postnatal Day 4 and on alternate days thereafter, for a total of 14 injections over 28 days.

Shenai reported that the vitamin A supplementation resulted in bronchopulmonary dysplasia being diagnosed in 45% of the infants, compared with 85% of the controls. The need for mechanical ventilation, supplemental oxygen and intensive care were also reduced in the infants given vitamin A supplements. Also, airway infection and retinopathy or prematurity were also less frequent in the supplemented group. Retinopathy is a noninflammatory degenerative disease of the retina.

The results of the study showed a total vitamin intake of between 1,500 and 2,000 IU/kg/day not only improved the vitamin A status in very low birth weight neonates, but also it appears to promote regenerative healing from lung injury, as evidenced by the decreased incidence of mortality and bronchopulmonary dysplasia.

Shenai went on to say that, while preventing prematurity may be the primary perinatal health goal, strategies for reducing the incidence of bronchopulmonary dysplasia among very low birth-weight survivors are clearly indicated, and vitamin A supplementation is a single approach that can help in this syndrome.

As reported in the New England Journal of Medicine, in 405 very low-birth weight infants, compared to 402 controls, intramuscular administration of 5,000 IU of vitamin A three times weekly for 4 weeks, reduced biochemical evidence of vitamin A deficiency and slightly decreased the risk of chronic lung disease in extremely low-birth weight infants, according to a research team from the University of Texas at Houston.[27]

According to an article in the Journal of Pediatrics, a research team evaluated 2,067 Indonesian neonates who received either 50,000 IU of vitamin A orally or a placebo on the first day of life.[28]

In the 2 groups studied, 74% and 51% more control infants were brought for medical treatment for cough and fever. Neonatal vitamin supplementation may reduce infant mortality rates, and the prevalence of severe respiratory infection, reported the researchers at the Department of International Health, Division of Human Nutrition, in Baltimore, Maryland.

In an earlier article in the Journal of Pediatrics, Sinasi Ozsoylu, M.D., of Hacettepe University in Ankara, Turkey, gave 200,000 IU of vitamin A orally, or a placebo, randomly to 57 (Group I) and 46 (Group II) children with chickenpox, who had no evidence of vitamin A deficiency.[29]

In addition, 8 of the siblings of the first group who had not had the disease received the same amount of vitamin A during the incubation period of varicella, 1 to 3 days before the appearances of eruptions in the patients.

Crusting of all lesions occurred earlier in the first group than in the second group. The main duration of disease was shorter in the 8 siblings than in those who were given the vitamin A during the incubation period of the disease, than in the group of children who initially had the disease.

Five of the children in the placebo group had complications, 1 was viral pneumonia. Two had conjunctivitis or associated infections such as gastroenteritis, but there was no complication in the vitamin A-supplemented group.

Ozsoylu suggests that normal children need no treatment of the benign and self-limited disease, however, vitamin A might be given on the first day of eruption to shorten the crusting period and protect against complications, since this protocol is much cheaper than antiviral treatment.

Vitamin A should be given to more children during the incubation period of the disease to be certain about its effect on chickenpox, Ozsoylu continued. The role of vitamin A in acute viral diseases may not be due to absolute deficiency, but rather to pharmacologic effect.

At Johns Hopkins Hospital in Baltimore, Maryland, Richard D. Semba, M.D., and colleagues, evaluated the profile of the anti-tetanus toxoid IgG subclasses in children receiving vitamin A supplements, or a placebo, in order to assess the potential utility of the enhanced anti-tetanus toxoid response, they reported in Clinical and Diagnostic Laboratory Immunology.[30]

In a double-blind clinical trial, the levels of the different anti-tetanus toxoid IgG subclasses were measured 2 weeks before and 3 weeks after immunization in 139 Indonesian preschool children, ranging in ages from 3 to 6.

Children who were given vitamin A prior to the immunization had significantly increased IgG-1 levels, regardless of whether they were undergoing primary or memory reactions.

In a group of children undergoing a second response to tetanus toxoid, vitamin A supplementation was associated with a modest, but significant, change in the level of anti-tetanus toxoid IgG-3.

There were only minor changes in the levels of anti-tetanus toxoid IgG-2 and IgG-4.

Since IgG-1 is a subclass that is associated with a protective response to tetanus toxoid immunization, these results suggest that vitamin A supplementation may be a safe and effective way to enhance the humoral response to tetanus toxoid and other vaccine antigens, the researchers added.

In evaluating 423 pregnancies exposed during the first 9 weeks of gestation to a high dose of vitamin A, defined as 10,000 IU/day or more, data were collected on 394 of the women, according to Teratology.[31]

Major structural malformation, excluding chromosomal and genetic diseases, were evaluated in 311 infants exposed to a median daily dose of vitamin A at 50,000 IU/day, ranging from 10,000 to 300,000 IU/day.

Three infants with a major malformation were reported, which included pulmonary stenosis, stenotic anus with fistula and bilateral inguinal hernia. Pulmonary stenosis is a narrowing of the opening into the pulmonary artery from the right ventricle. No congenital malformations were recorded among 120 infants exposed to more than 50,000 IU/day.

The study, in Rome, Italy, found no evidence of an association between major structural malformations and a high intake of vitamin A as preformed vitamin A supplements during the first 9 weeks of gestation. Most infants born after "high" vitamin A exposure are normal and without major malformations, the researchers said.

Of 35,727 pregnant women who had control infants without birth defects, 3,399, or 9.5%, were treated with vitamin A. Of 20,830 pregnant women who had offspring with nongenital abnormalities, 1,642, or 7.9%, were treated with vitamin A, reported the International Journal of Vitamin and Nutrition Research.[32]

The case-control pair analysis taken from a data set of Hungarian Case-Control Surveillance of Congenital Abnormalities between 1980 and 1994, showed a lower rate of vitamin A treatment during pregnancy, and in the first trimester of gestation in most congenital abnormality groups.

The use of low or moderate doses of vitamin A of less than 10,000 IU/day during the first trimester of pregnancy is not teratogenic (causing abnormal embryonic development), but may have some protective effects on the fetus, the researchers said.

The researchers added that a multivitamin preparation containing doses of vitamin A lower than 10,000 IU/day is safe, and important in the primary prevention of certain major congenital abnormalities, explained Andrew E. Czeizel, M.D.

Higher esposures later in pregnancy, which is after organogenesis (formation of organs), do not appear to be toxic, he continued. Widespread vitamin A deficiency may be of greater public health importance than the small number of cases of vitamin A overdose.

A research team at the Institute of Child Health in London, United Kingdom, conducted a randomized, controlled trial of vitamin A supplementation in 1,455 children, ranging in age from 6 to 59 months, in rural Northern Ghana, reported the American Journal of Clinical Nutrition.[33]

For 4 months, oral doses of either 60 mg (200,000 IU) of retinol or 30 mg (100,000 IU) to children between 6 and 11 months, in the form of retinyl palmitate, plus 40 IU of vitamin E, or a placebo, were given.

The study lasted for 1 year, and there was a tendency for vitamin A supplemented children, but not placebo children, to have elevated acute phase proteins in association with vomiting and severe diarrhea.

The unsupplemented children failed to mount an acute phase response, which may have contributed to their increased morbidity from gastrointestinal symptoms, the researchers said.

At the Medical College of Georgia in Augusta, Joseph H. Clark, M.D., and colleagues, reported on the case of an 8-year-old boy who developed a limp and periorbital swelling. He was found to be hypocalcemic (low levels of calcium in the blood), and he had radiographic evidence of rickets. His serum vitamin A level was undetectable, and his blood levels of vitamin D were low. His diet consisted mostly of French fried potatoes and water for several years. Periorbital refers to around an orbit.[34]

There was considerable improvement with dihydrotachysterol at 0.25 mg twice daily; 50 mg of calcium per kg; and 50,000 IU of vitamin A for seven days. The vitamin A supplement was decreased to 5,000 IU/day, and serum vitamin A and retinol-binding protein concentrations remained normal.

Ophthalmologic examination after 10 weeks was entirely normal, and his total and ionized calcium normalized within several days.

His rickets healed radiographically within 10 weeks, however, after 2 months, all supplements were stopped. He refused to eat any food, in spite of 3 months of intensive psychotherapy. He was eventually discharged to a chronic-care facility, where he was given 40 ounces of nasogastric Pediasure daily.

Diabetes disrupts vitamin A metabolism by a still unknown mechanism, according to an article in the Journal of Clinical Biochemistry and Nutrition. In insulin-dependent diabetes mellitus (Type 1 diabetes), there is lower blood levels of retinol and retinol-binding protein.[35]

In addition, increased levels of free retinol in the liver may be due to increased activity of the enzyme retinyl ester hydrolase, even though this has not yet been proven.

High levels of free retinol in the liver may be due to its lower release into the circulation, the researchers said. Since retinoids are potent modulators of cell growth and differentiation, a significant alteration in the circulatory level of retinol, along with changes in insulin and glucose homeostasis (balance), may lead to proliferation changes in target organs, such as diabetic retinopathy (disease of the retina), the researchers added.

As reported in the American Journal of Clinical Nutrition, a research team evaluated the effect of a single high dose or daily low dose of vitamin A on diarrhea, acute lower respiratory tract infections, and all-cause fevers in 900 hospitalized pre-school children.[36]

Children were given either 200,000 IU of vitamin A orally on the day of admission (100,000 IU if the child was under 12 months of age), or a low-dose treatment of vitamin A at 5,000 IU/day until discharge, or a placebo.

Low-dose vitamin A supplementation significantly reduces the incidence of severe diarrhea in severely malnourished children, the researchers said.

In this group of malnourished and subclinically vitamin A-deficient children, daily low doses of vitamin A appeared to be more beneficial for severely malnourished children.

A research team at the University of Alabama in Birmingham, evaluated the association between serum retinol and diarrhea in 137 Peruvian children, of whom 77 had diarrhea. Controls consisted of 65 illness-free children.[37]

It was found that blood levels of retinol were lower in the children with diarrhea. These results suggest that diarrhea may lead to lower circulating retinol concentrations, and perhaps to its depletion. Diarrhea could be a major contributing factor to vitamin A deficiency in children in developing countries, the researchers added.

As reported by Mauricio L. Barreto, M.D., and colleagues, at the Department of Preventive Medicine, Canela, Brazil, they evaluated 1,240 children, 6 to 48 months of age, who were assigned to vitamin A or placebo groups at a dose of 100,000 IU, if they were under 12 months of age, and 200,000 IU, if they were older than 12 months. These amounts were given every 4 months for 1 year, according to The Lancet.[38]

It was found that the incidence of diarrhea was significantly lower in the vitamin A supplemented group, compared to controls. The benefit was greater in those with the more severe cases of the illness.

Also, the incidence was 20% lower in the vitamin A group than in the placebo group. But there was no effect on the incidence of acute lower-respiratory tract infection.

It is believed that vitamin A's ability to lower mortality may be due to its effect on reducing the severity of diarrhea, the researchers continued.

According to an article in Archives of Ophthalmology, researchers evaluated a 5-year-old boy with autism and a history of bilateral corneal ulceration. His eyes had been red and sensitive to light for several weeks. He was also clumsy, falling over furniture in the home.[39]

Further examination revealed a central ulcer in the right eye, a culture of which revealed Streptococcus pneumoniae (a parasite that inhibits the respiratory tract). He was given intensive antibiotic drop therapy, and it was found that he had a poor diet, eating only bacon, an occasional blueberry muffin and Kool-aid.

Since he refused vitamin supplements, it was found that his vitamin A stores measured less than 50 mcg/1, with the normal reading being 360 to 1,200 mcg/1.

The boy was given a vitamin A palmitate injection of 100,000 USP units intramuscularly, and this was repeated 2 months later with 50,000 IU, also intramuscularly.

Three months later an eye exam showed the surfaces of the eyes to be normal. This was a case of vitamin A deficiency with secondary xerophthalmia (dry eyes), which is uncommon in developed countries, the researchers said.

As reported in the American Journal of Clinical Nutrition, 133 children, 6 to 13 years of age, with marginal plasma retinol concentrations, were randomly assigned and supplemented with either zinc at 25 mg/day, vitamin A at 1,500 retinol equivalents per day; zinc plus vitamin A; or placebo for 6 months.[40]

Zinc supplementation resulted in imporvement in vision restoration in dim light. Vitamin A and zinc synergistically normalized conjunctival epithelium, as measured by conjunctival impression cytology.

It was found that both vision restoration time and conjunctival impression cytology showed significant correlations with plasma zinc and vitamin A, respectively. Cytology studies the chemistry of a cell.

This data suggests that functional improvements of populations with suboptimal vitamin A and zinc nutriture can be achieved by supplementation with less than 2 times the RDA of the 2 nutrients, the researchers added.

A study in the British Medical Journal evaluated 256 children receiving retinyl palmitate at a dose of 200,000 IU, and 254 children who were given beta-carotene at a dose of 1.2 million IU for vitamin A deficiency documented by abnormal eye cytology.[41]

Seven weeks after supplementation, 51.2% of the children given vitamin A and 50% of those taking beta-carotene had recovered to normal eye cytology.

These treatments were statistically significant, and C. Cartier, M.D., and colleagues, conclude that beta-carotene supplementation is a promising modality to reduce vitamin A deficiency. It can be given either as a high-dose capsule or through increased dietary intake.

Indonesian children with a history of diarrhea or respiratory disease were more likely than those without to develop xerophthalmia within the next 3 months, which may be due to decreased intestinal absorption, reported Suzanne M. Filteau and Andrew Tomkins, of the Institute of Child Health in London, United Kingdom, in the Royal Society of Tropical Medicine and Hygiene.[42]

It was also reported that serum retinol normalizes as malaria parasites are removed. Vitamin A supplements can reduce mortality rates even in populations with a low prevalence of xerophthalmia.

In addition, vitamin A appears to have a greater and more consistent beneficial effect on mortality from diarrhea than from respiratory disease. The World Health Organization has recommended large doses of vitamin A for all children with measles in areas where vitamin A deficiency is recognized as a public health problem, or where the measles can cause fatality of more than 1%, the researchers said.

At the Wilmer Eye Institute in Baltimore, Maryland, a research team conducted a double-blind trial in rural Nepal to evaluate the side effects of high-dose vitamin A in neonates and infants, reported the Bulletin of the World Health Organization.[43]

The dosages used were vitamin A at 15,000 RE (50,000 IU), and 30,000 RE (100,000 IU), or 75 RE (250 IU); and 150 RE (500 IU). There were 1,461 children in the vitamin A group and 1,370 controls.

The researchers reported that neonates exhibited no excess risk of adverse side effects after receiving 15,000 RE. Compared with controls, the older infants who ingested 30,000 RE had a 1.6 excess rate of vomiting, and a 0.5 excess rate in the occurrence of bulging fontanelles (one of several membranous intervals at the angles of the cranial bones in infants).

The researchers said that the control distribution of a single

15,000 RE dose of vitamin A has no apparent risk in young infants. A 30,000 RE dose is associated with a minimum risk of transient acute side effects.

As reported in The Lancet, blood levels of vitamin A were compared to physiological, nocturnal (during darkness), and stimulated growth hormone secretion in 68 short, prepubertal children. Fasting plasma vitamin A correlated with nocturnal growth hormone secretion, but not the stimulating growth hormone secretion, according to Daniele Evain-Briton, M.D., and colleagues, of Infantile Hopital Robert Debre in Paris, France.[44]

It was found that total dietary vitamin A intake was lower in children with abnormal nocturnal growth hormone secretion than the intake in the normal children, and the endocrinologically-normal short children.

In 9 of 12 children who were supplemented with 3,000 mcg/day of vitamin A for 3 months, normal growth hormone secretion increased. It appears that vitamin A is involved in the regulation of nocturnal growth hormone secretion, Evain-Briton said.

The researchers added that a preliminary study of short children with impaired nocturnal growth hormone secretion showed that vitamin A supplementation may, in part, restore nocturnal growth hormone secretion.

At the Aga Khan University Medical Center in Karachi, Pakistan, a research team evaluated vitamin A status in 532 children, ranging in age from 6 to 60 months, who lived in the slums of Karachi. The mean vitamin A intake estimated from food questionnaires was inadequate, according to Ayesha Molla in the American Journal of Tropical Medicine and Hygiene.[45]

Serum retinol levels were deficient in 12 children, and low levels of retinol between 10 and 19 mcg/dl were seen in 46%, while 51% had adequate levels greater than 20 mcg/dl.

The data revealed that a significant number of children in these communities are low in vitamin A, and they may be at high risk for blindness and infection, Molla added.

In evaluating the eyes of 22,335 children who were between 7 and 71 months of age, from 100 sites in Bangladesh, after 6-month of massive dosing of preschool-aged children with oral vitamin A at 200,000 IU of retinyl palmitate, and 40 IU of vitamin E, almost half of the rural target population, and less than 20% of the urban slum population, were being tested, reported the American Journal of Clinical Nutrition.[46]

Risk of night blindness was cut in half for children who were given the high dose of vitamin A.

Risk of corneal ulcers or keratomalacia was 2.7 times higher in children not given the vitamin. The researchers added that the efficacy of protection against potentially blinding corneal lesions was 63%. Keratomalacia is dryness with ulceration and perforation of the cornea.

The authors recommend that massive dosing with vitamin A should be given at less than 6-month intervals in combination with other nutrition and health approaches.

Researchers at the University of Bergen in Norway, evaluated 105 children from Bangladesh, who were said to have night blindness, and compared them with matched controls. The mean blood levels of vitamin A were lowest among children identified as night blind, and highest among those who were not affected, reported the Bulletin of the World Health Organization.[47]

Using a luxometer, in addition to parent histories for night blindness, increased the sensitivity of diagnosis. Therefore, blood levels of vitamin A should be identified, the researchers added.

In 86 children who were between 0.9 and 20 years of age with solid tumors—neuroblastoma, germinal tumors, and osteocarcinoma—it was found that vitamin A, selenium, and vitamin E concentrations were much lower in newly diagnosed tumor patients than in healthy controls, or in tumor-free patients who had recovered.[48]

As reported in the New England Journal of Medicine, a randomized controlled trial for 1 year in Southern India involved 15,419 preschool-aged children, who were given 8,333 IU of vitamin A, 20 mg of vitamin E, or vitamin E alone, in a weekly dosage.[49]

The vitamin A group had less than half the risk of death as compared to the controls. The benefit was most apparent under the age of 3, and among those who had stunted growth suggestive of chronic undernutrition.

Vitamin A supplementation contributed substantially to these children's survival in these deficient areas, according to Barbara A. Underwood, Ph.D., of the National Eye Institute in Bethesda, Maryland.

In all, vitamin A supplementation reduced mortality by 54%. Weekly supplementation at lower doses aided in monitoring and avoidance of potential overdose.

Impression cytology of the conjunctiva is a very highly sensitive way of detecting vitamin A deficiency early in the preclinical stage, according to a research team at the Postgraduate Institute of Medical Education and Research in Chandigarh, India.[50]

This procedure is noninvasive and does not require sophisticated equipment.

In the study, 26 of 37 children with diarrhea greater than 14 days were found to have abnormal cytology suggestive of a vitamin A deficiency. Controls had no abnormal impression cytology (study of the anatomy).

The children were given 100,000 IU of vitamin A in a single dose, and then reassessed weeks to several months later. It was found there was a remarkable increase in mucous glycoprotein-goblet cells in the conjunctiva (the mucous membrane in the anterior surface of the eyeball and the posterior surface of the lids).

There were no ill effects from the therapy, and the article suggests that vitamin A deficiency is often present in persistent diarrhea. This has special significance for children in developing countries with persistent diarrhea, the researchers added.

As reported in the American Journal of Epidemiology, over 1,700 children, between the ages of 1 and 8 in Thailand, were evaluated for the role of mild vitamin A deficiency and the occurrence of diarrhea and respiratory disease.[51]

Children with a history of these conditions had lower blood levels of retinol and retinol-binding protein. Deficient serum retinol was associated with a 4-fold risk of respiratory distress.

In 166 children, 1 through 5, who were given oral doses of 200,000 IU of vitamin A and 40 IU of vitamin E, it was found that after 2 months the control group—which did not receive the vitamins—had a 2.9 times higher incidence of respiratory disease, and 3.1 times the incidence of diarrhea.

The study supports a greater risk of respiratory disease and diarrhea with mild vitamin A deficiency, and that supplementation reduces the incidence of both diarrhea and respiratory disease for at least 2 months.

The authors noted the association between vitamin A deficiency and infectious diseases, and suggests that this data requires us to pay attention to mild vitamin A deficiency.

Mild vitamin A deficiency leads to patchy keratinization of the epithelial linings of the respiratory, genitourinary, and gastrointestinal tracts, which are the first barriers of the protection mechanism against infection, the researchers said.

In spite of effective and inexpensive treatment, diarrhea claims the lives of about 1.5 million children younger than 5 years annually, reported Joan Stephenson, Ph.D., in the November 18, 2009 issue of the Journal of the American Medical Association.[52]

The report was released in October 2009 by the United Nations Children's Fund and the World Health Organization.

It is estimated that only 39% of children with diarrhea in developing countries currently receive the recommended treatment of fluid replacement using low-osmolarity oral dehydration salts and zinc supplements.

The report describes a 7-point plan that, in addition to the just-named strategies, recommends 5 preventive strategies to reduce diarrhea-related deaths:

1. Immunization for rotavirus and measles. A rotavirus is a reovirus that has a double-layered capsid (outer protein shell) and causes diarrhea.
2. Promotion of early and exclusive breastfeeding and vitamin A supplementation.
3. Promotion of hand washing with soap.
4. Improvement of water quality and quantity.

5. Promotion of community-wide sanitation.

The ingestion of a sufficient amount of vitamin A is a persistent challenge for populations subsisting on a largely plant-based diet, according to Judy D. Ribaya-Mercado, and colleagues at the Jean Mayer-US Department of Agriculture Human Nutrition Research Center at Tufts University in Boston, Massachusetts. Hypovitaminosis A is endemic primarily in societies that rely on provitamin A carotenoids (carrots, spinach, etc.) as the source of dietary vitamin A.[53]

Nicaragua instituted a national program of vitamin A fortification of its domestic sugar supply beginning with the 1999-2000 sugarcane harvest. The vitamin A status of Nicaraguan schoolchildren improved during the year after the initial distribution of vitamin A-fortified sugar in Nicaragua.

Reporting in the American Journal of Clinical Nutrition, Laura E. Caulfield, and colleagues at Johns Hopkins University in Baltimore, Maryland, said that their findings underscore the need to make the improvement of the nutritional status of children a priority.[54]

"In addition to reducing growth faltering, investments in child nutrition programs would support and complement disease-specific prevention and control programs in developing countries," they said. "In round numbers, this means that 1 million pneumonia deaths, 800,000 diarrhea deaths, 500,000 malaria deaths, and 250,000 measles deaths could be prevented by eradication of child undernutrition."

They added that, although the potential for nutrition programs to reduce diarrhea morbidity and mortality was previously recognized, the result that a large proportion of child deaths as a result of malaria could be prevented by child nutrition interventions is noteworthy.

"Zinc supplementation in populations that have a moderately high prevalence of zinc deficiency has had similar effects on reducing infectious disease morbidity in children who were classified to be undernourished or not, and vitamin A supplementation reduces mortality in vitamin A-deficient populations regardless of athropometric status," they continued. The latter word refers to the branch of science concerned with the physical, social, and cultural relationships of humans.

References

1. Surles, Rebecca L., et al. "One-Time Graded Doses of Vitamin A to Weaning Piglets Enhance Hepatic Retinol But Do Not Always Prevent Vitamin A Deficiency," American Journal of Clinical Nutrition 86: 1045-1053, 2007.
2. World Health Organization. "Immunizations, Vaccines, and Biologicals. Vitamin A Supplementation. Updated May 2003.
3. Ross, D.A. "Recommendations for Vitamin A Supplementation," Journal of Nutrition 131: 2902S-2906S, 2002.
4. Wieringa, F.T., et al. "Redistribution of Vitamin A After Iron Supplementation for Indonesian Infants," American Journal of Clinical Nutrition 77:651-657, 2003.
5. Bahl, R., et al. "WHO/CHD Immunization-Linked Vitamin A Group. Vitamin A supplementation of Women Postpartum and of Their Infants As Immunization Alters Breast Milk Retinol and Infant Vitamin A Status," Journal of Nutrition 132:3243-3248, 2002.
6. Rahman, M.M., et al. "Administration of 25,000 IU Vitamin A Doses of Routine Immunization in Young Infants," European Journal of Clinical Nutrition 49: 439-445, 1995.
7. Sommer, A, and Davidson, P.R. "Assessment and Control of Vitamin A Deficiency: The Annency Accords," Journal of Nutrition 132: 2845S-2850S, 2002.
8. Labadarios, D. "Vitamin A—Time of Action," South African Medical Journal 84: 1-2, January 1994.
9. Feinstein, Alice, editor. Prevention's Healing with Vitamins. Emmaus, PA: Rodale Press, Inc., 1996, pp. 322-323.
10. Zimmerman, Michael B., et al. "Vitamin A Supplementation in Iodine-Deficient African Children Decreases Thyrotropin Stimulation of the Thyroid and Reduces the Goiter Rate," American Journal of Clinical Nutrition 86: 1040-1044, 2007.
11. Hadi, H., et al. "Vitamin A Supplementation Selectively Improves the Linear Growth of Indonesian Preschool Children: Results from a Randomized Controlled Trial," American Journal of Clinical Nutrition 71: 507-513, 2000.
12. Diness, Birgitte R., et al. "Effect of High-Dose Vitamin A Supplementation on the Immune Response to Bacille Calmette Guerin Vaccine," American Journal of Clinical Nutrition 86: 1152-1159, 2007.
13. Becker, Katja, et al. "Antioxidant Vitamins in Malnourished Nigerian Children," International Journal for Vitamin and Nutrition Research 4:306-310, 1994.

14. Glaszion, P., et al. "Vitamin A Supplementation in Infectious Disease: A Meta-Analysis," British Medical Journal 306: 366-370, 1993.

15. Kucukbay, H., et al. "Serum Vitamin A and Beta-Carotene Levels in Children with Recurrent Acute Respiratory Infections and Diarrhea in Malaya" Journal of Tropical Pediatrics 43: 337-340, December 1997.

16. Fawzi, Wafaie W., et al. "Dietary Vitamin A Intake and the Risk of Diarrhea and Respiratory Infection Among Sudanese Children," Journal of Nutrition 125: 1211-1221, 1995.

17. Pinnock, C.B., et al. "Vitamin A Status in Children Who are Prone to Respiratory Tract Infections," Australian Pediatric Journal 22: 95-99, 1986.

18. Nesheim, M.C. "Human Nutrition Needs and Parasitic Infections," Parasitology 107: S7-S18, 1993.

19. Robbins, Sandra T., R.D., and Fletcher, Anne B., M.D. "Early Versus Delayed Vitamin A Supplementation in Very-Low-Birth-Weight Infants," Journal of Parenteral and Enteral Nutrition 17(3): 220-225, May-June 1993.

20. Underwood, Barbara A. "Editorial: The Timing of High-Dose Vitamin A Supplementation in Children," American Journal of Public Health 85(9): 1200-1201, September 1995.

21. Semba, Richard D., M.D., et al. "Depressed Immune Responses to Tetanus in Children with Vitamin A Deficiency," Journal of Nutrition 122: 101-107, 1992.

22. Shenai, Jayant P., M.D., et al. "Vitamin A Supplementation and Bronchopulmonary Dysplasia Revisited," Journal of Pediatrics 121(3): 399-401, September 1992.

23. Fukul, Yuichi, M.D., "Vitamin A Status in Biliary Atresia: Intestinal Absorption and Liver Storage of Retinol," Journal of Pediatric Surgery 28(11): 1502-1504, November 1993.

24. Porcelli, Peter J., M.D., et al. "Retinol (Vitamin A) and Riboflavin (Vitamin B2) Administration and Metabolism in Very Low Birth Weight Infants," Seminars in Pediatrics 16(3): 170-180, June 1992.

25. Inder, T.E., et al. "Vitamin A and E Status in Very Low Birth Weight Infants: Development of an Improved Parenteral Delivery System," Journal of Pediatrics 126: 128-131, 1995.

26. Shenai, Jayant P., M.D. "Does Vitamin A Reduce the Risk of Bronchopulmonary Dysplasia in Infants," Journal of Respiratory Diseases 14(18): 895-900, August 1993.

27. Tyson, J.E. "Vitamin A Supplementation for Extremely Low-Birth-

Weight Infants," New England Journal of Medicine 340(25): 1962-1968, 1999.

28. Humphrey, Jean H., Sc.D., et al. "Impact of Neonatal Vitamin A Supplementation on Infant Morbidity and Mortality," Journal of Pediatrics 128 :489-496, April 1996.
29. Ozsoylu, Sinasi, M.D. "Vitamin A for Varicella," Journal of Pediatrics 125(6): Part I: 1017-1018, December 1994.
30. Semba, Richard D., M.D., et al. "Effect of Vitamin A Supplementation of Immunoglobulin Subclass Response to Tetanus Toxoid in Children," Clinical and Diagnostic Laboratory Immunology 1(2): 172-175, March 1994.
31. Mastroiacovo, P., et al. "High Vitamin A Intake and Early Pregnancy in Major Malformations: A Multicenter Prospective Controlled Trial," Teratology 59: 7-11, 1999.
32. Czeizel, Andrew E., M.D., and Rockenbauer, M. "Prevention of Congenital Abnormalities by Vitamin A," International Journal of Vitamin and Nutrition Research 68: 219-231, 1998.
33. Filteau, Suzanne M., et al. "Vitamin A Supplementation: Morbidity and Serum Acute-Phase Proteins in Young Ghanian Children," American Journal of Clinical Nutrition 62: 434-438, 1995.
34. Clark, Joseph H., M.D., et al. "Symptomatic Vitamin A and D Deficiencies in an Eight-Year-Old with Autism" Journal of Parenteral and Enteral Nutrition 17(3): 284-286, May-June 1993.
35. Vidro, E., et al. "Insulin-Dependent Diabetes Mellitus and Vitamin A Metabolism," Journal of Clinical Biochemistry and Nutrition 26(2): 155-160, 1999.
36. Donnen, P., et al. "Randomized, Placebo-Controlled Clinical Trial of the Effect of a Single High Dose or Daily Dose of Vitamin A on the Morbidity of Hospitalized, Malnourished Children," American Journal of Clinical Nutrition 68: 1254-1260, 1998.
37. Salazar-Lindo, Eduardo, et al. "Association of Diarrhea and Low Serum Retinol in Peruvian Children," American Journal of Clinical Nutrition 58: 110-113, 1993.
38. Barreto, Mauricio L., M.D., et al. "Effect of Vitamin A Supplementation on Diarrhea in Acute Lower-Respiratory-Tract Infections in Young Children in Brazil," The Lancet 344: 228-231, July 23, 1994.
39. Steinemann, Thomas L., M.D., and Christiansen, Stephen P., M.D.

"Vitamin A Deficiency and Xerophthalmia in an Autistic Child," Archives of Ophthalmology 116: 392-393, March 1998.

40. Udomkesmalee, Emorn, et al. "Effect of Vitamin A and Zinc Supplementation on Nutriture of Children in Northeast Thailand," American Journal of Clinical Nutrition 56:50-57, 1992.

41. Cartier, C., M.D., et al. "A Randomized Controlled Trial to Test Equivalence Between Retinyl Palmitate and Beta-Carotene for Vitamin A Deficiency," British Medical Journal 307: 1106-1110, 1993.

42. Filteau, Suzanne M., and Tomkins, Andrew. "Micronutrients and Tropical Infections," Transactions of the Royal Society of Tropical Medicine and Hygiene 88: 1-3, 26, 1994.

43. West, K.P., Jr., et al. "The Tolerance of Young Infants to a Single, Large Dose of Vitamin A: A Randomized Community Trial in Nepal," Bulletin of the World Health Organization 70(6): 733-739, 1992.

44. Evain-Briton, Daniele, M.D., et al. "Vitamin A Deficiency in Nocturnal Growth Hormone Secretion in Short Children," The Lancet 343: 87-88, January 8, 1994.

45. Molla, Ayesha, et al. "Vitamin A Status in Children in Urban Slums of Karachi, Pakistan, Assessed by Clinical, Dietary and Biochemical Methods," American Journal of Tropical Medicine and Hygiene 48(1): 89-96, 1991.

46. Cohen, N., et al. "Impact of Massive Doses of Vitamin A on Nutritional Blindness in Bangladesh," American Journal of Clinical Nutrition 45(5): 970-976, 1987.

47. Hussein, A., et al. "Diagnosis of Night Blindness and Serum Vitamin A Levels: A Population-Based Study," Bulletin of the World Health Organization 73(4): 469-476, 1995.

48. Cser, M.A., et al. "Selenium, Lipid, Vitamin A and Vitamin E State in Children Suffering from Solid Tumors," Met. Ions. Bind. Med. 5: 597-602, 1998.

49. Rabmathullah, Laxmi, M.D., et al. "Reduced Mortality Among Children in Southern India Receiving a Small Weekly Dose of Vitamin A," New England Journal of Medicine 323(14): 929-935, 1990.

50. Usha, W., et al. "Early Detection of Vitamin A Deficiency in Children with Persistent Diarrhea," The Lancet 335:422, February 17, 1990.

51. Bloom, Martin W., et al. "Mild Vitamin A Deficiency and Risk of Respiratory Tract Disease and Diarrhea in Preschool and School Children in Northeastern Thailand," American Journal of Epidemiology 131(2): 332-339, 1990.

52. Stephenson, Joan, Ph.D. "Diarrhea Deaths in Children," JAMA 302(19): 2083, 2009.
53. Ribaya-Mercado, Judy D., et al. "Use of Deuterated Retinol-Dilution Technique to Monitor the Vitamin A Status of Nicaraguan Schoolchildren One Year After Initiation of the Nicaraguan National Program of Sugar Fortification with Vitamin A," American Journal of Clinical Nutrition 80: 1291-1298, 2004.
54. Caulfield, Laura E., et al. "Undernutrition As An Underlying Cause of Child Deaths Associated with Diarrhea, Pneumonia, Malaria, and Measles," American Journal of Clinical Nutrition 80: 193-198, 2004.

8

VITAMIN A AND THE ELDERLY

Aging is associated with higher levels of oxidative stress, which are likely to play an important role in the development of cardiovascular disease, and cancer, reported Brian Buijsse, and colleagues, at the National Institute for Public Health and Environment in Bilthoven, Netherlands.[1, 2, 3, 4, 5]

Oxidative stress is lower among those with a high antioxidant status. Therefore, elderly people with a high antioxidant status may have a lower risk of these chronic diseases, the researchers said.

In the study, blood levels of carotene and vitamin E (alpha-tocopherol) were measured in 1,168 elderly men and women. Following a follow-up of 10 years, 388 of the volunteers had died.

Plasma carotene concentrations were associated with a lower mortality risk for an increment of 0.39 micromol/l. This lower mortality risk was observed for both cancer and cardiovascular disease.

The lower risk of cardiovascular death was confirmed in those with a body mass index of less than 25. However, plasma concentrations of vitamin E were not associated with all-cause or cause-specific mortality.

"This prospective study suggests that high plasma concentrations of carotene are associated with lower-mortality from all causes, and with cancer in the elderly," the researchers added. "For cardiovascular mortality, the inverse association was confined to elderly with a body mass index less than 25. (Those with a body mass index above 27 are considered dangerously overweight).

Dementia of the Alzheimer's type and Parkinson's disease are characterized by a transmitter-specific loss of neurons, which progress to several neuronal systems over the course of the illness, explained P. Riederer, M.D., and colleagues at a psychiatric clinic in Warburg, Germany.[6]

Oxidative stress has been proposed as a means of neurodegeneration in these dementias, and there is evidence of increased free radical oxygen activity and impaired defenses in dementia of the Alzheimer's type.

Several antioxidant vitamins—including vitamins A, C, and E—may have beneficial free-radical scavenging mechanisms for dementia of the Alzheimer's type, the researchers added. And the effects of selegiline, an MAO-B inhibitor, has shown a slowing of the progression of Parkinson's disease, which has also been used in dementia of the Alzheimer's type.

The researchers said that pharmacologic drugs/supplements—desferrioxamine, alphalipoic acid, Ginkgo biloba, etc.—showing effects on oxygen free radical mediated mechanisms, also have other pharmacologic properties which might be beneficial in the treatment of dementia of the Alzheimer's type.

With aging, there may be a reduction in the absorption of vitamins A, B1 (thiamine), folic acid, and B12, and reduced exposure to sunlight may be associated with low vitamin D levels. Reduced food intake in the elderly may also be further compromised by drugs that impair appetite and absorption, reported the International Journal of Vitamin and Nutrition Research.[7]

Anticonvulsant drugs and medications that impair appetite and absorption induce hepatic (liver) microsomal enzyme activity, accelerate vitamin D metabolism, and can aggravate postmenopausal bone loss. Acid inhibiting agents increase achlorhydria and reduce vitamin B12 absorption.

High doses of vitamin C can reduce renal (kidney) clearance of acidic drugs, such as acetylsalicylic acid and barbituric acid, while vitamin B6 reduces the therapeutic benefit of L-dopa.

As reported in Aging Clinical and Experimental Research, J. Haller, M.D., reviewed the role of vitamins in reducing disability and improving the quality of life in the elderly. People over 65 account for almost 29% of personal health expenditures.[8]

A number of intervention studies of the elderly have included giving antioxidant mixtures containing beta-carotene, vitamins C, E, and the B Complex of vitamins.

Various studies have shown that antioxidant vitamins with or without selenium and/or other vitamins and minerals can improve age-associated memory impairment or various aspects of dementia.

In one study, the Hamilton Depression Scale score was shown to be inversely related with vitamin B6 plasma levels. Carotene, vitamin B2, and hematocrit were negatively associated with the score.

However, the more severe the depression, the lower was the vitamin status. The Mini-Mental Total Score was positively correlated with vitamin C plasma levels, suggesting the higher the cognitive score, the higher the plasma vitamin C levels. The worse the Activity of Daily Living Score, the lower the carotene and vitamin B12 status.

There was also a large number of inverse associations between the Sandos Clinical Assessment Geriatric Scale and vitamin A, vitamins B1, B2, C and folic acid.

Supplementing the diet with antioxidants improves cell mediated immunity in the elderly institutionalized patients, reported N. Penn, M.D., and colleagues, in Age and Ageing.[9]

Volunteers were divided into either dietary supplement or placebo groups. The supplemented seniors were given 100 mg/day of vitamin C; 8,000 IU/day of vitamin A; and 50 mg/day of vitamin E. Nutritional status and immunocompetence were evaluated before the study began, and after the 28-day study.

The research team reported that those who supplemented their diets with antioxidant nutrients had improved cell-mediated immune function, including an increase in the number of T-cells, T4 subsets, T4 and T8 ratios, and the proliferation of lymphocytes. There were no significant changes in the controls.

The researchers concluded that supplementing the diets of elderly patients with vitamins A, C, and E, might improve immune response, perhaps by stabilizing cell membranes and preventing free-radical damage to immunological tissues and cells.

Almost 80 to 90% of bone mineral content is comprised of calcium and phosphorus, with other components including protein, magnesium, zinc, copper, iron, fluoride, and vitamins A, C, D, and E, reported the Journal of the American College of Nutrition.[10]

With the increasing elderly population, osteoporotic fractures are expected to reach epidemic proportions, according to Jasminka Z. Ilich, Ph.D., and colleagues.

Although nutrition inadequacy represents a potential health threat to the entire elderly population, the risk of poor nutrition is greater among some subgroups of community-dwelling older adults, according to researchers at the University of North Carolina at Chapel Hill, and Duke University at Durham.[11, 12]

"These include women, minorities, those with limited income and education, and those who are homebound," the researchers said. "Previous studies showed an increased interest in the nutritional status of the elderly, but few researchers targeted the increasing homebound elderly populations for study."

They added that, for the rapidly growing elderly population, the achievement and maintenance of good nutritional status are critical to health, functioning, and quality of life.

After adjusting for various variables, women had significantly lower intakes of total energy, protein, phosphorus, B1, B2, B3, selenium, iron, and vitamin A. A less than adequate intake of calcium was reported by 96% of the patients, and of vitamin D by 99% of the subjects.

For vitamin A, 33.3% of the men consumed low levels of the vitamin, as did 36.9% of the women.

In evaluating 228 institutionalized elderly, 61 to 101 years of age, 98% showed beta-carotene levels less than acceptable in that 85.2% were deficient; 12.9% were at medium risk; and only 1.85% had acceptable levels, according to Ismael Lares-Asseff of the National Institute of Sciences and Technology in Colonia Insurgentes Cuicuiloco, C.P., Mexico.[13]

However, it was reported that 92% had acceptable levels of retinol.

The antioxidant capacity of plasma may be an important factor in preventing various diseases, according to the Journal of Nutrition.[14]

In the study, the authors investigated the antioxidant effect of dietary beta-carotene supplementation on the peroxidation potential of plasma in a randomized, double-blind study.

The researchers supplemented the diets of 12 healthy women, 62 to 80 years of age, with 90 mg/day of beta-carotene or placebo capsules for 3 weeks. The research team measured blood concentrations of beta-carotene, vitamin E, vitamin C, urate, bilirubin, and in vitro production of phosphatidylcholine (PC) hydroperoxides and other parameters before and after supplementation. Bilirubin is a yellow pigment in bile and blood, which causes jaundice if in excessive amounts.

The research team reported that plasma beta-carotene increased in the supplemented but not in the placebo-treated women, with no significant changes in the plasma concentrations of other antioxidants in either group.

During the study, it was found that plasma vitamin C concentrations were depleted first, followed by loss of bilirubin and vitamin E, and then by the sequential loss of vitamin E, urate, and beta-carotene.

The authors concluded that beta-carotene supplementation increases the plasma antioxidant capacity in older women.

Many elderly adults are afflicted with age-related chronic disease, which significantly diminishes quality of life, reported Regan L. Bailey, et al, of the National Institutes of Health in Bethesda, Maryland, and colleagues at Pennsylvania State University in University Park.[15, 16]

However, they added, poor health is not necessarily an inevitable consequence of aging. High-quality diets are associated with reduced risk of major chronic diseases, and are associated inversely with mortality.

"Thus, early detection of those with compromised dietary intakes may be an effective strategy to prevent nutritional risk and to lessen the burden of chronic disease within the older segment of the population," they said. "Proactive screening of older adults in the community is an effective public health strategy for targeting individuals who could make dietary improvements for primary or secondary prevention of disease, and thus reduce medical expenditures."

In their study, they found dietary intakes of vitamin A, vitamin E, and vitamin B12 were significantly lower in the at-risk group when compared with the not at-risk individuals. Dietary intakes of vitamin B6, folic acid, and zinc were lower in the at-risk group compared with both the possible-risk and not-at-risk groups.

They also found that dietary intakes of vitamin K, vitamin C, calcium, magnesium, and potassium were significantly different among all 3 risk groups with the at-risk groups at the lowest intakes of these nutrients. The at-risk subjects also had the lowest Mean Adequacy Ratio (MAR).

"Many of the diseases common in aging, including obesity, diabetes, cancer, and heart disease, are influenced by diet," the researchers continued. "However, dietary assessment in the clinical treatment of older adults is not a routine practice. Older adults are vulnerable to nutritional risk, therefore, effective and evidence-based screening strategies are essential to help combat age-related chronic disease, and reverse declines in the quality of life associated with nutritional risk."

They added that the clinical setting provides an ideal environment for dietary screening of older adults. Their study shows that the dietary screening tool (DST) is a practical and effective tool for dietary screening of older adults in a clinical setting.

No rapid methods currently exist to screen the overall dietary intakes of older adults. However, the researchers reported on a dietary screening tool that is capable of characterizing the overall dietary patterns of older adults.

Two dietary patterns were devised, in which one pattern was represented by more healthful foods, including fruit, vegetables, and lean proteins, and the other pattern was represented by less optimal food choices such as sweets, processed meats, and salty snacks.

References

1. Buijsse, Brian, et al. "Plasma Carotene and Alpha-Tocopherol in Relation to 10-Year All-Cause and Cause-Specific Mortality in European Elderly: The Survey in Europe on Nutrition and the Elderly, a Concerted Action (SENECA)," American Journal of Clinical Nutrition 82: 879-886, 2005.
2. Finkel, T., et al. "Oxidants, Oxidative Stress and the Biology of Aging," Nature 408: 239-247, 2000.
3. Griendling, K.A., et al. "Oxidative Stress and Cardiovascular Disease," Circulation 96: 3264-3265, 1997.
4. Klaunig, J.E., et al. "The Role of Oxidative Stress in Carcinogenesis," Ann, Rev. Pharmacol. Toxicol. 44: 239-267, 2004.
5. Block, G., et al. 'Factors Associated with Oxidative Stress in Human Populations," American Journal of Epidemiology 156:274-285, 2002.
6. Frolich, L., and Riederer, P. "Free Radical Mechanisms in Dementia of the Alzheimer's Type and the Potential for Antioxidative Treatment," Drug Research 45(1): 443-446, 1995.
7. Schumann, K. "Interactions Between Drugs and Vitamins at Advanced Age," International Journal of Vitamin and Nutrition Research 69(3): 173-178, 1999.
8. Haller, J., M.D. "Vitamins for the Elderly: Reducing Disability and Improving Quality of Life," Aging Clinical and Experimental Research 5(Supp. 1): 65-70, 1993.
9. Penn, N., M.D., et al. "The Effect of Dietary Supplementation with Vitamins A, C, and E on Cell-Mediated Immune Function in Elderly Long-Stay Patients: A Randomized Controlled Trial," Age and Ageing 20: 169-174, 1991.
10. Xlich, Jasminka Z., Ph.D., et al. "Nutrition in Bone Health Revisited: A Story Beyond Calcium," Journal of the American College of Nutrition 19(6): 715-737, 2000.
11. Sharkey, Joseph R., et al. "Inadequate Nutrient Intakes Among Homebound Elderly and Their Correlation with Individual Characteristics and Health-Related Factors," American Journal of Clinical Nutrition 76: 1435-1445, 2002.
12. Institute of Medicine. "The Role of Nutrition in Maintaining Health in the Nation's Elderly." Washington, DC: National Academy Press, 2000.
13. Lares-Asseff, Ismael, et al. "Nutritional State of Beta-Carotene and Retinol in Institutionalized Elderly Individuals in Mexico City," International Journal of Vitamin and Nutrition Research 65: 236-240, 1995.

14. Meydani, M., et al. "Beta-Carotene Supplementation Increases Antioxidant Capacity of Plasma in Older Women," Journal of Nutrition 124(12): 2397-2403, 1994.

15. Bailey, Regan L., et al. "Dietary Screening Tool Identifies Nutritional Risk in Older Adults," American Journal of Clinical Nutrition 90: 177-183, 2008.

16. Caskins, N.D., M.D., et al. "Poor Nutritional Habits: A Modifiable Predecessor of Chronic Illness? A North Carolina Family Medicine Research Network Study," Journal of the American Board of Family Medicine 20: 124-134, 2007.

9

EYE PROBLEMS

The eye is one of the most important organs of the body, since a large portion of our information is acquired through vision. The remainder is provided by such senses as hearing, smelling, tasting, and touching, reported The Book of Health.[1]

The eye is frequently compared to an extremely delicate camera, the publication continued. Like a camera, the eye contains a lens which focuses light on a light-sensitive area, the retina, which is analogous to the film in the camera.

"The working parts of the eye are the lens, which focuses the picture, the retina which receives it, and the optic nerve which transmits an impression of the picture to the brain," the publication continued.

The eye is located in a socket formed by the bones of the head, thereby protecting it from heavy blows. It rests on a soft pad of fatty tissue which further minimizes damage.

The eye is equipped with a lid, a thin flap of skin which completely covers and protects the organ. The lashes and brows help to filter dust particles and microorganisms from the air, as well as help to screen out perspiration.

"The conjunctiva is a membrane which covers the inner side of the lid and folds back onto the front of the eyeball," the publication added. "Near the upper and lateral folds of the conjunctiva, there are many small glands (accessory lacrimal glands), which secrete tears. They are spread over the surface of the conjunctiva to lubricate and protect it.

The eyeball is protected by its tough outer layer, the sclera, a completely opaque layer, except in the transparent central region which is called the cornea. The conjunctiva and sclera protect the eye from dust, invading bacteria, and foreign matter.

The eye is subject to a variety of disorders, such as:

1. Conjunctivitis is the general term given to any inflammation or infection of the conjunctiva.
2. Hordeolum (sty) is a common infection of one or more of the glands of the eyelids, usually caused by staphyloccoci.
3. Dacryocytitis is an infection of the lacrimal sac.
4. Keratitis is an inflammation of the cornea caused by infection, trauma, or chemical irritation.
5. Cataract is a cloudy or opaque discoloration of the lens of the eye.
6. Glaucoma is an increase of pressure within the eyeball.
7. Strasbismus is best described as cross-eyes or well-eyes.
8. Blindness is caused by pressure on the optic nerve, caused by tumors, eye injuries, various eye diseases, etc.
9. Night blindness is caused by a vitamin A deficiency, in which the person has difficulty seeing at night.
10. Macular degeneration, which affects the central part of the retina.

Writing in Archives of Ophthalmology, Edward A. Maumenee, M.D., of Point Clear, Alabama, reviewed vitamin A's use and potential clinical benefits in ophthalmological disorders.[2]

Ancient Egyptians treated night blindness by administering the juice of compressed liver onto the surface of the eye. This may have been possible if the juice were applied frequently enough that the liver extract, which contained vitamin A, could have passed the nasolacrimal (nasal) duct and into the digestive system in sufficient amounts. It was also reported that cod liver oil could cure both night blindness and Bitot's conjunctival spots. These spots were named after Pierre A. Bitot (1822-1888), a French physician.

Egg yolk extract was found to contain fat-soluble material that was later isolated as vitamin A, Maumenee continued. In 1913, with animal experiments of diets devoid of meat, in which lard had been substituted as the sole source of fat, resulted in a nutritional deficiency that could be corrected with the addition of butter, egg yolks, and cod-liver oil.

In 1925, a vitamin A deficiency in rats led to keratinized cells in many tissues of the body, and, in 1953, mucous membranes from the noses of chicks would grow feathers when placed in a vitamin A-deficient culture. These cells in tissue culture would reconvert to "mucous membrane" with globlet cells and cilia when vitamin A was added.

Research at the National Cancer Institute has shown that retinoic acid can reverse the keratinization of the tracheal mucous membranes in vitamin A-deficient cultures, the author continued. Retinoic acid can also act directly on monoeoplastic cells to suppress the process of malignant transformation induced by chemical carcinogens, by radiation, or by transforming growth factors.

Etretinate, a retinoid used to treat psoriasis, has resulted in reduction in the degree of bronchial metaplasia in heavy smokers, and 13-CIS-retinoic acid (isotretinoin) was found to be effective in the treatment of 4 patients with reflective cutaneous T-cell lymphoma.

In 1930, the chemical structure of beta-carotene was determined, and, in 1931, the structure of vitamin A (retinol) was discovered. Vitamin A was purified in 1942 and eventually synthesized in 1946 and 1947. Approximately 1,000 to 1,500 analogs of vitamin A exist.

In children with a vitamin A deficiency, keratinized conjunctiva can be more rapidly transformed when all-trans retinoic acid was placed in 1 eye versus the placebo, even though these patients were receiving 100,000 to 200,000 IU of vitamin A systematically.

The isomer 13-cis-retinoia retinoic acid is very effective in the treatment of cystic acne and other diseases such as pustular psoriasis, Darier's disease, pityriasis rubra pilaris, lichen planus, and other keratinizing skin diseases. This isomer is associated with increased incidence of birth defects when given during pregnancy.

The author has used all-trans retinoic acid in the treatment of a boy with Stevens-Johnson syndrome, who had developed severe keratinization of the tarsal conjunctiva. Within 2 weeks the keratinization had disappeared along with his photophobia (fear of light). There are 2 other cases of keratinization in those with Stevens-Johnson syndrome improving within a few weeks, and have been sustained several years later.

Stevens-Johnson syndrome involves mucous membranes and large areas of the body. Albert M. Stevens (1884-1945), was an American physician, and Frank C. Johnson (1894-1934), was an American pediatrician.

A 74-year-old women with severe Sjögren's syndrome, who was wearing bandage contact lenses, and, despite using drops of saline every 15 minutes, was very uncomfortable. She had marked keratinization of the conjunctiva from drying. She was placed on all-trans retinoic acid, and, within a few weeks, she was able to remove her soft contact lens and use the drops only once or twice a day to moisten her eyes.

In a study of most Sjögren's disease patients from 10 different medial institutions, it was found that keratinization improved with the therapy of all-trans retinoic acid, but there was little influence on the formation of tears.

Sjögren's syndrome results in dryness of mucous membranes, purpuric spots on the face, parotid (salivary gland) enlargement, seen in menopausal women, rheumatoid arthritis, Raynaud's phenomenon, dental caries, and other disorders. Henrik C. Sjögren, a Swesish ophthalmologist, was born in 1899.

Night blindness : Although a complex problem, doctors now know that it can result from nutritional factors, genetics, uncorrected nearsightedness, or an eye disease such as cataracts, macular degeneration, or retinitis pigmentosa, according to Prevention's Healing with Vitamins. Anything that affects vitamin A metabolism, such as liver disease, intestinal surgery, malabsorption, or alcoholism, can also cause the problem.[3]

"On the retina are rods and cones that house 4 kinds of pigments, one of which binds to an eye-friendly form of vitamin A," explained Elias Reichel, M.D., of Tufts University School of Medicine in Boston, Massachusetts. "When you enter a sunny room and light enters the eye, the pigment transforms. Instantly, the vitamin A in your eye changes shape, and in the process, excites nerve endings to start transmitting chemical impulses to your brain to let it know what's going on—that you've entered a sunny room."

However, when you enter a dark room, the vitamin A changes shape again and helps your eyes realize that you've entered a dark room.

"But nothing is ever completely light or completely dark," Reichel added. "That's why you have over 130 million light - and dark-sensing eye structures that make the minute adjustments necessary to perceive light and dark. And they're all dependent on vitamin A to do their jobs."

While night blindness is rather rare, it can often be reversed within an hour with injections of vitamin A. Most people with night blindness have eyes that mobilize vitamin A so slowly that it takes time to adjust to the dark, such as driving at night or going into a darkened theater.

While vitamin A is effective in treatment for deficiency-induced night blindness, it may slow night blindness that is induced by several hereditary conditions, such as retinitis pigmentosa, Reichel continued.

"People with retinitis pigmentosa usually develop a loss of daytime side (peripheral) vision in young adulthood that progresses to tunnel vision and eventually to loss of vision in midlife," Reichel said. "Without treatment, most people with retinitis pigmentosa will have significantly reduced day vision between the ages of 50 and 80."

He added that a study of almost 600 people, 18 to 49, researchers at the Massachusetts Eye and Ear Infirmary in Boston reported that 15,000 IU of vitamin A in supplement form each day, added to the approximate 3,000 IU a day generally available in a well-balanced diet, could slow the progression of retinal degeneration that can cause night blindness as a result of retinitis pigmentosa.

The Boston study, headed by Eliot L. Berson, M.D., of the Harvard Medical School, found that those who had the lowest intakes of vitamin A had the most progression of retinal degeneration, while those who had intakes of 18,000 IU/day had the least retinal degeneration. The 18,000 IU came from both supplements and food.

In a study of children who were between 0 and $4\frac{1}{2}$ years of age in West Bengal, 200,000 IU of vitamin A every 4 months eliminated night blindness and prevented the development of new cases of Bitot's spot in a statistically significant number of children, reported the American Journal of Clinical Nutrition[4].

Bitot's spots, caused by a vitamin A deficiency, are small, lusterless, grayish-white deposits adjacent to the cornea in the area of the palpebral (eyelid) fissure of both eyes. They are named after Pierre A. Bitot (1822-1888), a French physician.

The significance of massive doses of vitamin A in 4-month intervels was confirmed in this village study.

Night blindness occurred in a patient 4 years after jejunoileal bypass, according to the International Journal of Obstetrics. Daily supplements of 30,000 IU of vitamin A normalized vitamin A levels and retinal-binding protein, and the patient's night blindness improved but the retinopathy remained. The jejunum is a portion of the small intestine. Jejunoileitis also involves the ileum, a third portion of the small intestine.[5]

As reported in the Journal of Nutrition, weekly supplementation with 7,000 mcg of retinol equivalents as preformed A or beta-carotene versus a placebo were given over a 3-year period to about 29,000 women of childbearing age, who were living in 171 wards, and who delivered 9,912 first pregnancies.[6]

Results revealed that vitamin A supplementation reduced the incidence of night blindness during pregnancy from 10.7% among controls to 6.7% in those who took vitamin A. Beta-carotene had less of an effect.

Among the women who took 95% of their vitamin A supplements during pregnancy, the incidence of night blindness was reduced by 67%.

The incidence of night blindness during the first 3 months postpartum was 11.3 in the controls, versus 4.3 in the vitamin A group, and 8.7 in the beta-carotene group.

In the second 3 months of postpartum, both vitamin A and beta-carotene reduced night blindness by about 50%.

Xerophthalmia (excessive dryness of the conjunctiva and cornea) in 75 patients with this disorder and 74 matched controls, the preschool children were randomized to 1 of 3 oral regimens of vitamins: Peanut oil only; 7,500 mcg retinol equivalent of vitamin A; or 60,000 mcg retinol equivalent; followed in all cases by 60,000 mcg retinol equivalent for 1 week.[7]

Results showed that xerophthalmic children reversed to biochemical deficiency after therapy ,than non-xerophthalic children. A small or large priming dose might extend the protection conferred by a 60,000-mcg retinol equivalent dose, supporting the use of repeated spaced doses of vitamin A for treating the disease.

The 60,000 mcg retinol equivalent prophylactic dose recommended by the World Health Organization need not be increased, the researchers reported in the Journal of Nutrition.

Xerophthalmia is caused by an insufficient supply of vitamin A in the eye, which causes conjunctival serosis, corneal serosis, corneal ulceration, and keratomalacia. Night blindness is a secondary sign of the disease.

It is estimated that 20,000 to 100,000 children in developing countries develop blindness due to xerophthalmia annually.[8]

The initial treatment is 100,000 IU of vitamin A intramuscularly, and 200,000 IU orally on the following day. This dose should be reduced by half for children less than 1 year of age.

Prior to discharge from the clinic, another dose of 200,000 IU of vitamin A should be given orally, and, for the children under 1 year of age, the recommended dosage is 100,000 IU, the researchers said.

As reported in Archives of Ophthalmology, in a randomized, controlled, community-based study involving 25,000 preschool children in 450 villages in northern Sumatra, 200,000 IU of vitamin A given biannually resulted in a dramatic decline in xerophthalmia prevalence.[9]

When prevalence rates are low, night blindness is not an accurate reflection of vitamin A status, the researchers added. Bitot's spots should be used to diagnose new cases of the disease.

As reported in World Health Forum, supplementing with vitamin A, iodine, and iron could help to prevent community and national losses in human potential in preventing xerophthalmia, goiter, and anemia, respectively.[10]

Forty million children under the age of 5 are physiologically deficient in vitamin A, the researchers said. Of these, about 400,000 will die of severe vitamin A deficiency each year, and over 250,000 will become partially or completely blind. Vitamin A deficiency should be studied in both mothers and children under the age of 6.

At Johns Hopkins Hospital in Baltimore, Maryland, Richard D. Semba, M.D., and colleagues, evaluated 55 children, 3 to 6 years of age, of whom 30 had xerophthalmia while 25 did not. Acutely malnourished children were excluded from the study.[11]

The research team evaluated helper suppressor ratio and the proportion of circulating CD4 naive, CD4 memory, CD8, CD45RA, and CD8, CD45RO T-cell subsets.

It was found that children with conjunctivitis had lower helper suppressor ratios, lower proportions of CD4 naive, T-cells, and higher proportions of CD8, CD45RO T-cells than those without xerophthalmia.

In the study, 26 of the children were given 60 mg retinol equivalents of vitamin A supplementation, while 29 received placebos.

Five weeks after supplementation, the vitamin A group had higher CD4/CD8 ratios, higher proportions of CD4 naive T-cells, and lower porportions of CD8, CD45RO T-cells than in the placebo group.

The authors suggested that vitamin A-deficient children have an underlying abnormality of T-cell subsets, and that these abnormalities are reversible with vitamin A supplementation.

In evaluating 81 rural Nepali households with a 1- to 6-year old child with a history of xerophthalmia, compared to controls, the control households and children were more likely to consume vitamin A-rich foods during July-September and October-December than the xerophthalmia children, reported a research team from Johns Hopkins Hospital.[12]

Those with the eye condition were less likely to consume preformed vitamin A-rich foods throughout the year. Infrequent intake of beta-carotene and preformed vitamin A-rich foods begins early in life and clusters among siblings within households, the researchers added.

In developing countries where there is a significant vitamin A deficiency, counseling for children with xerophthalmia should be extended to their younger siblings. Preformed vitamin A intake may be as important, or more so, as carotenoid-containing food consumption in protecting children and others in the household from vitamin A deficiency, the researchers concluded.

Cataract : As reported in the British Medical Journal, 493 cataracts were extracted during 470,302 person-years of follow-up. Intake of carotene and vitamin A were inversely associated with cataracts, according to Susan E. Hankinson, M.D., and colleagues.[13]

Women in the highest intake, including supplementation, had a 39% lower risk of cataract relative to women in the lowest fifth. Neither vitamin B2 nor vitamins C and E were associated with cataract in multivariant analysis.

Among specific food items, spinach (rather than carrots) was the greatest source of beta-carotene, and it was the most consistent with a lower relative risk. The risk was 45% lower among women who used vitamin C supplements for 10 years or more.

Oxidative stress has long been implicated in the development of age-related cataract, according to a research team at the University of Sydney in Australia, and colleagues at other Australian facilities.[14,15]

Hydrogen peroxide found in the aqueous can give rise to reactive oxygen species (ROS), such as superoxides and hydroperoxides, which can damage lens components, such as crystallin proteins, lens fiber membranes, and lipids, which lead to lens opacities. Aqueous refers to watery.

In the study, during 1992-1994, 3,654 people over the age of 49 attended baseline examinations in the Blue Mountain Eye Study, which is a population-based study of vision, common eye, and systemic conditions in a population living in a region west of Sydney.

Of this number, 2,464 people were followed after the beginning of the study at either 5 or 10 years. At each exam, lens photography was performed and questionnaires were collected, including a 145-item semiquantative food-frequency questionnaire.

The participants were evaluated for antioxidant intake, including beta-carotene, zinc, and vitamins A, C, and E. Those with the highest quintile of total intake, from diet and supplements, of vitamin C, had a reduced risk of incident nuclear cataract. An above-median intake of combined anfioxidants (vitamins C and E, beta-carotene, and zinc) was associated with a reduced risk of incident nuclear cataract.

The researchers concluded that, "higher intakes of vitamin C or the combined intake of antioxidants, had long-term protective associations against development of nuclear cataract in this older population."

Vitamin E and lutein, from both foods and supplements, may reduce a woman's risk of developing cataracts, according to Nicholas Bakalar in the February 12, 2008 issue of the New York Times.[16]

The study, which originally appeared in the January 2008 issue of Archives of Ophthalmology, followed 35,000 women for an average of 10 years.

After adjusting for smoking, alcohol use, body mass index, and other variables, the research team, headed by William G. Christen, M.D., of Brigham and Women's Hospital in Boston, Massachusetts, found that the more vitamin E and lutein the women used, the less likely they were to have cataracts, when compared with the one-fifth of women who consumed the least amount of the antioxidants.

The one-fifth of the women who consumed the most antioxidants reduced their risk for cataracts by 14% with vitamin E and 18% with lutein.

Macular degeneration : Age-related macular degeneration (AMD) blurs the sharp, central vision you need for "straight ahead" activities such as reading, driving, etc., according to the National Eye Institute, Bethesda, Maryland. AMD affects the macula, the part of the eye that permits you to see fine detail.[17]

"In some cases, AMD advances so slowly that people notice little change in their vision," the Institute said. "In others, the disease progresses faster and may lead to a loss of vision in both eyes. AMD is a leading cause of vision loss in those 60 years of age and older."

The macula is located in the center of the retina, the light-sensitive tissue at the back of the eye. The retina converts light, or an image, into electrical impulses. The retina then sends these impulses, or nerve signals, to the brain.

There are two forms of AMD:

1. Wet AMD occurs when abnormal blood vessels behind the retina start to grow under the macula. These vessels can leak blood and fluid, which raise the macula from its normal place at the back of the eye, quickly damaging the eye.

Wet AMD, the more advanced form of the disease, begins when straight lines appear wavy. That is when you need to see an eye-care specialist to have a comprehensive dilated eye exam.

2. Dry AMD begins when the light-sensitive cells in the macula slowly break down, gradually blurring central vision in the affected eye. As AMD progresses, you may see a blurred spot in the center of your vision. Over time, as less of the macula functions, central vision in the affected eye can be lost gradually.

One of the most common early signs of dry AMD is drusen, which are yellow deposits under the retina.

Dry AMD has three stages, all of which may occur in one or both eyes, the Institute added.

1. *Early AMD*. These patients have either several small drusen or a few medium-size drusen. At this stage, there are no apparent symptoms and no vision loss.

2. *Intermediate AMD*. These patients have either many medium-size drusen or one or more large areas. There may be a blurred spot in the center of the vision, and more light may be needed for reading and other tasks.

3. *Advanced dry AMD*. In addition to drusen, these patients have a breakdown of light-sensitive cells and supporting tissue in the central retinal area. This causes a blurred spot in the center of vision. Over time, the blurred spot may get bigger and darker, taking more of your central vision. You may have difficulty reading or recognizing faces unless they are very close to you.

These are the major risks of AMD:

1. Being middle-aged and older.
2. Smoking.
3. Obesity.
4. Race. Caucasians are more likely to lose vision from AMD than African-Americans.
5. Family history.
6. Gender. Women appear to be at a greater risk than men.

During an eye exam, you may be asked to look at an Amster grid. The pattern of the grid resembles a checkerboard. You cover one eye and stare at a black spot in the center of the grid. You may notice that straight lines appear wavy, and that some of the lines are missing. These may be signs of AMD.

For wet AMD, your eye-care professional may suggest a fluorescein angiogram, in which a special dye is injected into the arm. Pictures are taken as the dye passes through the blood vessels in the retina. Any leaking blood vessels may warrant treatment.

The National Eye Institute's Age-Releated Eye Disease Study (AREDS) found that taking a high-dose formulation of antioxidants and zinc significantly reduces the risk of advanced AMD and its associated vision loss. Slowing AMD's progression can save the vision of many people, the Institute said.

The daily amounts of antioxidants and zinc used by study researchers were: (a) 500 mg of vitamin C; (b) 400 IU of vitamin E; (c) 15 mg of beta-carotene—often labeled as equivalent to 25,000 IU of vitamin A; (d) 80 mg of zinc and zinc oxide; and (e) 2 mg of copper as copper oxide. Copper was added to the formulation containing zinc to prevent a copper deficiency anemia, a condition associated with high levels of zinc intake.

"High levels of vitamins and minerals are difficult to obtain from diet alone," the Institute added. "However, previous studies have suggested that people who have diets rich in green leafy vegetables have a lower risk of developing AMD. A daily multivitamin alone does not provide the same high levels of antioxidants and zinc as the AREDS formulation."

The Institute added that, if you are already taking daily vitamins and your doctor suggests you take the high-dose AREDS formulation, review all of your supplements with your doctor. Multivitamins contain many important vitamins not found in the AREDS formulation, so you may want to take a multivitamin along with the AREDS formulation. As an example, those with osteoporosis need to be concerned about vitamin D, which is not in the AREDS formulation.

The prevalence and effects of age-related macular degeneration and cataract are increasing dramatically as the proportion of elderly in our population continues to rise, reported a research team from the Massachusetts Eye and Ear

Infirmary, Harvard Medical School, in Boston, Massachusetts.[18, 19, 20, 21]

In 1984, in the Epidemiology Unit of the Infirmary, researchers began to explore whether diet or supplements could prevent or slow the progressions of AMD and cataract.

"Our hypothesis involved oxidative mechanisms whereby daily insults such as pollution, smoking, sunlight, and even normal metabolic processes that lead to free radicals and oxidation could damage the retina, and could theoretically be blocked by antioxidants such as those that occur in foods and supplements," the researchers said. "There was also much discussion at the time about the potential effects of vitamins on other chronic diseases such as cancer and heart disease."[22]

After reviewing the various studies, the researchers reported that, a multivitamin-multimineral supplement with a combination of vitamin C, vitamin E, beta-carotene, and zinc (with cupric oxide) is recommended for AMD but not cataract. Observational studies for cataract only provide weak support for multivitamins or other supplements.

They added that the results of observational studies suggest that a healthy lifestyle with a diet containing foods rich in antioxidants, especially lutein, zeaxanthin, and omega-3 fatty acids appears beneficial for AMD and possibly cataract. Lutein is a cousin of beta-carotene.

In the First National Health and Nutrition Examination Survey, conducted between 1971 and 1972, the frequency of consumption of fruits and vegetables rich in vitamin A, in those 45 and older, was inversely related to AMD, according to the American Journal of Epidemiology.[23]

In 135 cases of age-related macular degeneration, foods rich in carotene—especially spinach, broccoli, carrots and winter squash—were inversely associated with AMD, and, to a lesser extent, higher vitamin C intake was associated with a lower AMD risk.[24]

In 102 patients with macular degeneration, who consumed vitamin C at 500 mg/day; vitamin E at 400 IU/day; beta-carotene at 10,000 IU/day; and sodium selenite (selenium) at 250 mcg/day over 7 to 12 years, 60% of the patients had stabilized their disease or improved.[25]

In 176 patients with diabetes and diabetic macular edema, who were followed for 7-12 years, the just-named therapy showed that 50% of the diabetics with macular edema had stabilized or improved, according to the Southern Medical Journal.

A number of research studies have suggested that diets high in lutein and zeaxanthin may be associated with a reduced risk of age-related macular degeneration, according to Investigative Ophthalmology and Visual Science.[26]

In the study, researchers evaluated lutein and zeaxanthin levels in the retinas from 56 eye donors with AMD, and 56 eye donors without the disease. Each eye was divided into three concentric sections centered around the fovea, the central part of the retina where the largest amount of lutein and zeaxanthin are found.

The research team said that, on average, lutein and zeaxanthin levels were lower in all three concentric sections in the retinas from those with AMD. In studying the most reliable region of the retina, the researchers found that eyes containing the largest amount of the two carotenoids were 82% less likely to have AMD.

The research team said that their study is consistent with research suggesting that high levels of the two carotenoids in the retina greatly reduce the risk of AMD, and that low levels are not a consequence of the disease.

Antioxidant carotenoids help to protect plants from dangerous free radicals, which can be generated by oxygen and light. This protective benefit is thought to carry over to people when they consume carotenoid-rich vegetables, and fruit, reported Archives of Biochemistry and Biophysics.[27]

In a detailed review, researchers described the roles of lutein and zeaxanthin in the eyes. Both carotenoids form the yellow "macular pigment" at the center of the eye's retina, and this macular pigment filters out harmful blue wavelength light and may also reduce levels of free radicals.

The researchers added that increased intake of lutein-containing foods or lutein ester supplements increase blood levels of lutein, thereby leading to a subsequent increase in macular pigment density.

This research suggests that supplemental lutein—some of which may be converted to meso-zeaxanthin—may reduce the risk of age-related macular degeneration due to the association between age-related macular degeneration and macular pigment density.

The research team added that blood levels associated with the normal diet are below the maximal levels achieved with supplements. Therefore, lutein ester supplements—a common form of lutein—could be used to optimize levels of the nutrient in the eye.

Retinitis pigmentosa: At the Massachusetts Eye and Ear Infirmary in Boston, 601 patients, 18 to 49 years of age, with retinitis pigmentosa, were given 1 of 4 treatments: (1) 15,000 IU/day of vitamin A; (2) 15,000 IU/day of vitamin A plus 400 IU/day of vitamin E; (3) trace amounts of both vitamins; and (4) 400 IU/day of vitamin E.[28]

The 2 groups given vitamin A had a slower rate of decline in retinal function than the 2 groups not given vitamin A. Out of 354 patients with higher initial amplitudes, the 2 groups given 15,000 IU of vitamin A were 32% less likely to have a reduction in the amplitude of 50% or more from baseline (beginning of the study) in a given year than those not receiving this dosage.

However, the 2 groups given 400 IU of vitamin E were 42% more likely to have a decline in amplitude of 50% or more from baseline than those not given this dosage.

Eliot L. Berson, M.D., and colleagues, conclude that there was a beneficial effect of 15,000 IU of vitamin A daily, and an adverse effect of 400 IU of vitamin E on the course of retinitis pigmentosa.

As reported in the American Journal of Clinical Nutrition, 4,500 retinol equivalents (RE)—15,000 IU/day—of vitamin A caused no toxic manifestations of hypervitaminosis A in young and middle-aged adults with retinitis pigmentosa, who were in generally good health, and who were followed for up to 12 years.[29]

UV-radiation damage : Carotenoids (beta-carotene, lycopene, etc.) deposit in the skin and eyes, where they may act as a visible-light filter by absorbing some of the sun's harmful UV rays, and prevent photooxidative reactions that cause free-radical damage to tissues, according to the International Journal of Vitamin and Nutrition Research.[30]

In the review, 2 researchers described the role of carotenoids in preventing photooxidative damage to the eyes and skin. These areas of the body are constantly exposed to oxygen and sunlight, which may increase the risk of sunburn, skin aging, skin cancer, macular degeneration, and cataracts.

The research team reported that several studies have found that supplemental beta-carotene can reduce sunburn; it may provide systemic protection in addition to topical sunscreens; and the sunburn-reducing effects are achieved after 10 weeks of supplementation.

Beta-carotene is thought to reduce sunburn by increasing protective antioxidant reserves on the skin. Another study reported that lycopene can also protect against sunburn.

As for eye health, lutein and zeaxanthin form the macular pigment, which may filter out harmful visible or "blue" light rays and reduce free-radical damage in the central retina, the researchers concluded.

Deficiencies in vitamin A and zinc can play a role in night blindness and hypogonadism in some chronic alcoholics, according to Alcoholism: Clinical Experimental and Research.[31]

Avoiding alcohol and supplementation with vitamin A and zinc may be of some benefit in these disorders.

As reported in the Australian Journal of Dermatology, researchers evaluated a 16-year-old male who developed night blindness 2 weeks after starting isotretinoin at a dose of 20 mg/day for cystic acne. The patient also had cystic fibrosis, complicated by hapatic cirrhosis.[32]

Although the young man had been on long-term vitamin A therapy, blood levels of the vitamin were found to be 0.3 micromol/l, with the normal range being 0.9 to 2.5 micromol/l.

Oral vitamin A supplementation was given, which resulted in resolution of his visual symptoms in 6 months. The isotretinoin therapy was continued without deterioration in liver function, however, the drug may interfere with the processing of endogenous vitamin A in the liver, the researchers added. Isotretinoin is 13-cis-retinoic acid, a retinoid used in the treatment of severe recalcitrant cystic acne.

Vitamin A supplementation in the treatment of xerophthalmia has been suggested to reduce not only blindness, but also to prevent mortality in young children, reported James M. Tielach, M.D., and Keith P. West, Jr., of Johns Hopkins University School of Medicine in Baltimore, Maryland.[33]

In their study, of over 21,000 Indonesian children, from 12 to 71 months, they were given either a placebo or vitamin A at 200,000 IU, a standard prophylactic dose for the prevention of xerophthalmia.

Vitamin A was given on 2 different occasions 6 months apart. It was reported that there was a 34% reduction in child mortality in the treatment vs. control group.

The vitamin reduced the incidence and severity of diarrhea and/or respiratory tract infections, which may be the mechanism for the reduction of mortality rates.

As reported in Johns Hopkins Magazine, Alfred Sommer, world renowned for the use of vittamin A in the prevention of night blindness, found that Third World Countries children's risk of death correlated less strongly with their general nutritional status than with the severity of vitamin A deficiency, as measured by their vision problems.[34]

Night blindness affects 16 to 52% of pregnant women in Nepal, and in some cases persists after vitamin A treatment, reported Joanne M. Graham, M.D., of the University of California at Davis, and colleagues at other facilities.[35]

Iron and riboflavin (vitamin B2) affect vitamin A utilization and photoreceptor function, respectively, and a pilot data in the study population showed a high prevalence of iron and B2 deficiencies.

Although vitamin A deficiency is the main cause of maternal night blindness in low-income populations in developing countries, iron and B2 deficiencies could increase the risk of night blindness by affecting both vitamin A metabolism and the process of dark adaptation, the researchers added.

In previous studies of pregnant women in the Terai region of Nepal, vitamin A supplements reduced the incidence of night blindness by 67%.

"Our preliminary studies in the same region showed a 40% prevalence of iron deficiency, and an 86% prevalence of B2 deficiency in pregnant women," they added. "These nutrient deficiencies often coexist with vitamin A deficiency when consumption of animal source foods is low."

Thus, they continued, the objectives of our study were to assess whether providing iron and B2, as compared with a placebo, would improve nutritional status and dark adaptation among nightblind women receiving vitamin A-fortified rice. The relation between pupillary threshold score and biochemical indicators of iron and riboflavin was also evaluated.

Night blindness is a debilitating disorder for pregnant women in Nepal, which negatively affects their quality of life (6), and increases the risk of mortality of their infants by 63% in the first month of life.[36]

Their study shows that nutrient deficiencies in addition to vitamin A deficiency must be involved, the researchers concluded.

"Iron deficiency may limit the efficacy of vitamin A programs in the treatment of night blindness in pregnant women," they added. "More research is needed to test different strategies for simultaneous delivery of multiple micronutrients, especially in combination with iron, appropriate micronutrient-rich foods, or both, for the prevention and treatment of night blindness during pregnancy."

Vitamin A and Retinitis Pigmentosa

When patients with retinitis pigmentosa take 15,000 IU/day of vitamin A, a review of the published literature shows that vitamin A supplements at that level are safe for healthy adult men and nonpregnant women, who eat a diet without an excessive intake of foods high in the vitamin.

Pregnant women need to have their vitamin A intake—from foods and supplements—monitored so as not to harm the fetus. As we know, vitamin A is stored in the liver, and a fetus's liver is quite small.

Annual monitoring of liver enzymes and triglycerides (fat) levels is recommended for those getting the vitamin A supplement.

Source: Semba, Richard D. "Safety of Daily Oral Vitamin A Supplements for Individuals with Retinitis Pigmentosa," Annals of Ophthalmology 34(3): 194-198, 2002.

The Number of Blind People in India

India is home to the world's largest number of blind people, reported *The Times of India*. Of the 37 million people worldwide who are blind, over 15 million live in India. Of these, 3 million—or 26%—are children, who suffer from corneal disorders.

Equally shocking, 75% of those are cases of avoidable blindness because of an acute shortage of optometrists and donated eyes for the treatment of corneal blindness. While India needs 40,000 optometrists, it only has 8,000, the newspaper said.

Although India needs 2.5 lakh—a year, the country's 109 eye banks—of which 5 are in Delhi—collect only about 25,000 eyes, of which 30% are unusable.

Ajeet Bhardwaj, M.D., outgoing president of the Asia Pacific Optometrists Organization, said that India has 12,000 ophthalmologists, but they have no time to conduct blindness-preventing strategies, since they are flooded with general eye check-up patients.

Dr. Bhardwaj added that 153 million Indians need reading glasses, but they do not have them. Optometrists are physicians trained in vision eye care, eye diseases, who prescribe eyeglasses, contact lenses, and medications to treat eye disorders. An ophthalmologist specializes in surgical care of the eyes.

Source: Niksharli, M., M.D. "India Has Largest Blind Population," The Times of India, October 11, 2007.

References

1. Clark, Randolph Lee, M.D., and Cumley, Russell W., Ph.D., editors. The Book of Health. New York: Van Nostrand Reinhold Co., 1962, pp. 558ff.
2. Maumenee, Edward A., M.D. "The History of Vitamin A and Its Ophthalmic Implications: A Personal Viewpoint," Archives of Opthalmology 111: 547-550, April 1993.
3. Feinstein, Alice, editor. Prevention's Healing with Vitamins. Emmaus, PA: Rodale Press, Inc., 1996, pp. 418ff.
4. Sinha, D.P., et al. "The Effect of Massive Doses of Vitamin A on the Signs of Vitamin A Deficiency in Preschool Children," American Journal of Clinical Nutrition 29(1): 110-115, 1976.
5. Yarborough, C. W., et al. "Retinopathy Following Jejunoileal Bypass Surgery," International Journal of Obstetrics 6(3): 253-258, 1982.
6. Christian, P., et al. "Vitamin A or Beta-Carotene Supplementation Reduces But Does Not Eliminate Night Blindness in Nepal," Journal of Nutrition 128(9): 1458-1463, September 1998.
7. Humphrey, J.H., et al. "A Priming Dose of Oral Vitamin A Given to Preschool Children May Extend Protection Conferred by a Subsequent Large Dose of Vitamin A," Journal of Nutrition 123(8): 1363-1369, August 1993.
8. "Gruntzig, J. "Xerophthalmia," Fortsch. Med. 97(24): 1107-1110, June 28, 1979.
9. Djunaedi, E., et al. "Impact of Vitamin A Supplementation on Xerophthalmia: A Randomized Controlled Community Trial," Archives of Ophthalmology 106(2): 218-222, February 1988.
10. Ramalingaswami, V. "Challenges and Opportunities—One Vitamin, Two Minerals," World Health Forum 13:222-231, 1992.
11. Semba, Richard D., M.D., et al. "Abnormal T-Cell Subset Proportions in Vitamin A-Deficient Children," The Lancet 341:5-8, January 2, 1993.
12. Shankar, Anita V., et al. "Chronic Low Intakes of Vitamin A-Rich Foods in Households with Xerophthalmic Children: A Case-Control Study in Nepal," American Journal of Clinical Nutrition 6: 242-248, 1996.
13. Hankinson, Susan E., M.D., et al. "Nutrient Intake and Cataract Extraction in Women: A Prospective Study," British Medical Journal 305: 335-339, August 8, 1992.
14. Tan, Ava Grace, et al. "Antioxidant Nutrient Intake and the Long-Term Incidence of Age-Related Cataract: The Blue Mountain Eye Study," American Journal of Clinical Nutrition 87: 1899-1905, 2008.
15. Ottonello, S., et al. "Oxidative Stress and Age-Related Cataract," Ophthalmologia 214: 78-85, 2000.

16. Bakalar, Nicholas. "Antioxidants May Gut Cataracts," The New York Times, February 12, 2008, p. F6.

17. "Age-Related Macular Degeneration. What You Should Know," National Eye Institute, NIH, Bethesda, Maryland, August 2006.

18. Seddon, Johanna M. "Multivitamin-Multimineral Supplements and Eye Disease: Age-Related Macular Degeneration and Cataract," American Journal of Clinical Nutrition 85(30): 304S-307S, 2007.

19. National Advisory Eye Council. Vision Research—a National Plan, 1999-2003. Vol. 1. A Report of the National Advisory Eye Council, Bethesda, Maryland, National Institutes of Health, 1999. (NIH Publication 98-4120).

20. "We the People: Aging in the United States," Internet, June 20, 2006.

21. Klein, R., et al. "Prevalence of Age-Related Maculopathy," Ophthalmology 99: 933-943, 1992.

22. Hung, S., et al. "The Relationship Between Nutritional Factors and Age-Related Macular Degeneration," In: A. Bendich, et al., editors. Preventive Nutrition, the Comprehensive Guide for Health Professionals. 2nd Edition. Human Press, Totowa, New Jersey, 2001. pp. 247-269.

23. Goldberg, J., et al. "Factors Associated with Age-Related Macular Degeneration: An Analysis of Data from the First National Health and Nutrition Examination Survey," American Journal of Epidemiology 128(4): 700-710, 1988.

24. Seddon, Johanna M., et al. "Dietary Antioxidant Status and Age-Related Macular Degeneration: A Multicenter Study," Investigative Ophthalmology and Visual Science 34: 1133, 1993.

25. Crary, E.J. "Antioxidant Treatment of Macular Degeneration of the Aging and Macular Edema in Diabetic Retinopathy," Southern Medical Journal 80(9): S 38, 1987.

26. Bone, R.A., et al. "Macular Pigment in Donor Eyes with and without AMD: A Case-Control Study," Investigative Ophthalmology and Visual Science 42: 235-240, 2001.

27. Landrum, J.T., and Bone, R.A. "Lutein, Zeaxanthin, and the Macular Pigment," Archives of Biochemistry and Biophysics 385: 28-40, 2001.

28. Berson, Eliot L., M.D. "A Randomized Trial of Vitamin A and Vitamin E Supplementation for Retinitis Pigmentosa," Archives of Ophthalmology 111: 761-772, 1993.

29. Sibulesky, L., et al. "Safety of Less Than 7,500 RE (Less Than 2,500 IU) Vitamin A Daily in Adults with Retinitis Pigmentosa," American Journal of Clinical Nutrition 69: 656-663, 1999.

30. Sies, H., and Stahl, W. "Non-Nutritive Bioactive Constituents of Plants: Lycopene, Lutein and Zeaxanthin," International Journal for Vitamin and Nutrition Research 73: 95-100, 2003.

31. McClain, C.J., et al. "Alterations in Zinc, Vitamin A, and Retinol-Binding Protein in Chronic Alcoholism: A Possible Mechanism for Night Blindness and Hypogonadism," Alcoholism: Clinical Experimental and Research 3(2): 135-141, April 1979.

32. Welsh, B.M., et al. "Night Blindness Precipitated by Isotretinoin in the Setting of Hypovitaminosis A," Australian Journal of Dermatology 40(4): 208-210, November 1999.

33. Tielach, James M., M.D., and West, Keith P., Jr. "Cost and Efficiency Considerations in Community-Based Trials of Vitamin A in Developing Countries," Statistics in Medicine 9: 35-43, 1990.

34. Edmunds, Levina. "The Magic Bullet", Johns Hopkins Magazine 41(4): 12-30, August 1989.

35. Graham, Joanne M., M.D., et al. "Supplementation with Iron and Riboflavin Enhances Dark Adaptation Response to Vitamin A-Fortified Rice in Iron-Deficient, Pregnant Nightblind Nepali Women," American Journal of Clinical Nutrition 85: 1375-1384, 2007.

36. Christian, P., et al. "Maternal Night Blindness Increases the Risk of Mortality in the First 6 Months of Life Among Infants in Nepal," Journal of Nutrition 131: 1510-1512, 2001.

10

CYSTIC FIBROSIS

Cystic fibrosis is an inherited disease that affects most of the body's endocrine glands, although with different degrees of severity, according to The Physicians' Manual for Patients. The endocrine glands—pancreas and sweat glands—are those that deliver their secretions through ducts to various organs and surfaces of the body, rather than pouring them directly into the bloodstream.[1]

The disease is characterized by persistent, serious lung infections; loose, pale stools that are foul-smelling and float in water; and a loss of weight.

"Cystic fibrosis is generally initially recognized in infancy or early childhood, however, it can escape detection until the teens," the publication said. "Among whites, the incidence is about 1 in 2,000 children; in blacks, about 1 in 17,000."

The disease is caused by a single defective gene, which is recessive. That is, it will occur only if both parents contribute to the gene that determines the disease to the fertilized ovum.

"About 1 person in 20 is a carrier for cystic fibrosis, usually without knowing it," the publication added. "These people are free of the disease, yet, since they carry the recessive gene responsible, they are capable of transmitting it to future generations."

The initial symptoms may occur shortly after birth, when the baby is unable to move his bowels, because they are obstructed with excessively sticky meconium (pasty, greenish material that fills the fetus's intestines and normally forms a newborn's first bowel movement).

This condition—meconium ileus—occurs because the baby's pancreas fails to produce the digestive enzymes that normally break up the meconium, making it soft and easily passed out of the bowel.

Initial symptoms may also be foul-smelling stools, a failure to gain weight, or the development of pneumonia. The pancreas does not produce sufficient quantities of enzymes that usually break down proteins, fats, and carbohydrates so they can be absorbed into the bloodstream. Thus, fats and other nutrients pass out of the body mostly unabsorbed.

"Treatments including giving extracts of animal pancreas to replace the missing or insufficient pancreatic enzymes," the publication continued. "A diet low in fat and high in protein is often prescribed, and the child will be given multivitamins, as well as additional amounts of vitamins A, D, and E, all fat-soluble vitamins."

In evaluating 35 cystic fibrosis patients with a mean age of 24.2 years, who were admitted to hospital with pulmonary exacerbations, there was a significant positive correlation found between plasma retinol/vitamin A concentrations at admission, and age, weight, body mass index, triceps-skinfold knee percentile, midupper arm circumference percentile, plasma vitamin E, and retinol binding protein concentrations, according to a research team at Children's Hospital in Boston, Massachusetts.[2] Retinol binding protein binds and transports retinol in the bloodstream.

When the patients were admitted, plasma retinol concentrations were negatively correlated with maximum body temperature, and C-reactive protein concentrations, which suggests that the body's acute phase response was associated with the depression in vitamin A concentrations. C-reactive protein is an inflammatory marker in the blood that is strongly associated with heart disease.

The authors concluded that plasma retinol concentrations are depressed in acute pulmonary exacerbations of cystic fibrosis.

In 31 cystic fibrosis patients with evidence of vitamin A deficiency, who were taking oral pancreatic enzyme replacement therapy and 5,000 IU/day of vitamin A, 10% of the patients were found to have frank conjunctival xerosis (dryness), and 19% had abnormal dark adaptation.[3]

The researchers added that vitamin A should be evaluated regularly in cystic fibrosis patients, along with ophthalmological assessment if serum levels fall below 30 ng/d1. Ng refers to nanogram or one-billionth of a gram.

At St. James University Hospital in Leeds, United Kingdom, researchers reviewed the importance of supplementation of fat-soluble vitamins in cystic fibrosis, especially since these patients have other severe medical conditions, and nutritional evaluation may be overlooked.[4]

Pancreatic insufficiency from birth can result in fat malabsorption of vitamins A, D, E, and K. Pancreatic enzyme replacement and routine vitamin supplemention eliminated many clinical deficiencies of the fat-soluble vitamins in those who were diagnosed and treated early.

The research team, headed by Rosemary J. Rayner, said that cystic fibrosis patients are at risk for vitamin deficiency if the diagnosis is made late, if part of the bowel has been resected (removed), or if fat-soluble vitamin supplements are not taken.

Rayner added that studies have found low levels of fat-soluble vitamins in those with cystic fibrosis. Example dosages of vitamins A, D, and E in children with cystic fibrosis or adults are 2.4 mg/day of vitamin A; 20 mcg/day of vitamin D; and 100 to 200 mg/day of vitamin E. Researchers list vitamin E dosages in International Units or milligrams; they have similar designations.

As the prognosis for these patients improves, clinical problems due to fat-soluble vitamin deficiencies will become more prevalent, Rayner continued. Those at greatest risk are those with severe malabsorption, poor compliance (they don't ingest enough of the vitamins), or those with liver disease.

In evaluating 15 patients with cystic fibrosis, between the ages of 8 and 34, 3 patients had serum concentrations of retinol below the reference range, and 7 patients had decreased serum levels of retinol-binding protein, according to the Journal of Pediatric Gastroenterology and Nutrition.[5]

The risk of a vitamin A deficiency in cystic fibrosis patients increases with age, the researchers said. And this data does not support the suggestion that cystic fibrosis patients are at risk for hypervitaminosis A (toxic levels) with long-term supplementation with the vitamin.

In addition, no correlation was found between the severity of liver disease and vitamin A content in the liver. Although vitamin A is largely stored in the liver, small amounts are collected in the lungs, body fat, and kidneys. As previously mentioned, vitamin A esters are transported through the blood in association with a retinol-binding protein. Carotenoids are associated with the lipid-bearing protein.

At Hopital d'Enfants in Dijon Codex, France, a research team evaluated levels of vitamin A in 10 stable cystic fibrosis teenagers, with a mean age of 14.3. It was found that retinol, alpha-carotene, and beta-carotene levels were below the lower limit of normal in all but 1 patient.[6]

Five out of 10 of the patients with a normal standard ophthalmological exam presented a poor or a pathological dark adaptation test.

Vitamin A supplementation at 20,000 IU/day for 1 year in the 2 patients who had pathological dark adaptation tests dramatically improved nocturnal vision.

Vitamin A levels are often low in clinically stable cystic fibrosis patients, and blood levels of the vitamin should be monitored in these patients, and dark adaptation tests should be performed when patients are deficient in the vitamin, the researchers added.

Malabsorption and poor consumption of vitamin A and vitamin E may result in low blood levels of the 2 vitamins, especially in patients with moderate to severe lung disease, according to Darcy Borowitz, M.D., and colleagues at Children's Hospital in Buffalo, New York.[7]

The authors recommend that health professionals should encourage the use of multivitamin supplements in patients with cystic fibrosis, even though all questions regarding optimal therapy have not been answered.

They added that primary care physicians who care for children with cystic fibrosis should inquire about the use of vitamins, and encourage them to be consistent in the use of this preventive modality. Physicians who care for these children should screen for vitamin A and vitamin E deficiency on a yearly basis, and should share this information with the patient and the primary care provider, the researchers said.

A study in the Journal of Human Nutrition and Dietetics reported on an 18-year-old caucasian male with cystic fibrosis, who developed a red, irritable, blurred, and photobiotic left eye. The latter refers to living or flourishing only in the light.[8]

Treatments with vitamin A and D capsules at a daily dose of 12,000 IU of vitamin A; vitamin E at 200 mg/day; ursodeoxycholic acid at 300 mg t.i.d. (3 times daily); and taurine at 500 mg. t.i.d., for cystic fibrosis-associated liver disease, and Creon 25000 at 40 capsules a day. Taurine is an amino acid or form of protein.

Vitamin A at 100,000 IU of retinol palmitate in oil-miscible preparation was given on 3 different occasions intramuscularly at 2-week intervals. Within the first 4 days of the first intramuscular dose, there was definite clinical improvement in the cornea. After 6 weeks of therapy, the corneal and conjunctival surfaces had almost returned to normal, the researchers reported.

Because of a low production of pancreatic enzymes, which are essential for digestion, patients with cystic fibrosis do not efficiently absorb fat-soluble vitamins and beta-carotene. Consequently, these patients suffer higher than normal levels of oxidative stress and free radical damage.[9]

As reported in Annals of Nutrition and Metabolism, a research team tested whether large doses of beta-carotene would reduce free radical damage and improve lung function in 24 children and teenagers with cystic fibrosis.

The patients were given 1 mg of beta-carotene per kg (2.2 lbs) of body weight, up to a total of 50 mg/day for 12 weeks. After that, the dosage was reduced to 10 mg/day.

In addition, the patients received 1 to 2 mg/day of vitamin A; 50 to 200 mg/day of vitamin C; and 110 to 380 mg/day of vitamin E, along with pancreatic enzymes.

Antioxidant supplementation, especially large doses of beta-carotene, significantly reduced levels of free radicals in the children. Also, the younger patients benefited from greatly improved lung function, since these patients often have chronic lung problems.

As reported in Ophthalmic Pediatrics, a 16-year-old with cystic fibrosis complained of night blindness. He was evaluated at an eye clinic in Columbus, Ohio, by Lawrence E. Leguire, Ph.D., and colleagues.[10]

Before vitamin A supplementation, the electro-oculogram Arden light/dark ratio was 1.27. Following 7 months of vitamin A supplementation, the Arden ratio had increased to 3.0. A vitamin A deficiency can cause an abnormal electro-oculogram, the researchers said.

They added that these findings are important for patient populations who are susceptible to vitamin A deficiency and night blindness, which includes those with cystic fibrosis, jejunal bypass surgery, and cirrhosis of the liver.

Supplementation with 25,000 IU of vitamin A returned blood levels to low normal range, and normalized the electro-oculogram. This device may be a beneficial diagnostic tool in vitamin A deficiency, the researchers continued. Oculography, in which electrodes are placed on the skin next to the eyes, measure changes in standing potential between the front and back of the eyeball as eyes move.

A clinical fat-soluble vitamin deficiency has been recognized in cystic fibrosis for many years, according to researchers at Southampton General Hospital in the United Kingdom.[11]

Cystic fibrosis seems to affect vitamin A metabolism since high liver vitamin A levels have been found in the face of low blood levels, the researchers said. This suggests a defect in mobilization or transport.

Vitamin A loss in stools of cystic fibrosis patients is accentuated even with good pancreatic supplementation, the researchers added. Vitamin A toxicity is always a concern, however.

Vitamin A in a water-miscible form has been shown to be well absorbed. Recommended dosage of vitamin A for cystic fibrosis patients range between 5,000 and 10,000 IU/day, the researchers continued. They also reviewed the importance of other vitamins in dealing with this illness.

At the University of Zurich in Switzerland, 35 cystic fibrosis patients, between 2.3 and 30.5 years of age, were given 0.5 mg/kg of beta-carotene daily for 16 months. Initially, beta-carotene concentrations were lower in patients with CF than in the controls.[12]

Following supplementation, beta-carotene levels rapidly reached a plateau after about 3 weeks, and they remained that way throughout the study. However, plasma retinyl palmitate did not increase during the therapy.

The researchers added that beta-carotene supplementation normalizes beta-carotene status in CF patients without any adverse side effects.

Supplementing CF patients with vitamin C in the early neonatal period may help prevent infections, according to a research team in Annals of Pediatrics (Paris).[13]

Supplementing with the antioxidants vitamin C, vitamin E, beta-carotene, and selenium may help to prevent against damage from reactive oxygen species, the researchers said.

In 210 cystic fibrosis patients compared with 42 controls, Italian researchers found that vitamin A and vitamin E levels were generally lower in the CF patients, according to the European Journal of Pediatrics.[14]

Vitamins A and E were significantly lower in the patients with pancreatic insufficiency, who were receiving enzyme and vitamin supplementation, than in the controls.

The authors added that CF patients have a clear tendency to vitamin A and E deficiency, irrespective of pancreatic function, body weight, and standard supplementation with pancreatic extract and liposoluble vitamins.

At the University of Hohenheim in Stuttgart, Germany, and other facilities in Tubingen and Bonn, Germany, a research team, headed by Evelyn I. Beck, investigated changes in antioxidant concentrations and oxidative stress in plasma, buccal mucosal cells (BMCs), and breath condensate in patients with cystic fibrosis in relation to age and disease progression[15,16,17]. Buccosal cells are adjacent or in the direction of the check.

The study involved 22 patients with cystic fibrosis and 35 healthy controls. Volunteers were in 4 age groups: (1) less than

6 years; (2) 6 to 11 years; (3) 12 to 17 years; and (4) over 18 years. The researchers evaluated carotenoid, vitamin E, vitamin C, protein cabonyls, thiobarbituric acid-reactive substances, and isoprotans.

In the patients with cystic fibrosis, blood levels of beta-carotene, beta-cryptoxanthin, and total lycopene, were significantly lower in patients than in controls in all age groups, the researchers said.

Also, vitamins E and C plasma concentrations, as well as vitamin E concentrations in buccal mucosal cells, were significantly lower in CF patients over 18 years of age, whereas all indicators of oxidative stress assessed were significantly higher than those same indicators in the controls.

"In a healthy organism, free radicals and reactive oxygen species are controlled by various enzymes and antioxidants in the body, and a balance exists between prooxidant and antioxidant processes," the authors added.

However, in patients with CF, this balance is disturbed because the availability of important dietary antioxidants, such as vitamin E and carotenoids, is diminished as a result of maldigestion, malabsorption, and increased turnover. Also, chronically stimulated immune cells as well as invading pathogens are able to produce free radicals, thus increasing the free radical load.

Thanks to therapeutic advances—improved antibiotic treatment—the life expectancy of patients with CF has increased, yet the just-mentioned imbalance is thought to contribute to disease progression in this disease, the researchers continued.

"Against this background, it seems important to strengthen the antioxidant defense to ensure health and well-being for an aging CF patient population," the researchers said. "The aim of our study was to assess whether potential changes in antioxidant systems and oxidative stress were attributable to disease progression in CF or merely an effect of age per se, that is, whether the same trends observed in patients with CF could be identified in a healthy reference population."

The authors went on to say that, adult patients with CF showed distinct vitamin deficits and elevated indicators of oxidative stress in plasma, BMCs, and breath condensate along with a progression of clinical status.

"We suggest that early in life dietary habits should be improved and that innovative supplementation strategies should be applied to optimize the antioxidant status of patients with CF," the authors added.

Cystic fibrosis patients have impaired absorption of antioxidants from the diet, and, therefore, may be more susceptible to oxidative injury to cells. They also experience recurring pulmonary infections, which subject them to more oxidative stress, according to Free Radical Biology and Medicine.[18]

The authors added that CF patients are more susceptible to oxidative-induced DNA damage, and suggest that this may be part of the explanation for the higher incidence of malignancy in CF when compared to healthy controls.

Cystic fibrosis patients are often severely deficient in beta-carotene due to exocrine pancreatic insufficiency, and so these patients present an opportunity to study the role of beta-carotene on lipid peroxidation, reported Free Radical Biology and Medicine.[19]

In the study, the authors investigated the effect of correcting beta-carotene deficiency in cystic fibrosis patients on 2 parameters of lipid peroxidation. Thirty-four CF patients were investigated before and after 3 months of oral beta-carotene supplementation, and were compared to 42 clinically healthy controls.

It was found that beta-carotene concentrations increased in plasma and in low-density lipoprotein cholesterol (LDL) without significant changes in vitamin E, either in plasma or LDL.

The authors conclude that excess lipid peroxidation occuring in beta-carotene deficiency can be limited and normalized during efficient beta-carotene supplementation in CF patients. Lipid peroxidation is an interaction of fats with oxygen, which can lead to the destruction of cells.

Patients with cystic fibrosis and pancreatic insufficiency (PI) are at risk of vitamin A deficiency because of steatorrhea in spite of pancreatic enzyme replacement, according to Rose C. Graham-

Maar, M.D. of the Children's Hospital in Philadelphia, Pennsylvania, and colleagues at other facilities. However, long-standing vitamin A supplementation may increase the risk of vitamin A toxicity, they added. Steatorrhea is excessive fat in the stool.[20]

Almost 90% of those with cystic fibrosis have PI, which increase the risk of vitamin A deficiency because of fat malabsorption, the researchers said. Vitamin A deficiency, which cause night blindness, xerophthalmia and immune dysfunction, has been documented in CF in spite of vitamin A and pancreatic enzyme supplementation.

In 1999, A.P. Feranchak, et al.[21] reported vitamin A deficiency in 4 to 11% of children with CF during a 10-year follow-up from newborn screening. The 2002 CF guidelines recommend vitamin A supplements for all children with CF and PI, specifically, 3,000 mcg retinol activity equivalents (RAEs) per day for children over 8 years of age.

CF-specific water-soluble preparations are widely used, including the fat-soluble vitamins—A, D, E, and K.

"Because children with CF and PI require fat-soluble vitamin replacement throughout their lives, they should be carefully monitored for excess vitamin A," the researchers added. "This task may prove difficult until noninvasive tests of vitamin A stores are developed."

They went on to say that, "until further information specific to CF patients is available, we recommend that this population receive the maximum vitamin A supplementation necessary to maintain normal serum retinol concentrations. In addition, we urge the dietary supplement industry to provide labels that state the content of vitamin A as micrograms RAE, the proportion of retinol and carotenoid compounds, and the fat or water solubility of their products."

Vitamin A and Cystic Fibrosis

Chronic malabsorption of vitamin A, as sometimes happens with cystic fibrosis, is one of the few instances in which injectable vitamin A is required, reported the Journal of the Royal Society of Medicine.

The majority of vitamin A deficient children, including third-world children with severe malnutrition, diarrhea, and keratomalacia (dryness in the cornea of the eye), respond as rapidly and successfully to oral as well as injectable vitamin A preparations. Oral therapy is obviously cheaper and safer.

Daily supplements with 5,000 to 10,000 IU of vitamin A is often inadequate for maintaining normal stores in cystic fibrosis patients, researchers say.

Consequently, 25,000 to 50,000 IU/day are often required.

Source: Sommer, Alfred. "Vitamin A Deficiency Today: Conjunctival xerosis of Cystic Fibrosis," Journal of the Royal Society of Medicine 82(1): 1-2, January 1989.

References

1. Subak-Sharpe, Genell J., editor. The Physicians' Manual for Patients. New York: Times Books, 1984, pp. 167ff.
2. Duggan, Christopher, et al. "Vitamin A Status in Acute Exacerbations of Cystic Fibrosis," American Journal of Clinical Nutrition 64: 535-539, 1996.
3. Neugenbauer, M.A., et al. "Nyctalopia and Conjunctival Xerosis Indicating Vitamin A Deficiency in Cystic Fibrosis," Eye 3(3): 360-364, 1989.
4. Rayner, Rosemary J. "Fat-Soluble Vitamins in Cystic Fibrosis," Proceedings of the Nutrition Society 51:245-250, 1992.
5. Linblad, Anders, et al. "Vitamin A Concentrations in the Liver Decreases with Age in Patients with Cystic Fibrosis," Journal of Pediatric Gastroenterology and Nutrition 24: 264-270, 1997.
6. Huet, F., et al. "Vitamin A Deficiency and Nocturnal Vision in Teenagers with Cystic Fibrosis," European Journal of Pediatrics 156: 949-951, 1997.
7. Borowitz, Darcy, M.D., et al. "Preventive Care for Patients with Chronic Illness: Multivitamin Use in Patients with Cystic Fibrosis," Clinical Pediatrics, December 1994, pp. 720-725.
8. Campbell, D.C., et al. "Vitamin A Deficiency in Cystic Fibrosis Resulting in Xerophthalmia," Journal of Human Nutrition and Dietetics 11: 529-532, 1998.
9. Rust, P., et al. "Long-Term Oral Beta-Carotene Supplementation in Patients with Cystic Fibrosis—Effects on Oxidative Status and Pulmonary Function," Annals of Nutrition and Metabolism 44: 30-37, 2000.

10. Leguire, Lawrence E., Ph.D., et al. "Electro-Oculogram in Vitamin A Deficiency Associated with Cystic Fibrosis," Ophthalmic Pediatrics 13(3): 187-189, 1992.

11. Peters, S.A., and Rolles, C.J. "Vitamin Therapy and Cystic Fibrosis: A Review in Rationale," Journal of Clinical Pharmacy and Therapeutics 18: 33-38, 1993.

12. Winklhofer-Roob, B.M., et al. "Response to Oral Beta-Carotene Supplementation in Patients with Cystic Fibrosis: A 16-Month Follow-Up Study," Acta Pediatrica 84: 1132-1136, 1995.

13. Laurens, M., et al. "Vitamins and Trace Elements in Cystic Fibrosis Patients," Annals of Pediatrics (Paris) 43(3): 218-223, 1996.

14. Lancellotti, L., et al. "Deficiency of Vitamin E and Vitamin A in Cystic Fibrosis is Independent of Pancreatic Function and Current Enzyme and Vitamin Supplementation," European Journal of Pediatrics 155: 281-285, 1996.

15. Beck, Evelyn I., et al. "Antioxidant Deficiency in Cystic Fibrosis. When Is the Right Time to Take Action?" American Journal of Clinical Nutrition 80: 374-384, 2004.

16. Sies, H., et al. "Vitamins E and C, Beta-Carotene, and Other Carotenoids As Antioxidants," American Journal of Clinical Nutrition 62: 1315S-1321S, 1995.

17. Lancellotti, L., et al. "Deficiency of Vitamins E and A in Cystic Fibrosis Is Independent of Pancreatic Function and Current Enzyme and Vitamin Supplementation," European Journal of Pediatrics 155: 281-285, 1996.

18. Brown, R.K., et al. "Oxidative Damage to DNA in Patients with Cystic Fibrosis," Free Radical Biology and Medicine 18(4): 801-806, 1995.

19. Winkhofer-Roob, B.M., et al. "Enhanced Resistance to Oxidation of Low-Density Lipoproteins and Decreased Lipid Peroxide Formation during Beta-Carotene Supplementation in Cystic Fibrosis," Free Radical Biology and Medicine 18(5): 849-859, 1995.

20. Graham-Maar, Rose C., M.D., et al. "Elevated Vitamin A Intake and Serum Retinol in Preadolescent Children with Cystic Fibrosis," New England Journal of Medicine 84:174-182, 2006.

21. Feranchak, A.P., et al. "Prospective, Long-Term Study of Fat-Soluble Vitamin Status in Children with Cystic Fibrosis Identified by Newborn Screen," Journal of Pediatrics 135: 601-610, 1999.

11

CARDIOVASCULAR DISEASE AND STROKE

Cardiovascular disease is the main cause of death in Western countries, and, while mortality has decreased in the past decades in many countries, these diseases still account for over 40% of total mortality, reported Sari Voutilainen, M.D., et al, of the University of Kuopio in Finland.[1] (The WHO has recently moved cancer to be the No. 1 killer).

Diets vary extensively between different populations. As an example, in the western part of Finland, the mortality rate was 10 times that found in Crete, where the population consumes a typical Mediterranean diet that is rich in plant foods and relatively poor in animal foods.

"A plant-dominated diet likely promotes health through multiple nutrients and mechanisms," the researchers said. "Carotenoids have been implicated as beneficial substances."

Most carotenoids, such as alpha-carotene, beta-carotene, and beta-cryptoxanthin have provitamin activation, and, in addition to their provitamin A activity, carotenoids have been considered to have many other biological functions.[2, 3]

They are proposed to be efficient scavengers of free radicals, and they have also been shown to protect low-density lipoprotein (LDL, the harmful kind), against oxidation in vitro.

"Antioxidant compounds found in fruit and vegetables, such as vitamin C, carotenoids, and flavonoids, may influence the risk of cardiovascular disease by preventing the oxidation of cholesterol in arteries," the researchers added.

Oxidation is the chemical reaction in which chemical energy is released from food to be used by cells. Unstable oxygen molecules (free radicals), which are generated by chemicals, tobacco smoke, pollution, etc., damage tissues and worsen many of our modern health problems, such as heart disease, cancer, arthritis, etc.

The researchers added that a higher intake of fruit and vegetables can help prevent the morbidity and mortality associated with heart disease, and that more information is needed to ascertain the association between the intake of single nutrients, such as carotenoids, and the risk of cardiovascular disease.

As reported in the American Journal of Cardiology, a research team, headed by Ram B. Singh, M.D., evaluated vitamin A at 50,000 IU/day; vitamin C at 1,000 mg/day; vitamin E at 400 mg/day; and beta-crotene at 25 mg/day for 28 days in 63 patients with myocardial infarction (heart attack) and 62 controls.[4]

The mean infarct size was significantly less in the antioxidant group, as measured by creatine kinase-MB.

Serum glutamic-Oxaloacetic transminase (GOT) decreased by 45.6 IU/dl in the antioxidant group when compared with 25.8 IU/dl in the controls. This serum, GOT, is an enzyme catalyzing the reversible transfer of an amine group from L-glutamic acid to oxaloacetic acid, which forms alpha-ketoglutaric acid and L-aspartic acid, which is a diagnostic tool for myocardial infarction.

The cardiac enzyme lactase dehydrogenase increased slightly in the antioxidant group, when compared with the placebos.

It was also reported that blood levels of lipid peroxides decreased over 5-fold in the antioxidant group, and angina pectoris (chest pain), total arrhythmias, and poor ventricular outcome occurred less frequently in the antioxidant group.

Antioxidant supplements of vitamins A, E, C, and beta-carotene in recent acute myocardial infarction may be protective against cardiac necrosis and oxidative stress, Singh said.

In evaluating 675 patients with myocardial infarction, compared with 725 controls, there was a strong inverse relationship between beta-carotene and heart attack incidence, which was dependent on polyunsaturated fatty acid intake, according to Arteriosclerosis and Thrombosis.

Beta-carotene showed a protective effect of heart attack risk in men, especially if there was a large amount of polyunsaturated fatty acids consumed.[5]

Researchers at the University of Tennessee at Memphis evaluated provitamin A activity and carotid artery plaques in 12,773 people in the Atherosclerosis Risk in Communities Studies, who were between the ages of 45 and 64, who had plaques examined by B-mode ultrasound of multiple carotid artery segments.[6] B-mode is a 2-dimensional diagnostic ultrasound procedure of echo-producing interfaces in a single plane, in which the intensity of the echo is represented by modulation of the brightness (B) of the spot.

It was reported that those in the highest quintile of carotid consumption had a lower prevalence of plaques compared to those in the lowest quintile of carotenoid consumption.

However, in women, the inverse association was especially strong for those who smoked. In men, no effect modification by smokers was seen. The inverse association was somewhat stronger in men between 55 and 64, compared to those 45 and 54.

The researchers added that carotid wall thickness is thought to occur early on in the disease, and they added that carotenoid intake was unrelated to average carotid artery wall thickness. Thus, carotenoids may exert their influence later rather than earlier in the atherosclerotic process.

Their findings supports the hypothesis that carotene-rich, plant-derived compounds may play a role in preventing arterial plaque formation.

Carotenoids, such as alpha-carotene and beta-carotene, are natural antioxidants that may reduce the risk of cardiovascular disease, reported Atherosclerosis.[7]

In the study, European researchers analyzed blood levels of various antioxidants and the thickness of carotid and femoral arteries among 392 men and women, who ranged in age from 45 to 65.

The researchers found that cardiovascular disease, as measured by the thickness of the carotid and femoral arteries, was inversely related to blood levels of alpha- and beta-carotene.

To assess the risk of cardiovascular disease, scientists measure the intima-media thickness (IMT) of the carotid artery. An increase in IMT suggests an abnormal thickening of the inner artery wall, which reduces blood flow and increases the risk of a heart attack or stroke. In studies, it has been found that lutein and other carotenoids may reduce the progression of IMT and protect against cardiovascular disease.[8]

As reported in Arteriosclerosis, Thrombosis and Vascular Biology, a research team used sophisticated ultrasound techniques to measure the IMT in the carotid artery of 573 middle-aged people who were free from symptomatic cardiovascular disease at the beginning of the study.

High blood levels of several carotenoids were strongly associated with reduced IMT progression over the 18-month trial. High blood levels of lutein, zeaxanthin, beta-cryptoxanthin, and alpha-carotene were associated with significant reductions in IMT progression.

Higher blood levels of all carotenoids, except zeaxanthin and vitamin C, were associated with lower blood levels of C-reactive protein, a marker for inflammation related to heart attack risk.

Existing research suggests that carotenoids may reduce the risk of heart disease, because carotene-rich foods quench the dangerous free radicals, and may reduce the oxidation of low-density lipoprotein cholesterol (LDL), an early step in the development of heart disease, according to the American Journal of Clinical Nutrition.[9]

Using a food questionnaire for carotenoid intake in 1984, researchers at Harvard University in Boston, Massachusetts, studied the eating habits and health of over 73,000 female nurses. During 12 years of follow-up, nonfatal heart attacks or fatal heart disease occurred in 998 of the women.

The researchers reported that women with the highest dietary intakes of beta-carotene and alpha-carotene were least likely to have fatal or non-fatal heart attacks. In fact, those with the highest intake of beta-carotene were 26% less likely to have coronary heart disease than those with the lowest intake, and those with the highest intake of alpha-carotene were 20% less likely to experience cardiovascular disease.

As reported in Biologia, a research team asked 48 healthy middle-aged men to take either a multi-antioxidant supplement or placebos daily for 3 months. The supplement contained 100 mg of vitamin E; 100 mg of vitamin C; 6 mg of beta-carotene; and 50 mcg of selenium. Vitamin E is usually listed in International Units (IU), but some researchers give milligrams, since the units are somewhat similar.[10]

At the beginning and end of the study, blood was taken from the volunteers and tested for LDL oxidation and levels of malondialdehyer (MDA), a marker for free radical activity.

Those taking the multi-antioxidant supplement had significant reductions in LDL oxidation and MDA levels. Tests indicated that their LDL was 11% more resistant to oxidation, and that plasma MDA levels decreased by 22%. There were no changes in the controls.

Carotenoids may help to reduce the risk of hardening of the arteries, lung disease, chronic inflammation, and neurological disorders, reported Archives of Biochemistry and Biophysics.[11]

A research team studied the interaction of peroxynitrite, a specific type of free radical, and numerous carotenoids within the LDL form of cholesterol.

While all of the carotenoids quenched the peroxynitrite radicals, the most effective carotenoids, in descending order, were lycopene, alpha-carotene, beta-carotene, beta-cryptoxanthin, zeaxanthin, and lutein.

The researchers suggest that a mix of carotenoids may be better than any single carotenoid in fighting free radicals. This is important because the oxidation of LDL is an early step in the development of heart disease, and the carotenoids protect LDL cholesterol from oxidation.

Stroke: A study in The Lancet evaluated 80 patients who were admitted to hospital because of a sudden focal neurologic deficit lasting over 3 hours. The deficit was due to acute ischemia in the territory of the middle cerebral artery, reported J. De Keyser, Ph.D., of the University of Brussels in Belgium.[12]

The patients who had serum vitamin A concentrations higher than the mean of 2.27 micromole/l were associated with a higher frequency of complete recovery within the first 24 hours, decreased mortality, and a better outcome as assessed by the Scale of Neurologic Deficit and the Barthel Index. There was no benefit from vitamin E. A micromole is one-millionth of a mole.

The authors added that high blood levels of vitamin A in stroke patients had a beneficial effect on early outcome. It seems that oxygen deficiency due to ischemia prevents oxidative phosphorylation and inhibits the production of adenosine 5′ triphosphate (ATP), the energy source of cellular ionic pumps.

This results in a rapid loss of potassium from the cell, and a subsequent depolarization of the cell membrane, allowing for uncontrolled calcium entry into the neurons, which impairs mitochondrial function and leads to further reduction of the ATP activated enzymes that deregulate proteins, nucleic acids, and phospholipids. It is apparently the phospholipid degradation that causes the neuronal damage, the researchers added.

To assess the risk of cardiovascular disease, researchers measure the intima-media thickness (IMT) of the carotid artery. Increased IMT represents an abnormal thickening of the inner artery wall, which reduces blood flow and increases the risk of heart attack and stroke, according to Arteriosclerosis, Thrombosis and Vascular Biology. It has been found that lutein and other carotenoids may reduce the progression of IMT and protect against cardiovascular disease.[13]

The research team used sophisticated ultrasound techniques to measure the IMT in the carotid artery of 573 middle-aged volunteers, who were free of symptomatic cardiovascular disease as the study began.

The people were also measured for blood levels of several antioxidant carotenoids, along with vitamins A, C, and E. After 18 months, the volunteers' IMT was again measured. Changes in IMT were correlated with the subjects' blood levels of individual antioxidants.

It was found that high levels of several carotenoids were strongly associated with reduced IMT progression over the 18-month study. High levels of lutein, zeaxanthin, beta-cryptoxanthin, and alpha-carotene were associated with significant reductions in IMT progression.

Also, higher blood levels of all carotenoids, except zeaxanthin, and vitamin C, were associated with lower blood levels of C-reactive protein, a marker of inflammation related to heart-attack risk.

It has been reported that elevated blood levels of C-reactive protein increase the risk of heart diseases by 4.5 times. C-reactive protein is regarded as both a predictor of heart disease risk and a substance that is toxic to blood vessel walls.[14]

Researchers reported in the American Journal of Epidemiology a relationship between blood levels of major dietary carotenoids—alpha-carotene, beta-carotene, beta-cryptoxanthin, lycopene, and lutein/zeaxanthin—and 3 markers of inflammation, including C-reactive protein.

It was found that all the carotenoids were significantly lower among those with high C-reactive protein levels, when compared to those with normal C-reactive protein amounts.

A variety of antioxidants and scavengers have been shown to reduce both cell damage and arrhythmias initiated by oxyradicals in ischemic and reperfused heart, reported Molecular and Cellular Biochemistry.[15]

In the study, the researchers tested the effect of vitamins A and E in reducing oxyradical effects and myocardial damage after ischemia-reperfusion in the rabbit heart.

The rabbits were pretreated with 150 mg of vitamin E and 60,000 IU of vitamin A 24 hours before the surgery. After reperfusion, full-thickness needle samples were obtained from 5 different myocardial areas. Controls received a different therapy.

In the vitamin-treated group, hydroperoxide-initiated chemiluminescence was decreased by 8% in the ischemic and non-reperfused ventrical areas and by 51-75% in the ventricular ischemic and reperfused areas.

The hearts of the animals displayed early signs of irreversible damage and infarction. The authors concluded that vitamins A and E reduce hydroperoxide-initiated chemiluminescence and myocardial cell damage during ischemia-reperfusion, at least in the rabbit. Chemiluminescence is light produced by chemical action at or below room temperature.

References

1. Voutilainen, Sari, et al. "Carotenoids and Cardiovascular Health," American Journal of Clinical Nutrition 82: 1265-1271, 2006.
2. Di Mascio, P., et al. "Lycopene As the Most Efficient Biological Carotenoid Singlet Oxygen Quencher," Archives of Biochemistry and Biophysics 274: 532-538, 1989.
3. Tapiero, H., et al. "The Role of Carotenoids in the Prevention of Human Pathogens," Biomedical Pharmotherapy 58: 100-110, 2004.
4. Singh, Ram B., M.D., et al. 'Usefulness of Antioxidant Vitamins in Suspected Acute Myocardial Infarction (The Indian Experiment of Infarct Survival-3,) The American Journal of Cardiology 77: 232-236, February 1, 1996.
5. "Antioxidants and Myocardial Infarction," The Nutrition Report, September 1995, p. 59.
6. Kritchevsky, S.B., et al. "Provitamin A Carotenoid Intake and Carotid Artery Plaques: The Atherosclerosis Risk in Communities Study," American Journal of Clinical Nutrition 68: 726-733, 1998.
7. D'Odorico, A., et al. "High Plasma Levels of Alpha- and Beta-Carotene are Associated with a Lower Risk of Atherosclerosis. Results from the Bruneck Study," Atherosclerosis 153: 231-239, 2000.
8. Dwyer, J.H. et al. "Progression of Carotid Intima-Media Thickness and Plasma Antioxidants: The Los Angeles Atherosclerosis Study," Arteriosclerosis, Thrombosis and Vascular Biology 24: 313-319, 2004.
9. Osganian, S.K., et al. "Dietary Carotenoids and Risk of Coronary Artery Disease in Women," American Journal of Clinical Nutrition 77: 1390-1399, 2003.
10. Nagyova, A., et al. "Plasma Antioxidant Status and LDL Oxidizability in Healthy Men After Dietary Supplementation with a Mixture of Antioxidant Nutrients," Biologia 58: 1095-1100, 2003.
11. Panasenko, O.M., et al. "Interaction of Peroxynitrite with Carotenoids in Human Low Density Lipoprotein," Archives of Biochemistry and Biophysics 373: 302-305, 2000.
12. De Keyser, J., Ph.D. et al. "Serum Vitamin Concentrations of Vitamins A and E and Early Outcome After Ischemic Stroke," The Lancet 339: 1562-1565, June 27, 1992.
13. Dwyer, J.H., et al. "Progression of Carotid Intima-Media Thickness and Plasma Antioxidants: The Los Angeles Atherosclerosis Study," Arteriosclerosis, Thrombosis and Vascular Biology 24: 313-319, 2004.
14. Kritchevsky, S.B., et al. "Serum Carotenoid and Markers of Inflammation in Nonsmokers," American Journal of Epidemiology 152: 1065-1071, 2000.
15. Llesuy, S., et al. "Effect of Vitamins A and E on Ischemia Reperfusion Damage in Rabbit Heart," Molecular and Cellular Biochemistry 145(1): 45-51, 1995.

12

IMMUNITY

The immune system is a collection of cells and proteins that work to protect the body from potential harmful, infections microorganisms (microscopic life-forms), such as bacteria, viruses, and fungi, according to the American Medical Association Home Medical Encyclopedia. The immune system also plays a role in the control of cancer, and it is responsible for the phenomena of allergy, hypersensitivity, and rejection problems when organs or tissues are transplanted.[1]

"A newborn child is, to some extent, protected against infection by barriers—such as the skin—by substances in the mouth, in the urinary tract, or on the eye surface that destroys microorganisms, and by antibodies and immunoglobulins (protective proteins) that have been passed to the child from the mother—including those received in breast milk," the publication added.

The acquisition of immunity, in response to an infection can take a few days or weeks to develop, and in the interim, a child or adult can become very ill and die.

Today, our chance of surviving, recovering, or totally avoiding infectious disease is much improved, partly as a result of better general health and nutrition—which bolsters the immune system—and partly through immunization against specific disease-causing microorganisms, the publication continued.

"If microorganisms are able to penetrate the outer layer of the skin or a mucous membrane, they soon encounter white blood cells called phagocytes (literally engulfing cells), which attempt to destroy them, and other types of white cells, such as natural killer (cytotoxic) cells," the publication added. "Microorganisms may also meet naturally produced substances (such as interferon), or a system of blood proteins known as the complement system, which act to destroy the invading microorganisms."

The immune system responds—whether hormonal or cellular—to an invading organism, and mounts an attack against an antigen (a protein that is foreign or different from any natural body protein).

"The hormonal response consists of the production of soluble proteins, called antibodies, or immunoglobulins, which are manufactured by cells called B-lymphocytes," the publication said. "Cellular responses center around the activities of the cells called T-lymphocytes."

Cellular immunity is especially important in the defense against viruses, some types of parasites that hide within cells, and, possibly cancer cells. The T-lymphocytes at the center of cellular immunity are of 2 types—helper cells and killer cells.

"The helper cells play a role in the recognition of antigens," the publication continued. "Along with various functions, they activate the killer cells. Killer lymphocytes lock onto cells that have been invaded by viruses or other parasites that have left recognizable antigens on the cell surfaces. The killer lymphocytes then destroy these parasitized cells. They may act in a similar way against tumor cells."

The immune system is a complicated and poorly understood defense mechanism in that it can destroy cancer, unless it is weakened by poor nutrition, emotional stress, or "locking factors" that are formed in advanced cancers, said Richard A. Passwater, Ph.D., in The Nutrition Superbook: The Antioxidants.[2]

He reviewed earlier research, and said that, in 1925, researchers initially noticed that there was a relationship between a deficiency in vitamin A and cancer. Several experiments from the 1930s through the 1950s confirmed this relationship, and, since then, we have learned that cancer-causing chemicals can react strongly with DNA in vitamin A-deficient cells; that cancers are hard to transplant into animals adequartely nourished with vitamin A; and that vitamin A is therapeutic in dealing with precancerous cells.

He added that scientific evidence about the effectiveness of vitamin A increased in 1974, when Dr. Frank Chytill of Vanderbilt University remarked that, "recent dramatic findings about vitamin A and its effects on cancer have opened up a whole new approach to cancer therapy. With vitamin A therapy, doctors may some day have a way to restore body cells to normal—rather than destroy them with surgery, chemotherapy, or radiation. We now have laboratory evidence that, under certain lab conditions, cancers such as breast, lung, and skin tumors can be cured by treatment with vitamin A. People can certainly cut their chances of getting cancer by making sure they are not deficient in vitamin A."

Passwater quoted Dr. David Ong, also of Vanderbilt University, as saying that, "We know that lack of vitamin A retards normal growth, weakens the mucous linings of the body, and causes night blindness. But when the proper level of vitamin A is restored, the body returns to normal. Preliminary evidence from Europe strongly indicates that vitamin A works the same way with cancer".

Passwater also quoted Dr. George Plotkin of the Massachusetts Institute of Technology as saying that, "A deficiency of vitamin A prevents a mucous coating from forming on the trachea, lungs, rectum, digestive system, and on the inside of the skin. A vitamin A deficiency doesn't cause cancer, but it makes these areas less able to resist cancer."

"Dr. E. Bjelke of the Cancer Registry in Norway found that 74% of the men with lung cancer were in the lowest third of the population, ranked by vitamin A intake," Passwater continued. "He also found that vitamin A especially helped smokers living in cities. Vitamin A-deficient city dwellers have 3 times the lung cancer rate of better-nourished city dwellers."

Dr. Michael Sporn was quoted as saying that, "Well over half of all human cancers start in epithelial tissue, the tissue that forms the lining of organs, forms glands such as mammary glands, skin, and passages in the body. The respiratory tract, the digestive tract, and the reproductive tract are all lined with epithelial tissue. And all of the specialized cells that form epithelial tissue depend on vitamin A for their normal development."

D.S.B. Wolbach of Harvard University was quoted as saying that, as far back as the 1920s, there was a relationship between vitamin A deficiency and cancer, since there are similarities between the cancerous process and what goes on in tissues that are vitamin A-deficient in terms of loss of control in cell differentiation. The problem that exists with cancer was pointed out many years ago. Wolbach added.

Dr. Sporn was quoted as saying that vitamin A works by strengthening the contention that cancer can be prevented or slowed with vitamins. As to whether vitamin A therapy actually arrests the development of cancer or whether this causes the precancerous cells to disappear from tissue, this is still being investigated.

"If all you do is just slow down this process of development of cancer so that instead of the typical 25-year latent period from the time people may develop cancer, you double that latent period, and there would be 20 additional years of good life that you would be offering people," Sporn said.

As often reported, vitamin A is especially important for growth, cellular differentation, and cell-cell or cell-substrate interactions, explained A. Catherine Ross, M.D., of the Medical College of Pennsylvania in Philadelphia.[3]

At the time of her article, she said that, in the previous 5 years, there had been an increase in interest in the role of vitamin A and immunity, based on 3 important advances: (1) there have been a variety of controlled studies demonstrating that vitamin A can decrease mortality in preschool children in populations at high risk for vitamin A deficiency; (2) vitamin A in the form of retinol or retinoic acid has been shown to stimulate the rejection of certain immunogenic tumors; and (3) there has been an increased interest in vitamin A's mechanism of action in almost all organ systems, as a result of the identification of nuclear receptors for retinoic acid, and the understanding that retinoic acid's role in gene regulation.

Historically, she continued, the potential relationship between vitamin A status and infectious disease has been noted since the 1900s. In experimental animals, vitamin A deficiency has a wide range of effects on immune function, including alterations in organ morphology, cell number, and response to specific pathogens and antigens, as well as nonspecific protection through phagocytic and cytotoxic mechanisms.

She added that, in almost all of the studies, vitamin A repletion has effectively reversed these adverse changes. In a variety of animal models, antibody production and phagocytosis has been found to be augmented in animals with normal vitamin A status. Although there have been studies showing vitamin A supplementation in high-risk populations to reduce the incidence of morbidity and mortality, more information is needed to determine whether vitamin A status in children in these populations is sufficiently low to compromise the response to vaccines or the ability to clear infectious agents.

In 20 patients with common variable immunodeficiency (CVI), with a median age of 42, 65% of the women when compared with 16 controls (median age of 41, which included 63% females), it was found that the majority of CVI patients had reduced vitamin A levels when compared with healthy controls.[4] CVI, of unknown origin, may occur at any age in either sex. The quantity of immunoglobulin is often less than 300 mg/dl, the number of B-lymphocytes is within the normal range, but there is a lack of plasma cells in lymphoid tissue. There is an increased susceptibility to infections as well as autoimmune disease.

Low vitamin A levels in the blood were associated with the occurrence of chronic bacterial infections and splenomegaly (enlarged spleen), as well as high neopterin levels. The latter is a pteridine (pigment) found in body fluids, and elevated levels result in immune system activation, malignant disease, and viral infections such as AIDS.

When vitamin A supplementation at 350,000 IU was given orally to 6 patients with low vitamin A levels, this resulted in increased interleukin-10 and a reduction in tumor necrosis factor levels. The study suggests that vitamin A supplementation may play a role in CVI, possibly by enhancing synthesis and downregulating inflammatory responses, reported the European Journal of Clinical Investigation.

Interleukin-10 is a cytokine derived from T-helper cells that inhibit gamma-interferon secretion by T-cell lymphocytes, as well as inhibiting mononuclear cell inflammation.

Writing in Clinical Infectious Diseases in 1994, Richard D. Semba, M.D., of Johns Hopkins Hospital in Baltimore, Maryland, reported that, at the time of his article, at least a dozen clinical trials had been done with vitamin A supplementation, and the trials had shown a reduction in severe morbidity and mortality from infectious diseases among children, who have acute measles, or who are from areas where a vitamin A deficiency is endemic.[5]

Vitamin A deficiency is an immunodeficiency characterized by alterations in immunity, changes in mucosal surfaces, impaired antibody responses, changes in lymphocyte subpopulations, and altered T- and B-cell function.

He added that vitamin A and its metabolites have immune enhancing properties, and they have been shown to potentiate antibody responses to T-cell-dependent antigens, increase lymphocyte proliferation responses to antigens and mitogens, inhibit apoptosis (cell death), and restore mucosal cell surfaces.

The specific immune-response genes that may be regulated by vitamin A through its metabolites have yet to be identified, since there is a gap in knowledge regarding the effect of vitamin A deficiency and treatment on the function as phagocytosis of natural killer cells, Semba continued.

At that time, he said that it is estimated that 124 million children are deficient in vitamin A, and, therefore, at a higher risk of death from infectious diseases. Improvement in vitamin A nutriture is expected to prevent 1.3 to 2.5 million deaths annually, and a periodic high-dose of vitamin A is now widely practiced in many countries where vitamin A deficiency is pronounced.

He goes on to say that high-dose vitamin A supplementation for children with acute measles is expected to contribute to a reduced mortality, and that measles is responsible for 2 million deaths annually.

Whether vitamin A will be able to reduce the severe morbidity and mortality from malaria and tuberculosis is yet to be discovered, he added. However, it is estimated that between 38 and 108 million people will be infected with HIV in the coming years. Vitamin A is inexpensive and it is one of the most cost-effective means of reducing childhood mortality, he said.

In an article in the Journal of Nutrition, Dr. Semba reviewed the history of the use of vitamin A as an "anti-infective agent," which was widely accepted by the 1940s, when the United States and Great Britain were very "vitamin conscious."[6]

During World War II, cod-liver oil was provided by the British Ministry of Food for children under 5 years of age, and for pregnant and breastfeeding women. As a source of vitamin A, the administration of cod-liver oil became part of the morning routine for millions of children in America and Europe. The oil is also a rich source of vitamin D, omega-3 fatty acids and other nutrients.

Controlled trials have evolved quite significantly since then, Semba continued, when vitamin A was called the "anti-infective" vitamin by Nellanby in 1934.

After a pause of almost 50 years, the value of vitamin A as an anti-infective therapy has been investigated in controlled trials, and there is compelling new evidence for the use of vitamin A as an important public health intervention, Semba continued.

In a study by Dr. Semba and his colleagues, as reported in Clinical and Diagnostic Laboratory Immunology, they evaluated the profile of the anti-tetanus IgG subclasses in children given vitamin A supplements or a placebo, in order to assess the potential use of the enhanced anti-tetanus toxoid response.[7]

In the study, the levels of the different anti-tetanus toxoid IgG subclasses were measured 2 weeks before and 3 weeks after immunization in 139 Indonesian preschool children ranging in age from 3 to 6.

The children who were given vitamin A prior to the immunization had significantly increased IgG-1 levels, whether or not they were undergoing primary or memory reactions.

In the children who underwent a secondary response to tetanus toxoid, vitamin A supplementation was associated with a modest, but significant, change in the level of anti-tetanus IgG-3. There were only minor changes in the levels of anti-tetanus IgG-2 and IgG-4. Because IgG-1 is a subclass that is associated with a protective response to tetanus toxoid immunization, these results suggest that vitamin A supplementation may be a safe and effective way to enhance the humoral response to tetanus toxoid and other vaccine antigens, the researchers added.

A vitamin A deficiency can compromise immune function, resulting in major morbidity and mortality, Dr. Semba reported in Nutrition Reviews. The role of vitamin A in infectious disease has been known for hundreds of years, and vitamin A supplementation in hospitals has been shown to reduce child mortality by 20 to 30%.[8]

Vitamin A capsule distribution is one of the most cost-effective interventions to improve health, and it ranks among vaccination and rehydration therapy in importance as a public health measure, Semba continued.

Vitamin A and related retinoids have therapeutic potential as immune modulators. Immune responses regulated by retinoids include keratinization (formation of hair, nails, etc.) mucin production (a substance of connective tissue); hematopoiesis (formation of blood cells); apoptosis (cell death); neutrofil function; natural killer cell function; monocyte/macrophage function; Langerhans cells function (in diabetes); T-lymphocyte function; cytotoxic T-lymphocyte function; B-lymphocyte function; immunoglobulin production; interleukin production; tumor necrosis factor production; and phospholipase A2 production. The latter enzyme has an important role in prostaglandin and leukotriene biosynthesis.

Over 22,000 male physicians were given beta-carotene at 50 mg on alternate days, or a placebo, for an average of 12 years. Those given beta-carotene had greater blood levels of beta-carotene than those taking a placebo, and they had significantly greater natural killer cell activity than those getting a look-alike pill, reported the American Journal of Clinical Nutrition.[9]

The study confirms that long-term beta-carotene supplementation significantly enhances natural killer cell activity in older men, when compared with controls.

Vitamin A and Vaccines

A vitamin A supplement given at birth is associated with decreased mortality in Asia, reported the American Journal of Clinical Nutrition.

In tuberculosis-endemic countries, researchers prescribe Bacille Calmette-Guerin (BCG) vaccine for newborn infants. Previous studies have shown that vitamin A supplements may influence the immune responses to the vaccines.

The researchers reported that vitamin A supplements and the BCG vaccination apparently do not interfere with long-term response to vitamin A supplements given with the vaccine.

However, the vitamin A supplements temporarily altered delayed-type hypersensitivity reactions to mycobacterium tuberculosis in boys 2 months of age, suggesting sex differences in the immunologic response to vitamin A supplements given with BCG.

Source: Diness, Brigitte R., et al. "Effect of High-Dose Vitamin A Supplements on the Immune Response to Bacille Calmette-Guerin Vaccine," American Journal of Clinical Nutrition 86(4): 1152-1159, October 2007.

Vitamin A and Childhood Infections

The World Health Organization has reported that pneumococcal infections are a leading cause of complications and death in young children worldwide, resulting in 650,000 infant deaths in the developing countries each year, according to the Journal of Nutrition.

Streptococcus pneumonia is a leading cause of fatal bacterial pneumonia, the most common cause of otitis media and sepsis—toxins in the blood. It is also a leading cause of meningitis, an inflammation of the brain and spinal cord.

Researchers recruited 464 infants, who were 2 months old, in South India, who were randomly assigned to be given 27,000 mcg (micrograms) retinol equivalent doses of vitamin A by mouth at birth. Nasopharyngeal—affecting the nose and throat—specimens were collected at ages 2, 4, and 6 months.

The risk of colonization with the bacteria among infants at 4 months of age, who were not colonized at 2 months, was significantly reduced in those given vitamin A compared to the controls. The odds of colonization were 27% lower in the treatment group.

The odds of colonization with penicillin-resistant isolates was 74% lower in the vitamin A group at 2 months of age.

The researchers said that neonatal vitamin A supplements may play a role in lowering morbidity rates associated with pneumococcal disease by delaying the age at which colonization occurs.

Source: Coles, Christian L., et al. "Vitamin A Supplements at Birth Delays Pneumococcal Colonization in South Indian Infants," Journal of Nutrition 131: 255-261, 2001.

Vitamin A and Infant Mortality

In a study involving 11,619 newborns in two rural districts of Tamil Nadu in southern India, researchers gave the infants 24,000 IU of vitamin A or a look-alike pill on days 1 and 2 following delivery, reported the British Medical Journal.

Infants in the vitamin A group had a 22% reduction in deaths, compared with those getting a placebo.

The vitamin had an impact on mortality between 2 weeks and 3 months following treatment, however, there was no reported benefits after 3 months.

Source: Rahmathullah, Lakshmi. "Impact of Supplementing Newborn Infants with Vitamin A on Early Infant Mortality: Commentary Based on Randomized Trial in Southern India," British Medical Journal 327: 254, 2003.

References

1. Clayman, Charles B., M.D., medical editor. The American Medical Association Home Medical Encyclopedia. New York: Random House, 1989, pp. 570-571.
2. Passwater, Richard A., Ph.D. "Antioxidants." The Nutrition Superbook: The Antioxidants. New Canaan, CT: Keats Publishing, Inc., 1995, pp. 5ff.
3. Ross, A. Catherine M.D. "Vitamin A Status: Relationship to Immunity and the Antibody Response," PSEMB 2000: 303-320, 1992.
4. Aukuret, P., et al. "Decreased Vitamin A Levels in Common Variable Immunodeficiency: Vitamin Supplementation In Vivo Enhances Immunoglobulin Production and Downregulates Inflammatory Responses," European Journal of Clinical Investigation 30(3): 252-259, 2000.
5. Semba, Richard D., M.D. "Vitamin A, Immunity and Infection," Clinical Infections Disease 19: 489-499, 1994.

6. Semba, Richard D., M.D. "Vitamin A As 'Anti-Infective' Therapy," Journal of Nutrition 129: 783-791, 1999.
7. Semba, Richard D., M.D., et al. "Effect of Vitamin A Supplementation on Immunoglobulin-G Subclass Response to Tetanus Toxoid in Children," Clinical and Diagnostic Laboratory Immunology 1(2): 172-175, March 1994.
8. Semba, Richard D., M.D. "The Role of Vitamin A and Related Retinoid Function," Nutrition Reviews 56(1): S38-S48, January 1998.
9. Santos, M.S., et al. "Beta-Carotene Induced Enhancement of Natural Killer Cell Activity in Elderly Men: An Investigation of the Role of Cytokines," American Journal of Clinical Nutrition 68: 164-170, 1998.

13

LUNG DISEASES

The main organ of the respiratory system, 2 lungs supply the body with oxygen and eliminate carbon dioxide from the blood, reported The Americal Medical Association Home Medical Encyclopedia.[1]

The trachea (windpipe) terminates in the chest into 2 main bronchi (air passages), which supply the left and right lungs. The main bronchi divide again into smaller bronchi, and then into bronchioles, which lead to air passages that open out into grapelike air sacs called alveoli. It is through the thin walls of the alveoli that gases diffuse into or out of the blood.

The lungs lie in the chest within the rib cage, and air entering the body by the nose and mouth travels down the trachea to the main bronchi. During espiration (breathing out), air leaves the body by the same route.

The lungs are continuously exposed to airborne particles, such as bacteria, viruses, and antigens, all of which can cause lung disorders, the publication said.

Some of the disorders of the lungs include:

1. Tracheitis, inflammation of the lining of the windpipe.
2. Bronchitis, inflammation of the bronchi.
3. Pneumonia, inflammation of the lungs.
4. Bronchial asthma, in which the muscles of the bronchi contract and obstruct the free passage of air.
5. Alergic alveoilitis, inflammation of the alveoli.
6. Lung cancer, usually associated with smoking.
7. Pulmonary embolism, in which blood clots formed elsewhere in the body break away and are carried to the lungs.

8. Emphysema, in which the walls of the alveoli seriously interfere with the oxygen supply.
9. Respiratory distress syndrome, often in newborns, which affects the oxygen supply.
10. Tuberculosis, caused by the tubercle bacillus, which mainly affects the lungs.
11. Chronic obstructive pulmonary disease (COPD), permanent or temporary narrowing of small bronchi in which forced expiratory flow is slowed.

Pneumonia: Vitamin A is stored in the liver and is transported to peripheral tissues through the blood by retinol binging protein (RBP). When liver stores fall below a critical level, serum retinol also decreases and can then be used as an indicator of liver stores, according to researchers at the School of Public Health, University of Alabama, in Birmingham.[2]

"The level at which this occurs varies among people, therefore, serum retinol is an inaccurate measure for identifying those with marginal vitamin A stores," the researchers said.

When serum retinol is less than 1.05 mol/l, stores are likely to be marginal, and concentrations of less than 0.70 micromol/l indicate that stores are probably depleted. Blood levels of less than 0.35 micromol/l are found in those with a clinical deficiency (xerophthalmia), when stores are essentially absent, the researchers added.

The objective of their study was to assess, with the relative-dose-response (RDR) test, the vitamin A status of children recovering from pneumonia. The trial used high-dose vitamin A supplements among children hospitalized with pneumonia in Lima, Peru. The researchers examined the association of treatment group, nutritional status, severity of the illness, and induction of the acute phase response—on the basis of serum C-reactive protein—on serum retinol and RDR test.

The researchers added that the RDR test was useful in assessing the vitamin A status of children recovering from pneumonia when C-reactive protein concentrations were less than 10 mg/1, but not when CPR concentrations were higher. CPR stands for cardiopulmonary resuscitation.

Serum retinol concentrations may decrease during acute infection, but typically rebound to preinfection concentrations within a few days, the researchers continued. This transient decrease does not reflect a depletion of liver stores, and, thus, it can interfere with the use of serum retinol as an indicator of vitamin A status.

Oral vitamin A and placebo preparations were given in a double-blind fashion, according to a randomized block design. No signs of toxicity were recorded.

The treatment involved a water-miscible preparation of retinol containing 50,000 IU/ml (15 mg/ml), and an identical placebo syrup. Children less than 1 year of age received 100,000 IU (2 ml, 30 mg) of vitamin A on admission to the study, and 50,000 IU (1 ml or 15 mg) on the second day of hospitalization.

Those over 1 year of age were given 200,000 IU (4 ml or 60 mg) on the second day. The controls received the appropriate volume of placebo syrup on both days.

At the just-named university, the same researchers evaluated 29 people with pneumonia and sepsis (infection), and found their mean excretion rate of vitamin A was 0.78 micromol per day. Those with fever excreted significantly more retinol than did those without fever.[3]

It was reported that 34% of the patients excreted over 1.75 micromol of retinol daily, which is equivalent to 50% of the RDA. This data suggests that vitamin A requirements are substantially increased during serious infections, because of the excretion of retinol in the urine.

Possible reasons for the association of acute infection with development of vitamin A deficiency include decreased intake of vitamin A-containing foods because of anorexia, decreased absorption of vitamin A during diarrhea, and increased metabolic requirements and impaired transport from the liver to target tissues during acute phase response.

The research team added that their study suggests that the excretion of vitamin A in the urine may also be an important link between infection and the subsequent development of vitamin A deficiency.

At Kokding Hospital in Denmark, researchers evaluated high-dose vitamin A—between 200,000 and 400,000 IU of retinol—in 592 children between 1 and 59 months of age, who were diagnosed with moderate and severe pneumonia, reported Acta Pediatrica.[4]

It was found that those who were given vitamin A and who were malnourished had a shorter time of hospitalization. The vitamin A was in peanut oil at a concentration of 200,000 IU retinol/ml. Each child was given 2 doses from the same bottle.

For children less than 1 year of age, the dosage was 0.5 ml on the day of inclusion and the day after. Those 1 to 4 years of age received 2 doses of 1.0 ml.

The researchers added that, in developing countries, supplementation with vitamin A in children with pneumonia could shorten the recovery rate in those who are undernourished, especially females greater than 1 year of age.

Bronchopulmonary dysplasia : In a study reported in Early Human Development, a dose of 5,000 IU of vitamin A 3 times a week was given to 91 very-low-birth-weight infants. There were no signs of clinical toxicity with the higher dosage, and blood levels of vitamin A.[5]

The authors encourage a trial of vitamin A supplementation at the 5,000 IU dose 3 times weekly to assess when vitamin A supplementation safely reduces the risk of bronchopulmonary dysplasia in very-low birth-weight infants. This disorder is chronic pulmonary insufficiency that arises from long-term artificial pulmonary ventilation, and it is often found in premature infants.

As reported in the American Journal of Perinatology, a research team evaluated 22 infants with a birthweight of less than 1,250 grams, who had baseline membrane disease that required mechanical ventilation with oxygen.[6]

Thirteen of the infants had 1 or more serum vitamin A concentrations less than 11 mcg/dl at greater than 10 days of age. In 9 infants, blood levels of vitamin A were greater than 11 mcg/d1 at greater than 10 days of age.

The incidence of severe bronchopulmonary dysplasia—which relates to bronchial tubes in the lungs—was significantly higher in the children with lower blood levels of vitamin A, and 3 of the children died.

The incidence of pulmonary air leak, the number of ventilator days, the number of days of postnasal glucocorticoid treatment for lung disease, the number of episodes of suspected sepsis (toxins in the blood), and the number of days of antibiotic treatment also were higher in the children with low blood levels of vitamin A, according to Rita Prasad Verma, M.D., and colleagues.

She went on to say that persistent marked vitamin A deficiency in low birth-weight infants is associated with a high incidence of severe bronchopulmonary dysplasia, delayed onset of enteral feeding, and low enteral intake of vitamin A.

Bronchial metaplasia : Bronchial biopsies from 49 asbestos workers found that those with metaplasia reported consuming significantly lower amounts of vitamin A—2,000 retinal equivalents/day—compared to those without metaplasia at 2,710 REs/day.[7] Metaplasia is the abnormal replacement of cells of 1 type by cells of another.

The researchers reported in the American Journal of Clinical Nutrition that higher intakes of retinol, provitamin A carotenoids, and total vitamin A were associated with a nonsignificant reduction in the odds ratio for metaplasia. A greater airway obstruction was associated with an increased odds ratio for metaplasia.

The researchers added that a higher intake of vitamin A from food reduces the risk of bronchial metaplasia in asbestos workers who have been exposed to the mineral.

COPD: At the Faculty of Medicine in Botucatu, Brazil, researchers evaluated the relationship between vitamin A status and the degree of lung airway obstruction in a cross-sectional study of 30 men between the ages of 43 and 74, who were healthy nonsmokers, healthy smokers, mild COPD patients, COPD-moderate-severe patients, and COPD moderate-severe patients with exacerbations.[8]

In 12 male smokers, between 45 and 61 with mild COPD, 6 men consumed vitamin A at 1,000 RE/day, and 6 men received a placebo for 30 days.

Low blood levels of retinol concentrations were found in the COPD-moderate-severe, and COPD-moderate severe with exacerbations group. It was also found that there was improvement in pulmonary function tests after vitamin A supplementation, which supports the assumption of a local vitamin A deficiency in patients with chronic obstructive pulmonary disease, the researchers added.

Vitamin A's critical value to the skin is but one aspect of its benefit to all epithelial tissues, according to Robert C. Atkins, M.D.[9]

"I have always used vitamin A as part of the Atkins Center protocol for emphysema, a form of chronic obstructive pulmonary disease (COPD)," he said. "Scientific studies show that those with severe pulmonary disease exhibit low levels of vitamin A, and the patients who take vitamin A supplements exhibit improved lung function."

Vitamin A deficiency affects 190 million preschool-aged children, and 19 million pregnant women worldwide, reported William Checkley, M.D., Ph.D., of Johns Hopkins University School of Medicine in Baltimore, Maryland, and colleagues at other facilities. It is the underlying cause of 650,000 early childhood deaths, and it has become recognized as an important problem among women of reproductive age in many developing countries.[10, 11, 12]

"The importance of vitamin A in regulating growth through cell proliferation and differentiation was recognized early in the 20th century," the researchers said. "Results from animal studies have since shown that vitamin A plays a key role in mediating fetal growth, morphogenesis (formation of tissues and organs), and maturation of multiple organ systems, including the respiratory system."

They added that since alveolarization (air conditioning cells of the lungs) begins in utero at about the 36th week of gestation, maternal vitamin A deficiency during pregnancy may have lasting effects of the lung maturation of their offspring.

Routine administration of vitamin A strengthens host defenses against infection, which can favor child survival in undernourished populations, the researchers continued. Randomized trials in Indonesia, India, and Bangladesh showed that oral supplementation with 50,000 IU of vitamin A in oil shortly after birth reduced the rates of death during the first year of life by 64, 23, and 16%, respectively. At sites in which specific causes of death were analyzed, the largest reductions were in diarrha-related deaths.

"In an area in which there was chronic vitamin A deficiency, maternal supplementation with vitamin A before, during, and after pregnancy was a critical determinant of lung maturation among offspring 9 to 13 years of age," the researchers said. "Early intervention involving vitamin A supplementation in communities where undernutrition is highly prevalent may have long-lasting consequences for lung health."

Vitamin A Is Important for Lung Function

Vitamin A is essential for the growth and development of cells and tissues, according to Molecular Aspects of Medicine. In its active form, retinoic acid, it controls the regular differentiation as a ligand—a molecule in a complex—for retinoic acid receptors, and it is involved in the integration of cell formation.

Vitamin A plays a significant role, especially in the respiratory epithelium and the lung. The epithelium is a thin layer of skin that covers glands and other surfaces.

During moderate vitamin A deficiency, the incidence for diseases of the respiratory tract is considerably increased, and repeated respiratory infections can be influenced therapeutically by moderate vitamin A supplements.

In addition to the importance of vitamin A for lung function, it is also responsible for the development of many tissues and cells in new-born infants.

Source: Biesaiski, H.K., and Nohr, D. "Importance of Vitamin A for Lung Function and Development," Molecular Aspects of Medicine 24(6): 431-440, December 2003.

Vitamin A and the Lungs

Vitamin A is a crucial antioxidant for pre-term infants, since it protects the lungs from oxidative damage induced by the supplemental oxygen given to them, researchers report.

Although all pre-term infants are born with smaller vitamin stores, the store of vitamin A in these children at risk for bronchopulmonary displasia (BDP) is often especially deficient.

In spite of increased blood levels of vitamin A achieved

through vitamin A supplements, only modest improvements in clinical outcomes and incidence of BDP have been reported in this population.

Source: Mentro, A.M. "Vitamin A and Bronchopulmonary Displasia: Research, Issues and Clinical Practice," Neonatal Netev. 23(4): 19-23, July/ August 2004.

References

1. Clayman, Charles B., M.D., medical editor. The American Medical Association Home Medical Encyclopedia. New York: Random House, 1989, pp. 650ff.
2. Stephenson, Charles B., M.D., et al. "Assessment of Vitamin A Status with the Relative-Dose-Response Test in Peruvian Children Recovering from Pneumonia," American Journal of Clinical Nutrition 76: 1351-1357, 2002.
3. Stephenson, Charles B., M.D., et al. "Vitamin A is Excreted in the Urine During Acute Infection," American Journal of Clinical Nutrition 60: 388-392, 1994.
4. Si, N.V., et al. "High-Dose Vitamin A Supplementation in the Course of Pneumonia in Vietnamese Children," Acta Pediatrica 86: 1052-1055, 1997.
5. Kennedy, Kathleen A., et al. "Vitamin A to Prevent Bronchopulmonary Dysplasia in Very-Low-Birth-Weight Infants. Has the Dose Been Too Low?" Early Human Development 49: 19-31, 1997.
6. Verma, Rita Prasad, M.D., et al. "Vitamin A Deficiency and Severe Bronchopulmonary Dysplasia in Very Low Birthweight Infants," American Journal of Perinatology 13(7): 389-393, October 1996.
7. Mayne, S.T., et al. "Dietary Vitamin A and Prevalence of Bronchial Metaplasia in Asbestos-Exposed Workers," American Journal of Clinical Nutrition 68: 630-635, 1998.
8. Paiva, Sergio A.R., et al. "Assessment of Vitamin A Status in Chronic Obstructive Pulmonary Disease Patients and Healthy Smokers," American Journal of Clinical Nutrition 64: 928-934, 1996.
9. Atkins, Robert C., M.D. Dr. Atkins' Vita-Nutrient Solution. New York: Simon & Schuster, 1998, p. 45.
10. Checkley, William, M.D., Ph.D., et al. "Maternal Vitamin A Supplementation and Lung Function in Offspring," New England Journal of Medicine 362: 1784-1794, 2010.
11. "Global Prevalence of Vitamin A Deficiency in Populations At Risk—1995-2005," WHO Global Database on Vitamin A Deficiency." Geneva, Switzerland: World Health Organization, 2009.
12. Zachman, R.D. "Role of Vitamin A in Lung Development," Journal of Nutrition 125: 1634S-1638S, 1995.

14

SKIN DISORDERS

The outermost covering of body tissue, which protects the internal organs from the environment, the skin is the largest organ in the body, reported the American Medical Association Home Medical Encyclopedia. Its cells are continually being replaced as they are lost through wear and tear.[1]

"The skin consists of a thin outer layer (epidermis) and a thicker inner layer (dermis)," the publication said. "Between the dermis is the subcutaneous tissue, which contains fat. The hair and nails are extensions of the skin and are composed mainly of keratin, which is the main constituent of the outermost part of the epidermis."

The skin is a sensory organ containing many cells that are sensitive to touch, temperature, pain, pressure, and itching. It also plays a significant role in keeping the body temperature constant.

When the body is warm, the sweat glands produce perspiration, which cools the body, and blood vessels in the dermis, which dilate (expand) to dissipate the heat. If the body gets cold, blood vessels in the skin constrict, thereby conserving the body's heat.

The skin is subject to a variety of infections and inflammation. Viral infections include cold sores, warts, chickenpox, herpes zoster, and others. Bacterial infections include boils, cellulitis, erysipelas, impetigo, etc. Inflammation of the skin involves dermatitis, eczema, psoriasis, and others. Acne is a hormonal disorder.

Psoriasis : As reported in Acta Dermatology Venerology (Stockholm), a research team evaluated vitamins A and E blood levels in 7 patients with erythrodermic psoriasis or psoriatic acral pustulosis that was associated or not with alcoholism. The same vitamins were studied in 5 patients with psoriasis vulgaris involving over 80% of the surface body area, and associated with chronic alcohol abuse, and 17 patients with psoriasis vulgaris involving over 50% of their skin without chronic alcoholism.[2]

Vitamin A levels were lower in all those with erythrodermia psoriasis/psoriatic acral pustulosis.

Vitamin E levels were below the normal range during acute psoriatic episodes in only 5 patients having a history of chronic alcohol intake.

The authors suggestion that attention should be paid to a vitamin A deficiency and erythrodermic or pustular psoriasis, and to vitamin E when these inflammatory diseases are associated with chronic alcoholism.

As reported in Cortland Forum, Jeffery Wiersum, M.D., said that he obtained beneficial results in treating over 30 patients with psoriasis with a daily regime of 25,000 IU of vitamin A in fish-liver oil; 800 IU of vitamin E in vegetable oil; and 50 mg of zinc.[3]

Vitamin E oil from capsules was applied to the lesions on even days, while oil from vitamin A capsules was applied on odd days.

Acne vulgaris : In 173 patients with acne, compared with controls, those with severe acne were found to have lower levels of retinol-binding protein than either patients with mild acne or healthy controls of the same age, according to the British Journal of Dermatology.[4] Retinol-binding protein is a blood protein that binds and transports retinol/vitamin A.

The males with severe acne had significantly lower blood levels of zinc than the controls.

Herpes : Although it is not a common treatment, some doctors recommend taking high doses of vitamin A to boost the immune system and prevent genital herpes from recurring, reported Prevention's Healing with Vitamins.[5]

"Vitamin A helps the immune system to fight viruses, so the symptoms are less and the number of infections is fewer," explained Jonathan Wright, M.D., a holistic physician in Kent, Washington.

Wright recommends 50,000 IU/day of vitamin A—which far exceeds the Daily Value of 5,000 IU—for the duration of the herpes outbreak. However, he recommends that you clear this with your doctor.

A form of vitamin A in breast milk seems to slow the growth of the herpes simplex virus, reported Medical Tribune. Retinoic acid, a derivative of vitamin A found in breast milk, after 48 hours dramatically slowed the growth rate among virus cells, compared with cells that had not been exposed to the vitamin A derivative.[6]

It is necessary to slow the growth of the virus, which allows the immune system a chance to overcome the virus and reduce the severity of the infection. Vitamin A has also been shown to help suppress the herpes virus in intestinal cells, and it may also perform similar effects in the vaginal cells, both of which are mucosal surfaces.

Eczema : In 10 children who were between 6 months and 10 years of age with chronic eczema, vitamin A was given at 50,000 IU twice daily in the older children, and 25,000 IU/day in the younger children.[7]

The dose in the older children was increased up to 100,000 IU twice daily for at least 6 months. Results revealed some improvement in dry skin and eczema, according to Annals of Allergy.

In 4 infants with intractable eczema associated with retarded development and malnutrition, the absorption of vitamin A from the intestinal tract was found to be impaired.[8]

In 24 systematically-treated people with nummular eczema, treatment included vitamin A at 30,000 to 75,000 USP units/day (therapeutic dose), and 25,000 USP units or less per day (maintenance dose); topical application of a bland ointment which contained some zinc oxide; the reduced use of soap and water for cleansing when active lesions were present, and, in some cases, intravenous injections of calcium gluconate and general irradiation with artifical sunlight, with avoidance of the parts affected by eczema.[9]

Results showed satisfactory results in 18 of the patients.

Nummular eczema is discoid or coin-shaped which denotes the thick mucous or mucopurulent sputum in certain respiratory diseases.

Chickenpox : At Hacettepe Children's Hospital in Ankara, Turkey, Sinasi Ozsoylu, M.D., gave 200,000 IU/day of vitamin A or a placebo to 47 (Group 1) and 46 (Group 2) children with chickenpox, who exhibited no clinical evidence of a vitamin A deficiency.[10]

In addition, 8 of the siblings of Group 1, who had not had the disease, were given the same amount of vitamin A during the incubation period of 1 to 3 days before the appearance of eruptions in the patients.

Crusting of all lesions occurred earlier in Group I than in Group 2. The mean duration of diseases was shorter in the 8 siblings than in those who were given the vitamin during the incubation period of the disease, than in the group of children who initially had the disease.

Five children in the placebo group (Group 2) had complications, but there were no complications in the vitamin A-supplemented group.

The author suggests that vitamin A might be given on the first day of eruption to shorten the crusting period and protect against complications, since it is much cheaper than antiviral medications.

Vitamin A should be given to more children during the incubation period of the disease to be certain about its effect on varicella. The role of vitamin A in acute viral disease may not be due to its absolute deficiency, but rather to its pharmacologic effect, Ozsoylu concluded.

Several studies have suggested that supplemental beta-carotene can reduce susceptibility to sunburn, because beta-carotene likely quenches free radicals, which can promote the inflammation and skin cell damage characteristic of sunburn, according to the Journal of Nutrition.[11]

During the 12-week study, a research team asked 12 young and middle-aged volunteers to take 24 mg of beta-carotene from a natural source of Dunaliella salina algae daily. Another 12 volunteers took a mixed-carotenoid supplement containing 8 mg each of natural beta-carotene, lutein, and lycopene daily. A third group of 12 received a placebo.

The volunteers' sensitivity in UV-simulated sunburn (erythema) on their backs was measured at the beginning of the study, after 6 weeks, and at the end of the study. Carotenoid levels in blood and skin were also measured.

Following 3 months of supplementation with either of the carotenoid supplements, the degree of sunburn was significantly less than the subjects had experienced at the beginning of the study. Both carotenoid supplements provided comparable protection. Blood and skin levels of carotenoids significantly increased after 6 and 12 weeks of supplementation. There were no changes in those given a placebo.

The research team concluded that, "The extent of protection with ingested carotenoids is not comparable to the use of sunscreen with a high sun protection factor, but the basal protection systematically contributes to the permanent defense against UV light-mediated skin damage."

Prescription-strength creams and washes containing the vitamin A derivatives tretinoin (Retin-A), tazarotene (Tazorac), or adapalene (Differin) speed the shedding of dead skin cells so that they cannot clog pores, reported Disease Free.[12]

They may also cool inflammation, easing redness and swelling. When researchers evaluated studies involving 900 people with acne, they found that tretinoin reduced the number of pimples by about 54%.

"In another study, tazarotene produced similar results," the publication said. "Other research suggests that retinoids may clear up 70% of blemishes."

Research suggests that diets high in sugar and refined carbohydrates may play a role in acne. In a study of 43 men with acne, those who followed a low-glycemic diet—foods that have a minimal impact on blood sugar levels—had 23% fewer blemishes after 12 weeks.

Vitamin A and Acne

High amounts of vitamin A were used to treat severe acne in teenagers, reported the Bastyr Center for Natural Health in Seattle, Washington.

Girls took up to 300,000 IU/day, while boys were given 500,000 IU/day.

Although the acne was lessened, the benefit diminished once the oral vitamin A therapy was discontinued.

Such high doses need to be monitored by a physician or health-care provider.

Source: Kligman, A.M., et al. "Oral Vitamin A in Acne Vulgaris: Preliminary Report," International Journal of Dermatology 20: 278-285, 1981.

Vitamin A Cousins and Acne

Derivatives of vitamin A (retinoids) are used to treat skin conditions such as acne.

Topical and oral prescription medications, such as tretinoin—Avitar, Renova, Retina-A, Retin A-Micro—and isotretinoin (Acutane) are available for the treatment of acne.

Isotretinoin may cause severe side effects, and should be used only for severe resistant acne. It must not be used by women who are pregnant or who plan to become pregnant because of possible birth defects.

These medications should be prescribed by a health-care provider, and vitamin A supplements should not be used simultaneously. Obviously, this would increase the intake of vitamin A, which could lead to possible toxicity.

Source: Mayo Clinic. com, Rochester, Minnesota, undated.

References

1. Clayman, Charles B., M.D., medical editor. The American Medical Association Home Medical Encyclopedia. New York: Random House, 1989, pp. 909ff.
2. Marrakchi, S., et al. "Vitamin A and E blood Levels in Erythrodermic and Psoriasis Associated with Chronic Alcoholism," Acta Dermatology Venerology (Stockholm) 74(7): 298-301, 1994.

3. Wiersum, Jeffery, M.D., "Psoriasis Ex: A Plus E Plus Zinc," Cortland Forum, May 1993, p. 31.
4. Michaelsson, G., et al. "Serum Zinc and Retinol-Binding Protein in Acne," British Journal of Dermatology 96: 283-286, 1977.
5. Feinstein, Alice, editor. Prevention's Healing with Vitamins. Emmaus, PA: Rodale Press, Inc., 1996, pp. 262-264.
6. Khan, Jason. "Vitamin A May Help Suppress Herpes Outbreaks," Medical Tribune, May 18, 1995, p. 10.
7. Stoesser, A.V., and Nelson, L.S. "Synthetic Vitamin A in Treatment of Eczema in Children," Annals of Allergy, Nov./Dec. 1952, pp. 703-704.
8. Di Sant'Agnesse, P.A., and Larkin, V. deP. "Vitamin A Absorption in Infantile Eczema," Proceedings of Experimental Biology and Medicine, 1943, pp. 343-344.
9. Gross, P. "Nummular Eczema: Its Clinical Picture and Successful Therapy," Archives of Dermatology and Syphilology 44: 1060-1077, 1941.
10. Ozsoylu, Sinasi, M.D. "Vitamin A for Varicella," Journal of Pediatrics 125(6): 1017-1018, 1995.
11. Heinrich, U., et al. "Supplementation with Beta-Carotene or a Similar Amount of Mixed Carotenoids Protects Humans from UV-Induced Erythema," Journal of Nutrition 133(1): 98-101, 2003.
12. Wait, Marianne, editor. Disease Free. Pleasantville, N.Y.: The Reader's Digest Association, Inc., 2009, pp. 72-73.

15

ULCERS AND WOUND HEALING

An open sore on the skin or a mucous membrane that results from the destruction of surface tissue, an ulcer may be shallow or deep and crater-shaped. It is usually inflamed and painful, explained the American Medical Association Home Medical Encyclopedia.[1]

Skin ulcers usually occur on the leg (leg ulcers) because of an inadequate blood supply to or drainage from the limb.

Ulcers on mucous membranes most commonly develop within the digestive tract, occurring in the mouth, stomach, or duodenum (peptic ulcer). They can also appear in the large or small intestine (ulcerative colitis).

The skin or mucous membranes of the genitalia may also be affected by ulcers. Ulcers can also appear on the cornea (corneal ulcers).

In evaluating 138 newly diagnosed cases of duodenal ulcer, those who had the highest intakes of vitamin A had a 54% lower risk of duodenal ulcers than those with the lowest intake, reported Medical Tribune.[2]

Men who had the highest intake of dietary fiber had a 45% lower risk for the ulcer, and duodenal ulcers were 33% less likely to develop in those who had 7 or more servings of fruits and vegetables per day than in those who had fewer than 3 servings per day.

In this study, apples, yams, and liver were the highest sources of vitamin A. Eating becon, hot dogs, or cold cereal was associated with an increased risk of ulcers.

In evaluating dietary factors and the risk of duodenal ulcer in a study of 47,000 men, ranging in age from 40 to 75, during a 6-year follow-up, there were 138 newly diagnosed cases of duodenal ulcer, reported Edward L. Giovannucci, M.D., of the Harvard School of Public Health in Boston, Massachusetts.[3]

It was found that a higher consumption of fruits and vegetables was associated with a lower risk of duodenal ulcer. Total dietary fiber was inversely related with the risk of this disorder. The soluble component of fiber was strongly associated with a decreased risk of duodenal ulcer.

Vitamin A from all sources combined, including supplements and multivitamins, was the only nutrient that was statistically significant after adjusting for variables in reducing the risk of developing a duodenal ulcer, Giovannucci said.

The duodenum is the first segment of the small intestine. Extending 12 fingerbreadths in length, it extends from the pylorus to the junction of the jejunum.

In 17 patients with chronic leg ulcers, compared to controls, those with leg ulcers had significantly lower blood levels of vitamins A and E, carotenes, and zinc, according to Nutrition Week.[4]

Supplementation with a multivitamin/mineral containing zinc and vitamins A and E, may help to reduce the risk of leg ulcers, the researchers said.

In 60 patients who took either 150,000 IU/day of vitamin A, plus an antacid; vitamin A plus an antacid and cyproheptadine; or an antacid alone; it was found that the number of patients with completely healed gastric ulcers was significantly higher in the groups with vitamin A than in the group taking antacid alone[5]. Cyproheptadine hydrochloride is Periactin and Pyrohep.

The extent of ulcer reduction was significantly higher in both of the groups which used vitamin A. The researchers added that vitamin A has a "true cytopreventive "effect" in patients with gastric ulcer.

Some of the just-named researchers reported in Lancet that, in a study of patients with gastric ulcer, 16 received antacids only, while 18 were given 50,000 IU 3 times daily of vitamin A. A third group was treated with the same protocol as Group 2, with the addition of cyproheptadine (an antihistamine) orally at a dose of 4 mg 3 times daily.[6]

All 3 groups showed significant reductions in ulcer size over the 4-week trial. However, the vitamin A groups had a significantly greater reduction than the group without the vitamin.

The researchers added that gastric ulcer can be thought of as a precancerous state, and there has been a significant negative correlation reported between serum levels of vitamin A and the development of urinary, bladder, lung, and epidermal cancers.

In evaluating 25 patients with ulcerative colitis, 9 patients with miscellaneous gastrointestinal tract disease, and 8 healthy controls, after an oral challenge of 100,000 USP units of vitamin A, results showed less a rise in vitamin levels in patients than in controls.[7]

There appears to be an impairment of absorptive power in the intestinal tract in those with ulcerative colitis, the researchers said.

Wound healing : Malnutrition increases the risk of wound-related complications, according to Jorge E. Albina, M.D., of Brown University School of Medicine in Providence, Rhode Island.[8]

Among his many recommendations, vitamin A increases the collagen content and breaking strength of experimental cutaneous wounds and colonic anastomosis in animal models. Anastomosis refers to and opening created by surgery, trauma, or disease between 2 or more organs.

Vitamin A deficiency usually occurs without symptoms and it is difficult to detect outside a hospital setting, according to Mary V. Mazzotta, Ph.D., of the California College of Pediatric Medicine in San Francisco, California.[9]

This deficiency is common when measured in hospital patients, and those who are severely injured or burned can become vitamin A deficient, which impedes wound healing, she said.

Vitamin A plays a significant role in each stage of wound healing, and it enhances the early inflammatory phase. In this deficiency, there is a reduction in fibronectin on the wound surface, with a subsequent decrease in chemotaxis, adhesion, and tissue repair. Fibronectins are glycoproteins. Chemotaxis is movement of cells.

She goes on to say that postoperative vitamin A supplementation for 7 days can increase collagen synthesis, the brusting strength of the scar, and lymphocyte activation.

A large supplemental dose of vitamin A can reverse the postoperative supression of immune responses, and improve healing retarded by stress, diabetes, and radiation.

Infrequent high doses of vitamin A are generally safe when given for vitamin A deficiency, she continued. Vitamin A can exhibit an anti-steroid activity, and wounds retarded by anti-inflammatory steroids are stimulated by retinoids for more than normal wounds.

To avoid anti-steroid activity, vitamin A can be applied topically to the wound or with sponge implants. Topical vitamin A increases the epithelization of wounds and improves the cosmetic appearance of the scars, she added.

Vitamin A has long been recognized for promoting wound healing, reported the Indian Journal of Pharmacology. Its effects on cyclophosphamide-induced suppression of healing was studied in two animal models. This is an anti-cancer, immunosuppressive drug that is sometimes called Cytexan and Neosar.[10]

In the study, the drug reduced tensile strength (incision wound), extended the epithelization period—which refers to the covering of the skin and glands—suppressed wound contraction, and increased the size of scar tissue.

Vitamin A at 5,000 IU on alternate days reversed the effects of the drug.

The researchers concluded that vitamin A reversed the wound-healing suppressant effect of the drug, as well as promoting the normal healing of surgical wounds.

Retinoids, a form of vitamin A, have long been associated with wound healing, since a deficiency of the vitamin retards repair, according to the Journal of the American Academy of Dermatology.[11]

Retinoids restore steroid-retarded repair to its normal state, since vitamin A tends to suppress fibroblasts—connecting tissues—in cell culture, along with stimulating steroid-treated macrophages—tissue cells that protect the body against infections—to initiate the repair of tissue.

The retinoids are especially important in macrophage inflammation, which play a significant role in wound healing, the researchers added.

Patients who take anti-inflammatory steroids should probably control their intake of retinoids, however, how this should be done is as yet unknown.

References

1. Clayman, Charles B., M.D., medical editor. The American Medical Association Home Medical Encyclopedia. New York: Random House, 1989, p. 1018.
2. Charnow, Judy A. "Vitamin A, Fiber May Cut Risk of Duodenal Ulcer," Medical Tribune, February 6, 1997, p. 15.
3. Aldoori, Walid H., et al. "Prospective Study of Diet and the Risk of Duodenal Ulcer in Men," American Journal of Epidemiology 145(1): 42-50, 1997.
4. Nutrition Week, Junuary 21, 2000, p. 7.
5. Patty, I., et al. "Cytoprotective Effect of Vitamin A and Its Clinical Importance in the Treatment of Patients with Chronic Gastric Ulcer," Int. J. Tiss. Renc. 5(3): 301-307, 1983.
6. Patty, I., et al. "Controlled Trial of Vitamin A Therapy in Gastric Ulcer," Lancet, October 16, 1982, p. 876.
7. Page, R.C., et al. "The Absorption of Vitamin A in Chronic Ulcerative Colitis," American Journal of Digestive Diseases 10(5): 174-177, May 1943.
8. Albina, Jorge E., M.D. "Nutrition and Wound Healing," Journal of Parenteral and Enteral Nutrition 18(4): 367-376, 1994.
9. Mazzotta, Mary V., Ph.D. "Nutrition and Wound Healing," Journal of the American Pediatric Medical Association 84(9): 456-462, September 1994.
10. Raju, S.S., and Kulkarni, D.R. "Vitamin A Reverses the Wound Healing Suppressant Effect of Cyclophosphamide," Indian Journal of Pharmacology 18(3): 154-157, 1986.
11. Hunt, T.K. "Vitamin A and Wound Healing," Journal of the American Academy of Dermatology 15(4): 817-821, October 1986.

16

CROHN'S DISEASE

Crohn's diseaase or ileitis is a chronic inflammatory condition in which the intestinal tract is ulcerated, according to Robert A. Ronzio, Ph.D. It is characterized by deep sores in the lower part of the small intestine and colon, as well as other regions of the digestive tract.[1]

Crohn's disease is one of 2 forms of inflammatory bowel disease, which most often effects people between the ages of 12 and 40. Symptoms include low-grade fever, cramps, gradual weight loss, anorexia, flatulence, weakness, malnutrition, persistent bouts of diarrhea, possibly arthritis, skin inflammation, abdominal tenderness, vaginal and urinary inflammation and rectal bleeding.

These patients typically consume more refined sugar and eat less fruit, vegetables, and fiber than healthy people, Ronzio said.

Vitamin and mineral deficiencies are also related to the disease, including vitamin A, vitamin D, vitamin K, calcium, magnesium, iron, zinc, selenium, vitamin C, vitamin B12, and folic acid, the B vitamin.

Fifteen patients with ulcerative colitis, 14 patients with active Crohn's disease, and 3 operated patients with current Crohn's disease were found to have serum retinol levels and retinol-binding protein significantly lower than controls, reported Jerzy Ostrowski, M.D., of Warsaw, Poland.[2]

Successful treatment of ulcerative colitis normalized serum retinol levels without vitamin A supplementation. In active Crohn's disease, low serum retinol levels are present, while in the inactive phase of the disease, vitamin A levels are normalized.

These results suggest that serum retinol levels in patients with active inflammatory bowel disease are secondary to decreased serum retinol binding concentrations, and probably depend on increased protein catabolism in these diseases. Catabolism is breaking down of complex chemicals into simpler ones.

The low retinol binding protein levels in these disorders could be from reduced release of vitamin A from the liver. Other theories of why there are low vitamin A levels in active Crohn's disease are: (1) decreased zinc levels; (2) previous poor intestinal absorption of fat; (3) previous bowel resection; and (4) localization of disease. Zinc plays a role in the synthesis of retinol binding protein, and, therefore, can influence vitamin A metabolism.

In an article in Lancet, a 31-year-old woman with Crohn's disease, who had moderate bouts of diarrhea twice daily, was given 50,000 IU of retinol palmitate 3 times daily, along with vitamin E at 100 mg, 3 times daily. This resulted in a healing of psoriatic lesions within 2 weeks, as well as a resolution of her diarrhea.[3]

The patient also reported that, after taking the vitamin A, she could eat food, including plums, without any adverse effects of diarrhea.

After stopping and starting the vitamin A several times, it became evident that the symptoms would recur within a few days of stopping the vitamin A, but the bowel would return to normal with reintroduction of the vitamin.

At the time the article was written, the patient was taking 100,000 IU/day of vitamin A. Vitamin E was of no benefit. Vitamin A levels were normal, and it was shown that the vitamin A supplementation improved intestinal-barrier function, the researchers said.

In a later issue of the magazine, it was reported that vitamin A allows for normal consumption of food, and stops diarrhea, in patients with Crohn's disease.[4]

Vitamin A supplementation may help the epithelial barriers of the gut in those with Crohn's disease. Vitamin A can also help in the production of mucous by goblet cells glycocalyx (filamentous coating) by epithelial cells, which can help to protect the intestinal barrier.

As reported in the Journal of the American Dietetic Association, in 23 men and 24 women with Crohn's disease, the mean daily intake of vitamin B6 and folic acid, also a B vitamin, by both genders, and of iron by women was less than the Recommended Dietary Allowance.[5]

In addition, according to Canadian Interpretative Standards, 50% of the women had inadequate intakes of iron (13%); vitamin B2 (21%); and vitamin A (21%).

The men consumed significantly less vitamin A and folic acid per 1,000 kcal than did the women. Blood levels of folic acid were low in 21% of the men, and 26% of the women. Low blood levels of folic acid were predictive of potential risk of nutritional deficiency for folic acid, vitamin B6, vitamin B12, and vitamin C.

According to an article in Gastroenterology, researchers evaluated 40 normal volunteers and 82 patients with Crohn's disease, and found that 65% of those with the disease had low blood levels of 25-hydroxyvitamin D, and 25% had deficient levels of the vitamin.[6]

Crohn'a disease patients are often deficient in vitamin A, according to The Whole Health Center in Houston, Texas.[7]

Although the information is anecdotal, they maintain that 50,000 IU/day of the vitamin may counteract this deficiency.

Confer with your doctor about whether or not to take this dosage, and for how long.

As reported in Gut, 52 patients—31 outpatients and 21 inpatients—were evaluated for a vitamin A deficiency. Eleven of the patients (12%) had low blood levels of the vitamin. As a group, the inpatients were more protein depleted than the outpatients.[8]

The researchers suggest that patients with extensive small bowel Crohn's disease, who weigh less than 80% of an ideal weight, should be checked for vitamin A concentrations.

Those with low levels of the vitamin run the risk of developing night blindness. Vitamin supplements should be given, and protein depletion should be corrected, they added.

References

1. Ronzio, Robert A., Ph.D. The Encyclopedia of Nutrition and Good Health. New York: Facts on File, Inc., 1997, p. 115.
2. Ostrowski, Jerzy, M.D., et al. "Metabolism in Vitamin A and Inflammatory Bowel Disease," Hepto-Gastroenterology 38: 391-395, 1991.
3. Skogh, M., et al. "Vitamin A in Crohn's Disease," Lancet, April 5, 1980, p. 766.
4. Dvorak, A.M. "Vitamin A in Crohn's Disease," Lancet, June 14, 1980, pp. 1303-1304.
5. Hodges, P., et al. "Vitamin and Iron Intake in Patients with Crohn's Disease," Journal of the American Dietetic Association 84(1): 52-58, January 1984.
6. Murray, Frank. Sunshine and Vitamin D. Laguna Beach, CA: Basic Health Publications, Inc., 2008, p. 105.
7. "Crohn's Disease," The Whole Health Center, Houston, Texas, internet, undated.
8. Main, A.N., et al. "Vitamin A Deficiency in Crohn's Disease," Gut 24(12): 1169-1175, December 1983.

17

DIABETES

It is estimated that roughly 21 million Americans have diabetes, including 6.2 million who don't know they have it, according to Diabetes Forecast, November 2007. An estimated 54 million more have pre-diabetes.[1]

"These numbers are stunning evidence that an epidemic is loose in our country, but, like other epidemics, this one does not honor borders," the publication added.

In fact, diabetes is a world-wide scourage, since approximately 5.9% of the world's population has diabetes. That breaks down to 246 million people, and the numbers keep growing.

At the same time, much of the world is ill-equipped to fight the disease. As Larry Deeb, past-president, Medicine and Science, of the American Diabetes Association, said in an address at ADA's Scientific Sessions in Chicago, Illinois, in 2007, "many countries not only lack insulin, but also they don't have the most basic refrigeration needed to store it."

Through the diligent work of diabetes advocates, spearheaded by Clare Rosenfelt, ADA's first National Youth Advocate, and in recognition of this worldwide health crisis, the United Nations passed a resolution in December 2006 creating United Nations World Diabetes Day, to spur member nations to take up the fight. It was officially observed for the first time on November 14, 2007.

Considerable epidemiological evidence exists that some carotenoids are potent antioxidants, and may play a protective role against the development of chronic diseases such as hardening of the arteries, stroke, certain cancers, and inflammatory diseases, reported a research team from the University of Queensland in Brisbane, Australia, and colleagues at other Australian facilities.[2]

While obesity and physical inactivity are known to be major risk factors for type 2 diabetes, evidence suggests that oxidative stress may also contribute to the pathophysiology of type 2 diabetes.[3]

Multiple factors have been implicated with increased oxidative stress in diabetes, including glucose autooxidation that results in the production of free radicals, an increase in protein glycation (glucooxidation), and a decrease in antioxidant defenses.

In their study, 1,597 adults over the age of 25, from 6 randomly selected cities and towns in Queensland, were evaluated between October and December 2000, including fasting plasma glucose, an oral-glucose tolerance test, and measurement of the serum concentration of 5 carotenoid compounds: alpha-carotene, beta-carotene, beta-cryptoxanthin, lutein/zeaxanthin, and lycopene.

Geometric mean concentrations for all serum carotenoids decreased, except for lycopene, with declining glucose tolerance status. Beta-carotene had the greatest decrease in those with normal glucose tolerance, impaired glucose metabolism, and type 2 diabetes, respectively.

"Serum or dietary vitamin A, E, and C concentrations have been hypothesized to be lower in those with impaired glucose tolerance, or with type 2 diabetes, than in those who have normal glucose tolerance," the researchers said. "However, there is conflicting evidence concerning these relations."

In their study, the research team evaluated the previously named carotenoids, and reported that serum carotenoids are inversely associated with type 2 diabetes and impaired glucose metabolism.

"Randomized trials of diets high in carotenoid-rich vegetables and fruits are needed to confirm these results, and those from other observational studies," the researchers continued. "Such evidence would have very important implications for the prevention of diabetes."

Diet has been implicated as a principal risk factor for type 2 diabetes, since a high intake of refined carbohydrates and sugar are associated with increased diabetes risk, reported the American Journal of Epidemiology.[4]

A research team analyzed blood levels of carotenoids in 1,665 people, ranging in age from 40 to 74. They reviewed correlations between carotenoid levels and the risk of diabetes and pre-diabetic symptoms.

The researchers reported that the highest beta-carotene levels were among those with normal glucose tolerance, but levels declined progressively among those with impaired glucose tolerance and diabetes. For example, those with impaired glucose tolerance had beta-carotene levels 13% below normal, and those with newly diagnosed diabetes had beta-carotene levels 20% below normal.

While this study did not demonstrate a direct protective effect of beta-carotene, the study is consistent with other research showing that antioxidants may reduce the risk of diabetes, since antioxidants may protect against insulin-damaging free radicals.

A number of studies have shown that those with diabetes often have low blood levels of antioxidants, according to the American Journal of Clinical Nutrition. Conversely, other research has found that high dietary intake or supplementation of antioxidants can improve various markers of glucose control.[5]

A research team evaluated 81 men and 101 women who were close relatives of people with type 2 diabetes. While the relatives were not diabetic, they were considered at increased risk of eventually developing the disease. Their levels of antioxidants were assessed by dietary intake and blood levels of vitamin E and carotenoids.

In men, higher dietary intake of mixed carotenoids (alpha-, beta-carotene, and lycopene) was associated with lower level fasting glucose levels. And their blood levels of beta-carotene were associated with a lower risk of insulin resistance, a prediabetic condition.

In women, higher dietary vitamin E intake was associated with lower fasting blood glucose levels, the researchers said.

Although it is not the perview of this book, researchers around the world are suggesting that vitamin D is essential for controlling diabetes. One of the reasons is that some people do not get enough of the vitamin from the sun, and there are so few foods that contain vitamin D.[6]

In other research, ampalaya—called karela or karella in India, and bitter melon in others—as a vegetable, tea, or capsule, has been shown to lower blood sugar levels in many patients, especially in the Philappines.[7]

Many diets in the Philippines are loaded with starch from white rice, along with sugar-sweet drinks, and this poses a problem for the pancreas to pump out enough insulin to deal with this unnecessary barrage of starches and sugars.

Diabetes in India and China

China is now the diabetes capital of the world, an ominous title once held by India, according to The Times of India.

*92.4 million adults in China are diabetic, and almost 150 million more Chinese will soon become diabetic.

*In 2009, the International Diabetes Federation (IDF) said that diabetes in India is expected to go from 50 to 87 million by 2030, or 8.4% of the adult population.

''I feel that India's burden will be a lot more than estimated at present,'' said Anoop Misra, M.D., director of Fortis Healthcare.

''While 50 million are known to be diabetic, 100 million are at the stage of pre-diabetes in India.''

''The aging population, urbanization, nutritional changes, and decreasing levels of physical activity, with the epidemic of obesity, have probably contributed to this rapid increase (in diabetes),'' added Yang Wenying, M.D., of China-Japan Friendship Hospital in Beijing.

''Around the world, diabetes is still largely undiagnosed,'' said David Whiting, M.D., of the IDF. ''In some poorer countries, 90% of the people with diabetes are undiagnosed, while even in high-income countries, 30% may be undiagnosed.''

Source: Sinha, Kounteya, The Times of India, March 28, 2010.

Vitamin A and Diabetes

The areas of greatest prevalence of endemic vitamin A deficiency are found in Indonesia, India, Indochina, central America, the Middle East, and the Philippines.

Vitamin A deficiency is the principal cause of blindness in the world, and this occurs mostly in tropical areas where carotenes (pro-vitamin A) that would prevent it are plentiful.

The chemical structure of beta-carotene and vitamin A were described in 1930, and the vitamin may be deficient in a diabetic diet.

Source: Akshya Kumar, Dr., Herbalist. "Diabetes Mellitus: Herbal Care," North East India News, undated.

References

1. "World Diabetes," Diabetes Forecast, November 2007, p. 41.
2. Coyne, Terry, et al. "Diabetes Mellitus and Serum Carotenoids: Findings of a Population-Based Study in Queensland, Australia," American Journal of Clinical Nutrition 82: 685-693, 2005.
3. Laight, D. W., et al. "Antioxidants, Diabetes and Endothelial Dysfunction," Cardiovascular Research 47: 457-464, 2000.
4. Ford, E.S., et al. "Diabetes Mellitus and Serum Carotenoids: Findings from the Third National Health and Nutrition Examination Survey," American Journal of Epidemiology 149: 168-176, 1999.
5. Ylonen, K., et al. "Dietary Intakes and Plasma Concentrations of Carotenoids and Tocopherols in Relation to Glucose Metabolism in Subjects in High Risk of Type 2 Diabetes: The Botnia Dietary Study," American Journal of Clinical Nutrition 77: 1434-1441, 2003.
6. Murray, Frank. Sunshine and Vitamin D. Laguna Beach, Calif.: Basic Health Publications, 2008.
7. Murray, Frank. Ampalaya: Nature's Remedy for Type 1 and Type 2 Diabetes. Laguna Beach, Calif.: Basic Health Publications, 2006.

18

MALARIA

A parasitic disease spread by the bite of Anopheles mosquitoes, malaria produces fever along with complications affecting the kidneys, liver, brain, and blood that can be fatal, according to the American Medical Association Home Medical Encyclopedia. Malaria kills about 1 million infants and children every year in Africa, however, those who survive can build up an immunity.[1]

The parasites responsible for malaria are single-celled protozoa organisms called plasmodia. Four species can cause disease in humans, namely, Plasmodium falciparum, Plasmodium vivax, Plasmodium ovale, and Plasmodium malariae. Each species spends part of its life cycle in humans and part in Anopheles mosquitoes.

Symptoms include shaking, chills, and a fever, and appear only when red blood cells, infected with parasites, rupture and release more parasites into the bloodstream.

In a number of studies, biologists have determined that the mosquito-borne parasite, P. falciparum, began killing a significant number of people within the past 12,000 years, reported Science News.[2]

At the National Institute of Allergy and Infectious Diseases in Bethesda, Maryland, a research team, headed by Xin-Zhuan Su, conducted a new analysis of the parasite's DNA, and determined a surprising variability within the genes, suggesting a much earlier origin.

As they reported in the July 18, 2002 issue of Nature, Su's team concluded that P. falciparum dates back 100,000 to 180,000 years.

"We have concluded that the P. falciparum population is quite ancient and diverse, a result that will be important in the development of drugs and vaccines," Su added.

Between September 2007 and October 2009, a team of experts from Egypt, Germany, and Italy, examined 11 royal mummies believed to be from King Tutankhamen's immediate lineage (1410 to 1324 BC), and 5 royal mummies from an earlier period (1550-1479 BC), in an effort to determine how King Tut died.[3, 4]

The scientists, headed by Zahi Hawass, Ph.D., of the Supreme Council of Antiquities in Cairo, Egypt, determined that many of the people, including King Tut, had malaria.

Thuya, a noblewoman, said to be the grandomother or great-grandmother of the king, and Yuya, a nobleman, thought to be the grandfather or great-grandfather, had malaria, but it is not known if it were fatal. Not everyone infected with P. falciparum became gravely ill, and the 2 lived to be about 50, rather old for the time.

It is possible that the 2 spent much of their time living in malaria-endemic areas close to the marshes of the Nile River, where partial immunization may have contributed to their survival.

King Tut (1324 BC), who was infected with malaria, had multiple disorders that contributed to his death, including Kohler's disease (he needed 2 canes to walk), a missing toe in the right foot, and a clubfoot on the left.

"A sudden leg fracture, possibly induced by a fall, might have resulted in a life-threatening condition when a malaria infection occurred," the researcher said. "Seeds, fruits, and leaves found in the tomb, and possibly used as medical treatment, support this diagnosis. The frail king died at 19.

From a nutritional standpoint, malaria is important for 2 reasons, reported Foods and Nutrition Encyclopedia. First, malaria survives in areas where the mosquito and the infected human population remain above a critical density for each. This situation often occurs in time of famine when people congregate, in which rains come and produce breeding grounds for the insects. Malaria then spreads rapidly among the weakened survivors of famine.[5]

Second, malaria attacks—chronic malaria—or repeated infections of malaria are taxing on the nutritional resources of the body.

"Good nutrition is essential to recovery," the publication added. "A high-calorie, high-protein, high fluid intake with vitamin supplementation is recommended."

A new survey reported in New Scientist suggested that between 125,000 and 277,000 people die from malaria in India annually, far higher than the 16,000 tabulated by the World Health Organization, according to United Press International, October 22, 2010.[6]

Estimates of malaria deaths in India are based on death rates recorded in clinics and corrected, in an attempt to account for people missed by the health system, UPI said.

However, researchers at the University of Toronto in Canada, and other universities, found that these numbers have been vastly underestimated.

The research team has been collaborating with the Indian government on a survey of 1.1 million households in India to improve the country's health statistics.

The researchers recorded "verbal autopsies," in which relatives described how family members died, to count deaths that were never officially diagnosed.

"Malaria deaths happen out in the countryside, and they are invisible to the health-care system", said Richard Peto of the University of Oxford in England, one of the researchers.

Added Bob Snow, also of Oxford University, "India has a space program, but cannot provide prompt access to malaria treatment in Orish state, where deaths are the highest. This study will surely be a wake-up call."

In a similar story in the New York Times on October 25, 2010, 3 malaria experts pointed out that several other countries have large malaria populations, but these are rural areas with little access to doctors, including Indonesia, Pakistan, Afghanistan, Bangladesh, and Myanmar (formerly Burma), so global estimates of malaria may be low.[7]

A vitamin A deficiency is a significant cause of blindness and death, especially in children and pregnant and lactating (breast-feeding) women, reported Resources, Fall/Winter, 2008.[8]

According to estimates from the World Health Organization, Geneva, Switzerland, 250 million pre-school age children in over 100 countries are deficient in vitamin A: Of these; between 250,000 and 500,000 lose their sight annually, and over half die within 12 months. A vitamin A deficiency also increases risk of dying from malaria and measles. This contributes to the death of 1.2 to 3 million children deaths annually.

About 7.2 million pregnant women in developing countries also suffer from vitamin A deficiency, which means their infants are likely to be born in an already compromised state, the publication said.

"Supplementation programs in India suffer from a lack of support from India's medical establishment, which, in spite of widespread evidence; has not uniformly endorsed vitamin A's link to mortality, and has displayed a preference for fortification of food-based approaches over supplementation," the publication continued.

Cooking oil from processed mustard seed is commonly used in northern India, where vitamin A is most widely prevalent, especially among the poor. Less than 1% of rice, tea, candy, etc., is fortified with vitamin A.

India's low meat and dairy consumption increases the likelihood that people will get enough vitamin A from their diet alone.

Once pressed, the biofortified mustard oil retains high levels of beta-carotene (pro-vitamin A), which gives the oil and rice its dark color.

The fortified oil provides more vitamin A per serving than through traditional means. However, after several years of lab work and limited trials, efforts to commercialize the technology has stalled, the publication reported.

Three studies confirmed that vitamin A supplementation is associated with a 23 to 35% reduced risk of slide-confirmed P. falciparum infection, reported Nutrition Research Newsletter.[9]

Considerable evidence from clinical trials show that vitamin A and zinc supplements are beneficial in preventing P. falciparum malaria in children in malaria-endemic areas, where there is a substantial burden of underlying micronutrient deficiencies.

A research team from the Institut de Recherche en Sciences de la Santa in Burkina Faso (formerly the Upper Volta), and other facilities, reported that vitamin A and zinc are crucial for the normal immune system to function, and they may play a synergistic role for reducing the risk of infection, including one from P. falciparum, reported the nutrition journal.[10]

In the study, 200,000 IU/day of vitamin A and zinc were given to children in the Sourkoudougou village in Burkina Faso.

Children 6 to 72 months were randomly assigned to be given the vitamin along with 10 mg/day of zinc for 6 days a week or a placebo for 6 months.

At the end of the study, there was a significant decrease in the prevalence of malaria in the supplemented group, the researchers said.

Anemia and iron deficiency during pregnancy are prevalent in the developing countries, but their causes are not always known, according to the Journal of Nutrition.[11]

The study assessed the prevalence and severity of anemia and iron deficiency, and their association with helminths, malaria, and vitamin A deficiency in a sample of 336 pregnant women in Nepal. Helminths are intestinal parasites.

The research team reported that 72.6% of the women were anemic; 19.9% had moderate to severe anemia; and 80.6% had iron deficiency.

It was noted that 88% of the cases with anemia were associated with iron deficiency. In addition, over half of the women (54.2%) had low blood levels of retinol (vitamin A).

The researchers added that the findings reinforce the need for programs to reduce the prevalence of hookworm, malaria infection, and vitamin A deficiency, as well as providing iron supplements to effectively control anemia.

Hookworm is the common name for bloodsucking nematodes of the family Ancyclostomatidae.

At Medical College and Hospital in Aligarh, India, and other facilities, researchers concluded that low levels of vitamin A are associated with P. falciparum malaria, and that vitamin A supplementation might help to reduce morbidity from malaria, reported the Journal of Infection in Developing Countries.[12]

The study involved 150 children, 2 to 5 years of age, versus 20 healthy controls.

Adil Raza, M.D., and colleagues said that the importance of vitamin A to health and visual acuity in children has been known since the 1920s.

Children 1 to 3 years are affected because of their fast rate of growth, and their higher physiological requirement for vitamin A at that age.

Gouado Inocent, M.D., and colleagues, reported in the African Journal of Biotechnology that P. falciparum uses vitamin A and calcium of its hosts for its proper metabolism, which leads to a decrease of these nutrients in the blood of the patients.[13]

A vitamin A deficiency makes children in Western Kenya vulnerable to infections, and influences the outcome of various health conditions, according to the East African Medical Journal.[14]

Retinal levels were significantly lower among children with high C-reactive protein, which is a beta-globulin that is found in the blood of people with certain inflammatory, degenerative, and neoplastic diseases.

The high prevalence of a vitamin A deficiency may have resulted from an acute phase response induced by infections, the researchers said.

In malaria-endemic areas, vitamin A supplements, which cost about 2 cents in U.S. currency, can help to reduce infections in children by one-third, according to a study in Malaria Journal.[15]

Peter Olumese, of the WHO's Global Malaria Programme, said that it is clear that vitamin A supplementation helps to prevent a range of infectious diseases in children.

"While waiting on results of further studies," he said, "vitamin A supplements can be used to decrease morbidity and mortality, including those at risk of malaria."

According to the World Health Organization, children under the age of 5 in Africa and South-East Asia had the highest levels of a vitamin A deficiency between 1995 and 2005.

UNICEF estimates that it reaches 70% of the children worldwide at risk of a vitamin A deficiency with supplements twice a year. But that means one-third of the children may not receive the minimum amount, Olumese added.

At a 2008 Malnutrition Conference at the Copenhagen (Denmark) Consensus Center, economists estimated that an annual $60 million investment in micronutrients, especially vitamin A and zinc, would yield annual benefits of more than $1 billion, including health-care cost savings, as reported by the Integrated Regional Information Networks (IRIN).

In a study reported in the Internet Journal of Tropical Medicine, 132 children, ranging in age from 6 to 60 months, were divided into 2 groups, and given varying amounts of iron and vitamin A or a look-alike pill.[16]

Approximately 40.15% of the children had malaria, along with moderate to severe vitamin A deficiency.

The study confirmed that vitamin A and iron could remarkably improve the treatment of malaria, when the supplements are given to infected children.

There are an estimated 70 to 80 million cases of P. vivax each year, accounting for over 50% of all malaria cases outside Africa, according to Toby Leslie, M.Sc., and colleagues, at the London School of Hygiene and Tropical Medicine in London.[17]

While rarely fatal, P. vivax infection is a major cause of illness, and it affects economic performance at individual and national levels, the authors reported in the May 23/30, 2007 issue of the Journal of the American Medical Association.

"Outside Africa, there is a significant overlap between P. falciparum and P. vivax, and in most areas they coexist, the researchers added. "Chloroquine (Aralen) usually remains effective against P. vivax malaria, especially where it has failed against P. falciparum."

They went on to say that this has resulted in divergent treatments for the 2 species, with artemisinin combination therapy being recommended for use in P. falciparum malaria cases. Where diagnostic services are good and species differentiation into P. falciparum and P. vivax malaria is reliable, this 2-drug policy is easy to maintain.

Equally in areas in which almost all malaria is caused by drug-resistant P. falciparum malaria, with little P. vivax, a policy that treats all patients with an artemisinin combination therapy should be cost-effective, the researchers said.

While that entire issue of JAMA was devoted almost entirely to malaria in the United States, Afghanistan, Pakistan, Uganda, Zambia, Kenya, Bahamas, and elsewhere, there was no mention of nutrition or vitamin and mineral supplements.

In an endemic area of P. falciparum in Papua, New Guinea, 480 children, ranging in age from 6 to 60 months, participated in a double-blind study, reported Lancet.[18]

Children were given vitamin A capsules containing 200,000 IU of vitamin A in 200 ml of peanut oil with 10 mg of vitamin E. Identical capsules containing only peanut oil as a placebo were given every 3 months for 13 months.

The number of P. falciparum episodes with a temperature of over 37.5°C., with a parasite count of 8,000 micrometer/l, was 30% lower in the vitamin A group than in the controls at the end of the study.

P. falciparum geometric mean density was lower in the vitamin A group than in the placebo group, as was the proportion with spleen enlargement.

Children between 12 and 36 months of age benefited the most, having 35% fewer fever episodes, 26% fewer enlarge spleens, and a 68% lower parasite density, the researchers said. The spleen is a large vascular organ lying between the stomach and the diaphragm.

As reported in The Lancet (also called Lancet), David A. Ross, M.D., and colleagues, reviewed 2 studies on vitamin A supplementation and the effects of clinical attendance, hospital admissions, and childhood mortality in northern Ghana.[19]

A total of 21,906 children, 6 to 90 months of age, were evaluated, and the children received either 200,000 IU of retinol equivalent or a placebo every 4 months. Children under the age of 12 months were given 100,000 IU of vitamin A.

It was reported that the vitamin A supplemented children had significantly fewer clinic attendances, hospital admissions, and deaths than children given a placebo. The mortality rate due to acute gastroenteritis was also lower in the vitamin A supplemented group than in the controls.

Mortality rates from other causes, except acute lower respiratory infections and malaria, were also in vitamin A clusters, but they were not significant.

The authors added that improving vitamin A nutriture in young children in populations where xerophthalmia—dryness or conjunctiva in the cornea—exists, should be a high priority for health and agricultural services in Africa and other developing countries.

Also, they said, it is important to gather information on local dietary and agricultural practices to assess the feasibility of improving the production, storage, and consumption of local vitamin A-rich foods, the introduction of new foods or fortification of healthful consumed foods.

Other options include vitamin A supplements to high-risk groups. In fact, supplementation may be the least cost-effective of all these strategies, but it is still a highly cost-effective child survivor invention, the researchers continued.

In October, 2007, at a scientific conference in Seattle, Washington, Bill and Melinda Gates, leaders of the world's richest charitable foundation, rocked the international health community by calling for the eradication of malaria, which kills some 1 million people annually, most of whom are women and children, reported Susan Okie, M.D., in the New England Journal of Medicine.[20]

History casts a shadow over any discussion of malaria eradication, because, 50 years ago, in the world's first coordinated disease-eradication effort, public health workers battled malaria for more than a decade with the insecticide dichlorodiphenyltrichloroethane (DDT) and the drug chloroquine, Okie said.

"They eliminated the infection from 24 countries and freed 1 billion people from malaria risk, yet the emergence of mosquito resistance to DDT and parasite resistance to chloroquine led to epidemic resurgence of malaria in some countries where it had been nearly vanquished," she continued.

Unfortunately, the campaign never included the tropical African countries with the most intense transmission, where about 90% of malaria deaths occur.

Consequently, calls for the eradication of malaria have been mixed reactions. Even the choice of target organisms is a matter of debate, since malaria can be caused by 4 species of plasmodia, although only P. falciparum and P. vivax commonly produce clinically significant disease.

Instead of targeting the 2 species for eradication, some malaria experts prefer to concentrate on prevention and treatment, Okie continued.

"In Zambia, for example," she continued," "where the Gates Foundation and other donors began 3 years ago to fund a national effort to reach 80% of the population with preventive measures, clinics literally were empty of malaria cases during this year's rainy season, reported Carlos C. (Kent) Campbell of the Malaria Control and Evaluation Partnership in African at the Program for Appropriate Technology in Health."

Some experts are concerned that money spent on elimination may be wasted in countries with neighbors that have intense malaria transmission and ineffective health-care systems, Okie said.

Arata Kochi, chief of the WHO's Global Program on Malaria, said that eliminating malaria from South-East Asia would have global benefits, because drug-resistant parasites usually evolve there first, but he noted that, because a mosquito vector there bites those who sleep outdoors in the forest, it is difficult to control malaria with bed nets and indoor spraying of insecticides.

Okie added that there is broad consensus that global eradication of falciparum malaria is not possible with current weapons, which differ little from those in the 1950s; that is, an insecticide (the pyrethroid compounds used to treat bed nets), and a medicine (artemisinin, given as part of the combination therapy), even though DDT and a few other insecticides are sometimes used.

"Resistance to the pyrethroids has already appeared in some African mosquito populations,"Okie continued, "and artemisinin resistance may be emerging near the Thai-Cambodian border."

Permanent elimination of malaria transmission from endemic regions may have to wait for new drugs and insecticides, and, perhaps, for a highly effective vaccine, Okie added.

At the time of the article, a vaccine developed by Glaxo-SmithKline Biologicals was being evaluated in trials in Africa, and could be on the market by 2012, but it appears to be less than 50% effective in preventing infection, although it may reduce the clinical severity of malaria.

An effective human malaria vaccine has been sought for over 70 years, but it has met with little success, reported William E. Collins, Ph.D., and John W. Barnwell, Ph.D., in the December 11, 2008 issue of the New England Journal of Medicine. A successful malaria vaccine used in conjunction with other control interventions would help reduce and eventually eliminate the considerable global disease burden caused by malaria.[21]

As the RTS,S vaccine headed into Phase 3 trials in 2009, large areas across Africa had moderate-to-intense malaria transmission.

"This is the first malaria vaccine to reach this stage of development, and it will be essential to learn how it performs in areas of more intense transmission," the researchers said. "Only then will we have a clear idea of what effect it will have on the well-being of children in Africa and elsewhere, and its role in malaria control."

A previous study of the malaria vaccine, RTS,S—which targets the circumsporozoite protein—was given an adjuvant system (ASO2A), showed a 30% rate of protection against clinical malaria in children 1 to 4 years of age, reported Philip Bejon, Ph.D., of the Centre for Geographic Medicine Research in Mombasa, Kenya, and researchers at various facilities.[22]

In this study, the researchers evaluated the efficacy of RTS,S given with a more immunogenic adjuvant system (ASOIE) in children 5 to 17 months of age, a target population for vaccine licensure.

"Our findings indicate that RTS,S/ASOIE vaccine should be further tested in a Phase 3 multicenter trial," the researchers said.

The use of RTS,S/ASO2D vaccine in infants had a promising safety profile, but it did not interfere with the immunologic responses to coadministered EPI antigens, and it reduced the incidence of malaria infection, according to Salim Abdulla, M.D., of the Bagamo Research and Training Centre of Ifakara Health Institute in Bagamoyo, Tanzania, and colleagues at other facilities. EPI stands for WHO's Expanded Program on Immunization.[23]

For centuries, the origin of the parasite that causes malaria has been elusive, reported Jon Cohen in the August 7, 2009 issue of Science.

However, an international research team has compelling evidence that the parasite, P. falciparium, evolved from a relative called P. reichenowki that affect chimpanzees. They suggest a provocative theory that, as human red blood cells evolved a way to dodge P. reichenowki, they became highly vulnerable to P. falciparum.[24]

The change may be linked to a change in human red blood cells 2 to 3 million years ago, said Jukian Rayner of the Wellcome Trust Sanger Institute in Hinxton, United Kingdom.

In 2005, working with Ajit Varki and Pascal Gagneux at the University of California at San Diego, Rayner reported a genetic mutation that protects people from P. reichenowki, but makes them more susceptible to P. falciparum.

"The mutation altered the surface of red blood cells, changing a sugar that P. reichenowki binds to during the infection process," Gagneux explained. "As a result, a new sugar adorned human red blood cells that P. falciparum favors."

"Varki now suggests that the chimp parasite might work as a vaccine against P. falciparum, much the way that cowpox immunizes against smallpox," Cohen said.

Researchers predict a global disaster if malaria parasites worldwide develop resistance against the new artemisinin-based combination therapies (ACTs) that have become the gold standard, according to Martin Enserink in the December 19, 2008 issue of Science.[25]

Large parts of the world would have no drugs to fall back on, and malaria cases and deaths could soar, erasing hope that the world might be on the verge of a huge reduction in the disease, he said.

However, resistance against ACTs is what now seems to be developing in western Cambodia, along the Thai border, according to studies given at the annual meeting of the American Society of Tropical Medicine and Hygiene (ADTMH) in New Orleans, Louisiana, in December 2008.

In a effort to eliminate malaria experts gathered in December 2008 in Phom Penh to discuss an implementation plan, which would be coordinated by the World Health Organization. The effort will be funded by the Bill and Melinda Gates Foundation in Seattle, Washington.

The main problem researchers have documented is a delay in clearing the parasites from the blood of some patients on artemininin drugs, Enserink continued. Researchers prefer to say that the parasite is "tolerant" rather than resistant to the drug, said Nicholas White of Mahidol University in Bangkok, Thailand.

"Cambodia's western border has long been the cradle of antimalaria drug resistance—chloroquine, sulphadoxine-pyrimethamine, and mefloquine—and all met their match there before becoming useless elsewhere," Enserink added. "Scientists believe this may have to do with the misuse of drugs there, as well as the widespread availability of underdose and counterfeit therapies. From Cambodia, gem miners and other migrants have carried resistant parasites to other South-East Asian countries."

With regard to ACTs, Cambodia has another problem, Enserink continued. These combination treatments rely on an artemisinin derivative for their powerful punch, and they contain a second drug to make it more difficult for the parasite to become resistant. However, in Cambodia, many artemisinin monotherapies are on the market.

Nailing down resistance is harder than it might seem, since treatment failures in individual patients—of which there have been several reports in the past 10 years—don't always signal resistance. Patients often do not get better because their blood levels of the drug are too low.

Testing parasites' sensitivity by exposing them to drugs in the test tube is possible, however, the results are difficult to interpret. Scientists have yet found unequivocal genetic markers of resistance to arteminsinin derivatives.

The newly developed containment plan calls for eliminating malaria from the areas where tolerance has been found, and greatly reducing transmission in a large surrounding area, Enserink continued. The plan, to be formulated by national malaria-control agencies in Cambodia and Thailand, with support from various research institutes, includes rapid and widespread treatment with ACTs, improved mosquito control, the distribution of long-lasting insecticide-impregnated bed nets, a ban on monotherapies in Cambodia, and an information campaign.

At the ADTMH meeting, scientists launched the Worldwide Antimalaria Resistance Network (WWARN), a global database that will collect information on resistance in vivo and in vitro, drug levels in patients' blood, and molecular markers. Based at Oxford University, United Kingdom, the network will be led by Philippe Guerin, an epidemiologist currently working for Doctors Without Borders.

As reported in the American Journal of Clinical Nutrition, 141 severely anemic children were given either 100,000 or 200,000 IU of vitamin A, depending on their age, or the drug sulfadoxine.

Seventy-two hours later, they were given the opposite therapy, plus daily hermatic syrup for 90 days.[26]

The researchers reported that vitamin A significantly decreased erythropoietin concentrations, which is a sialic acid-containing protein. The vitamin helped to reduce inflammation, and it mobilized iron from stores and stimulated the production of erythrocytes, which are red blood cells.

In evaluating 101 consecutively admitted children with cerebral malaria to a hospital, it was found that the whitening of the retina was associated with a mean blood level of vitamin A of 0.29 micromol/l, compared with a mean vitamin A level of 0.41 micromol/l in children without retinal whitening, according to Archives of Ophthalmology.[27]

The researchers stated that children with retinal whitening—referring to the sensory membrane that lines the eye—were 2.77 time more likely to have abnormal conjunctival impression cytology, when compared to those without whitening.

At the Hospital of Bicatre in France, 454 children, between 6 months and 6 years of age, were evaluated for their vitamin A status, and its relation to parasital or infectious disease.[28]

It was found that malaria, and to a lesser extent, vitamin A deficiency were responsible for a high morbidity and mortality rate in children.

Vitamin A was evaluated by impression cytology transfer (ICT), and plasma retinol concentrations. It was found that 28.6% were vitamin A deficient by the ICT method, and 37.5% were deficient by plasma retinol concentrations (less than 10 mcg/100 ml).

The authors conclude that there is a significant relationship between vitamin A deficiency and malarial access, which leads to increased illness and death.

In 19 patients, acute malaria hypozincemia—low levels of zinc—were found in 89% of the patients, according to Trace Elements in Medicine. Zinc levels returned to normal in 6 patients in 1 week with zinc supplements.[29]

Writing in the New England Journal of Medicine, Job C. J. Calis, M.D., and colleagues, of the Global Child Health Group in Amsterdam, The Netherlands, reported that several independent, yet over-lapping conditions, are associated with severe anemia in Malawian children. These include bacteremia, malaria, hookworm, HIV infection, and vitamin A and vitamin B12 deficiencies.[30]

Vitamin A deficiency was found in 92.3% of these patients and 65% in the controls, and it was considered severe—less than 10 mcg/deciliter—in 32.8% of case patients and 14.9% in the controls.

"Vitamin A deficiency was associated with malaria and bacteremia—the presence of bacteria in the blood—in the structural equation model," the researchers said. "Iron deficiency was found in 46.6% of the case patients and 69.8% of the controls."

The researchers added that, "our findings indicate that even in the presence of malaria parasites, additional or alternative diagnoses should be considered. Current treatment recommendations that promote iron and folic acid—a B vitamin—supplements ignore bacteremia, vitamin B12 deficiency, and, in young children, hookworm infections appear to be of limited applicability in our setting."

Recent immigrants and refugees constitute a substantial proportion of malaria cases in the United States, accounting for almost 1 in 10 imported malaria cases involving people with known resident status in 2006, according to the Journal of the American Medical Association.[31]

During June 27-October 15, 2007, 3 cases of P. falciparum malaria and 2 cases of P. ovale malaria were reported in King County, Washington.

The infections were diagnosed in Burundian refugees, who had recently arrived in the U.S., and 2 refugee camps in Tanzania.

"Since 2005, the Centers for Disease Control and Prevention in Atlanta, Georgia, has recommended presumptive malaria treatment with artemisinin-based combination therapy (ACT), that is, artemetherlumefantrine for refugees from sub-Saharan African before their departure for the United States," the publication said.

Resistance to the previous mainstays of treatment—chloroquine and sulfadoxinepyrimethamine—prompted the CDC to make the recommendation.

Up to 10,000 Burundian refugees from Tanzania were settled in the U.S. during 2007-2008. Health-care in the U.S. caring for refugee populations resettling from malaria regions should remain aware of the possibility of malaria in these groups, regardless of prior treatment, the publication said.

For thousands of years, Chinese herbalists have used leaves from the plant Artemisia annua to treat numerous illnesses, including malaria, reported Wilbur K. Milhous and Peter J. Weina of the University of South Florida in Tampa, and Walter Reed Army Institute of Research, in Silver Spring, Maryland, respectively.[32]

The plant's antimalarial compound—a sesquiterpene lactone and endoperoxide called artemisinin—is the most effective drug for combatting malarial infections, they said.

A major hurdle in using the compound to treat malaria has been producing enough artemisinin to meet the world's demand.

Now Ian A. Graham, et al.[33] have found a way of breeding varieties of the plant with highly desirable genetic traits that can improve agricultural yields, decrease production costs, ensure a steady global supply of the drug, and improve grower confidence in the crop.

"The next big hurdle for the molecule will be emerging resistance to the drug." the researchers said.

Artemisia is a group of aromatic herbs and shrubs like wormwood and sagebrush.

In 1992, Medical Tribune reported on an earlier article in Lancet, in which an extract of sweet wormwood (Artemether) cleared malaria parasites from children's bodies in 37 hours on average, compared with 48 hours among those given chloroquine in Africa.[34]

This poses an interesting question: Why don't researchers use the inexpensive herb, rather than going to the trouble of converting it into a drug?

If you are poor and living in Africa, it is not easy to buy the most effective drugs to fight malaria, where the local drugstore stocks a bewildering array of medicines, ranging in price from a few dimes to $10, usually with no information about which work and which don't, explained Martin Enserink in the November 21, 2008 issue of Science.[35]

Instead, there is a good chance you would choose a cheap treatment, and it would turn out to be totally ineffective, he added.

That is especially a problem with a new generation of malaria drugs called artemisinin-based combination therapies (ACTs). While they are cheap by Western standards, they are expensive to the world's poorest, and, in the private sector where most Africans buy their drugs, they face stiff competition.

Here is the situation concerning malaria drugs in Uganda:

* 174 different formulations and strengths of often outdated drugs are for sale.
* Fewer than 14% of private drug outlets sell ACTs.
* ACTs are up to 60 times more expensive than other drugs.

However, in 2008, Enserink continued, the Board of the Global Fund to Fight AIDS, Tuberculosis and Malaria voted to adopt a few financing systems aimed at bringing the best drugs to stores at rock-bottom prices—by letting the market do the work.

"ACTs combine a drug derived from Artemisia annua, with a second malaria drug to make it harder for the malaria parasite to develop resistance," Enserink added. "Highly effective, ACTs have revived hope that the enormous burden of malaria can be slashed, but their rollout has been slow and difficult."

An estimated half of patients get their drugs from private outlets, but drugstores often do not carry ACTs. If they do, they are more expensive than old, ineffective drugs like chloroquine, counterfeit drugs, and artemisinin monotherapies.

"Drug resistance to artemisinin-based drugs—already emerging in South-East Asia—is a huge worry, which is why global health leaders discourage the use of monotherapies," Enserink continued.

In 2004, a U.S. National Academies' Institute of Medicine panel suggested that pharmaceutical wholesalers in poor countries could buy ACTs from the manufacturer for pennies, rather than dollars, and various donors could pay the difference directly to the manufacturer.

In that way, drugs could be shipped through the supply chain and sold in even the remotest villages at the same price or for less than the undesirable drugs.

Commented panelist Ramanan Laxinanarayan of Resources for the Future in Washington, D.C., "If we only knew how Coca-Cola gets its cans into the most remote African villages, we could do the same for drugs."

Plans to Eradicate Malaria

When?	Who?	Goal:	What Happened?
1955	World Health Organization	Eradicate malaria	Campaign broke down
1998	Roll Back Malaria Partnership	Reduce cases and deaths by 50% by 2010	Little progress so far
2000	African heads of state (Abuja Declaration)	Reduce African malaria deaths by 50% by 2010	Little progress so far
2001	United Nations (Millenium Development Goals (MDG)	Have halted by 2015 and begun to reverse the incidence of malaria and other major diseases.	Appears feasible

Source: Roberts, Leslie. "New Malaria Plan Called Ambitious by Some, Unrealistic by Others." Science 322: 26-27, October 3, 2008.

References

1. Clayman, Charles B., M.D., medical editor. The American Medical Association Home Medical Encyclopedia. New York: Random House, 1989, pp. 659ff.
2. Travis, John. "Malaria Parasite Reveals Old Age," Science News 162(7): 110, August 17, 2002.
3. Hawass, Zahi, Ph.D., et al. "Ancestry and Pathology of King Tutankhamun's Family," JAMA 303(7): 638-647, 2010.
4. Markel, Howard, M.D. "King Tutankhamun, Modern Medical Science, and the Expanding Boundaries of Historical Inquiry," *ibid*, pp. 667-668.
5. Ensminger, Audrey, et al. "Foods and Nutrition Encyclopedia. Clovis, CA: Pegus Press, 1983, pp. 1344-1345.
6. "Malaria Deaths in India Underestimated," United Press International, October 22, 2010.
7. "India: Ambitious Study Indicates Malaria Deaths May be Underreported Across the World," New York Times, October 22, 2010.
8. Laxminarayan, Ramanan, et al. "A Recipe to Fight Vitamin A Deficiency in India: Add Mustard and Stir," Resources, Fall/Winter, 2008.
9. Hamer, Davidson H. "Vitamin A, Zinc and Pediatric Health," Nutrition Research Newsletter, 2008.
10. Zeba, Augustin N., et al. "Major Reduction of Malaria Morbidity with Combined Vitamin A and Zinc Supplements in Children in Burkina Faso: A Randomized, Double-Blind Trial," Nutrition Journal 7:7, 2008.
11. Dreyfuss, Michele L., et al. "Hookworms, Malaria and Vitamin A Deficiency Contribute to Anemia and Iron Deficiency Among Pregnant Women in the Plains of Nepal," Journal of Nutrition 130: 2527-2536, 2000.
12. Raza, Adil, et al. "Serum Retinol Concentration in Patients with Acute Falciparum Malaria in Aligarth, India," Journal of Infection in Developing Countries 3(11): 865-868, 2009.
13. Inocent, Gouado, et al. "Vitamin A Supplements Ameliorate the Adverse Effect of HIV-1, Malaria and Diarrheal Infections in Child Growth," African Journal of Biotechnology 6(7): 871-876, April 2, 2007.
14. Nabakwe, E.C., et al. "Vitamin A Deficiency and Anaemia in Young Children Living in Malaria Endemic District of Western Kenya," East African Medical Journal 86(6): 300-306, 2005.

15. "Vitamin A Supplements Can Reduce Malaria Cases in Children by One-Third, Study Finds," Malaria Journal 3:2, June 29, 2009.

16. Mofor, Claudine Teugwa, M.D., et al. "Effects of Vitamin A and Iron Supplementation on the Treatment of Malaria in Children," The Internet Journal of Tropical Medicine 3(1): 2006.

17. Leslie, Toby, M.Sc., et al. "Sulfadoxine-Pyrimethamine, Chlorproguanil-Dapsone, or Chloroquine for the Treatment of Plasmodium Vivax in Afghanistan and Pakistan: A Randomized Controlled Trial," JAMA 297: 2201-2209, 2007.

18. Shankar, A.H., et al. "Effect of Vitamin A Supplementation in Morbidity Due to P. Falciparum in Young Children in Papua, New Guinea: A Randomized Trial;" Lancet 354: 203-209, July 17, 1999.

19. Ross, David A., M.D., et al. "Vitamin A Supplementation in Northern Ghana: Effects on Clinic Attendance, Hospital Admissions, and Childhood Mortality," The Lancet 342:7-12, July 3, 1993.

20. Okie, Susan, M.D. "A New Attack on Malaria," New England Journal of Medicine 358: 2425-2428, 2008.

21. Collins, William E., Ph.D., and Barnwell, John W., Ph.D. "A Hopeful Beginning for Malaria Vaccines," New England Journal of Medicine 356:2599-2600, 2008.

22. Bejon, Philip, Ph.D., et al. "Efficacy of RTS,S/ASO1E Vaccine Against Malaria in Children 5 to 17 months of Age," New England Journal of Medicine 359:2521-2532, 2008.

23. Abdulla, Salim, M.D., et al. "Safety and Immunogenicity of RTS,S/ ASO2D Malaria Vaccine in Infants," *ibid*, pp. 2533-2544.

24. Cohen, Jon. "Key Malaria Parasite Likely Evolved from Chimp Version," Science 325: 663, August 7, 2009.

25. Enserink, Martin. "Signs of Drug Resistance Battle Experts, Trigger Bold Plan," Science 322: 1776, December 19, 2008.

26. Cusick, Sarah E., et al. "Short Term Effects of Vitamin A and Anti-Malarial Treatment of Erythropoiesis in Severely Anemic Zanciberi Pre-School Children," American Journal of Clinical Nutrition 82(2): 406-412, August 2005.

27. Lawellen, Susan, M.D., et al. "Association Between Measures of Vitamin A and Ocular Fundus Findings in Cerebral Malaria," Archives of Ophthalmology 116:293-296, March 1998.

28. Amedee-Manesme, O., and Samba-Dinard, C. "Vitamin A Deficiency in Acute Assess of Malaria in Children," International Journal of Vitamin and Nutrition Research 60:210-211, 1990.

29. Enk, C., M.D., et al. "Transient Hypozincemia and Endotoxinemia in Human Malaria," Trace Elements in Medicine 7(3): 131-133, 1990.

30. Calis, Job C. J., et al. "Severe Anemia in Malawian Children," New England Journal of Medicine 358: 888-899, 2008.

31. "Malaria in Refugees from Tanzania—King County, Washington, 2007," JAMA 300(22): 2602-2604, 2008.

32. Milhous, Wilbur K., and Weina, Peter J. "The Botanical Solution for Malaria," Science 327: 279-280, January 15, 2010.

33. Graham, Ian A., et al. "The Genetic Map of Artemisia Annua L. Identifies Loci Affecting Yield of Antimalerial Drug Artemisinin," *ibid*, pp. 328-331.

34. "Chinese Herb Curbs Malaria," Medical Tribune, February 27, 1992, p. 12.

35. Enserink, Martin. "Malaria Drugs, the Coca-Cola Way," Science 322: 1174, November 21, 2008.

19

TUBERCULOSIS

For centuries, tuberculosis (TB) was one of the most feared of all diseases, reported Reader's Digest Book of Facts. The disease, also known as consumption, attacks the lungs. At one time TB and its complications played a part in 1 in 5 deaths worldwide.[1]

The disease's characteristic lesions—named tubercles in the 17th century—have been identified in Neolithic skeletons in Europe and in mummies of Egyptians who lived in 3700 B.C.

In spite of all of their efforts, doctors were powerless against TB until Robert Koch (1843-1910), a self-trained German bacteriologist, identified the rodlike tubercle bacillus in 1882, the publication said.

The next advance came in 1922, when an effective vaccine—originally developed in 1906 by 2 French scientists—Albert Calmette and Camille Guerin—was first given to children. The vaccine was named BCG (bacille Calmette-Guerin).

"The final step was a treatment that could cure the disease, and this came in 1944 with the discovery of streptomycin, the first effective antituberculosis drug, by Selman Waksman (1888-1973), a Ukranian-born scientist who did much of his pioneering research while a professor at Rutgers University in New Jersey," the publication added. "For his discovery of streptomycin, derived from soil microorganisms, he received the Nobel Prize in medicine in 1952."

On a personal note, I happen to know that streptomycin was actually discovered by a friend of mine, Prof. Albert Schatz, while an undergraduate student at Rutgers. As a student, he was not eligible for the Nobel Prize, but, fortunately, in the last 20 years or so, he has received the recognisition that he rightfuly deserved, although not the encomiums. As a professor at Temple University in Philadelphia, Pennsylvania, he was a strong opponent of water fluoridation.

The spread of an especially virulent form of tuberculosis in South Africa illustrates a breakdown in the global program that is supposed to keep the disease, one of the world's deadliest, under control, reported Lawrence K. Altman, M.D., in the March 20, 2007 issue of the New York Times.[2]

The worldwide program was supposed to detect TB cases, make sure patients were taking their antibiotics, test patients for resistance to these drugs and monitor the spread of the disease.

"International experts say the system is in deep trouble for an array of reasons, including misuses of antibiotics, other bad medical procedures, like failing to segregate high-risk patients in hospitals and clinics, and cut in government spending for such basics as adequate supplies of drugs and labs to do the testing," Altman added.

Mycobacterium tuberculosis, the microbe that causes the disease, was discovered 125 years ago, but, today, the bacteria infects 8.8 million people annually and causes 1.6 million deaths. The microbe is spread in tiny droplets when patients cough.

The extent of the disease was highlighted when an outbreak of extremely drug-resistant tuberculosis—XDR-TB—killed 52 of its 53 victims in a South African province. All of the patients were also infected with HIV.

"The outbreak was detected in 2005, but it did not receive international attention until it was reported at the international AIDS conference in Toronto, Canada, in August 2006," Altman said.

The World Health Organization calls XDR-TB "a grave public health threat" because of its potential explosiveness among the millions of HIV-infected people in poor countries. XDR-TB is resistant to the 2 most important anti-TB drugs—isoniazid and rifampin—along with 2 other drugs—a member of the fluoroquinolone class and at least 1 of the 3 others—capreomycin, kanamycin, and amikacin.

Also of interest is MDR-TB, which is a step lower on the resistance scale, Altman continued. An outbreak of that form struck in New York City in the early 1990s, and it cost at least $1 million in emergency measures to control and manage TB patients.

An outbreak of XDR-TB is not confined to Africa, according to Paul Nunn, M.D., of the World Health Organization. One or more cases have been detected in 28 countries. He estimated that two-thirds of those cases were in China, India, and Russia.

At a meeting of global health leaders at the United Nations in New York City, Margaret Chan, M.D., of the World Health Organization, told the group that drug-resistant forms of tuberculosis are on an increasingly deadly colision course with HIV infection, reported Rebecca Voelker in the August 6, 2008 issue of the Journal of the American Medical Association.[3]

Chan added that any further spread of XDR-TB would be a setback of epic proportions in global efforts to control the spread of TB and HIV.

"If we allow XDR-TB to spread, we are, in effect, going back to the pre-antibiotic era," she said.

About one-third of the world's 33.2 million people with the HIV infection are also infected with TB.

"There is far too little awareness that TB is a raging infectious disease made more serious and widespread by the epidemic of HIV/AIDS," added Jorge Sampaio, the former president of Portugal, who is now the UN special envoy to stop the spread of HIV/AIDS.

From 1993 to 2006, the number of tuberculosis cases in the United States decreased by 45%, from 25,107 to 13,779, reported the July 23/30, 2008 issue of the Journal of the American Medical Association.[4]

"This decline has occurred disproportionately among the US-born population, for whom the number of cases has declined by 66%, while the number of TB cases among foreign-born persons in the U.S. increased by 5%," according to Kevin P. Cain, M.D., and colleagues, at the Centers for Disease Control and Prevention in Atlanta, Georgia.

As long as TB is a major problem globally, additional strategies will need to be implemented to improve TB control in the US-foreign-born population, Cain added.

There are 3 strategies that can presently be implemented:

1. We could enhance overseas preimmigration screening of immigrants and refugees for TB disease by adding TB culture to current screening practices. Currently, chest radiography is performed overseas for all US-bound immigrants and refugees more than 15 years of age, and a sputum-smear microscopy for acid-fast bacilli is obtained from those with an abnormal chest radiograph or symptoms of TB disease. Those entering the U.S. who are not immigrants or refugees, such as students, workers, and visitors, along with undocumented migrants, are not routinely screened. About 30% of all foreign-born people in the U.S. fall into 1 of these unscreened categories.

2. We could find and treat cases of LTBI among foreign-born people, including those already living in the U.S., and newly arriving migrants at elevated risk for TB could be tested and treated for LTBI after arrival in the U.S., or prior to U.S. entry.

3. We could make financial aid and technical investments in global TB control.

Researchers at a medical school in northern India found an incidence of about 17 new cases of active TB per 1,000 medical residents per years, as compared with about 2 cases per 1,000 in the general population and 0.05% in the general U.S. population, reported Vikram Paralkar, M.D., of Temple University Hospital, in the March 13, 2008 issue of the New England Journal of Medicine.[5]

He reported that John Keats, the British poet, accurately diagnosed himself with TB in 1820, and died soon afterward at age 25.

A century ago, he continued, TB posed substantial challenges even in wealthy countries, as Thomas Mann pointed out in The Magic Mountain, which was set in an affluent sanatarium in the Swiss Alps before World War I.

Before the advent of effective pharmacologic agents, Mann described the cutting-edge therapies of the day—enforced rest, fresh air, morning walks, and even artificial pneumothoraxes, in which air or gas, such as nitrogen, was injected into the pleural space to collapse the lung.

Africa is facing the worst tuberculosis epidemic since the advent of the antibiotic era, according to Richard E. Chaisson,

M.D., and Neil A. Martinson, M.B., in the March 13, 2008 issue of the New England Journal of Medicine. Chaisson is at Johns Hopkins University School of Medicine in Baltimore, Maryland, and Martinson is with the University of Witwaterstrand, Soweto, South Africa.[6]

Driven by a generalized HIV epidemic and compounded by weak health care systems, inadequate laboratories, and conditions that promote transmission of infection, this devastating situation has steadily worsened, exacerbated by the emergence of drug-resistance strains of TB, they said.

Africa, home to 11% of the world's population, carries 29% of the global burden of TB cases, and 34% of related deaths, and the challenges of controlling the disease in the region have never been greater, they continued.

The World Health Organization estimates that the average incidence of TB in Africa more than doubled between 1990 and 2005, from 149 to 343 per 100,000 population.

In 1990, Mali and Togo had an incidence of TB greater than 300 per 100,000 by 2005; 25 countries had reached that level; and 8 of them had an incidence at least twice that high.

While most of the TB research rightfully zeroes in on drugs, it is unfortunate that more research is not directed at nutrition, since a strong immune system can help patients to cope with the disease, as well as to counteract the many side-effects of the drugs.

While TB remains a major public health concern throughout the world, most of the causes of death from the illness occur in developing countries, reported a research team from the University of Indonesia in Jakarta, and colleagues in the Netherlands and Germany.[7]

For example, in Indonesia, the prevalence of TB is 0.24% on the basis of positive sputum smears, and the disease is regarded as a priority disease requiring proper treatment.[8]

"Malnutrition is frequently found in those with pulmonary tuberculosis," the researchers added. "Several studies reported that those with active pulmonary tuberculosis are malnourished as indicated by reductions in visceral proteins, anthropometric indexes, and micronutrient status."[9, 10]

In this study, patients with newly diagnosed TB were divided into 2 groups. One group of 40 received 1,500 retinol/ vitamin A equivalents (5,000 IU) as retinyl acetate; and 15 mg of zinc (as zinc sulfate) daily for 6 months. A second group of 40 served as controls.

Both groups received the same antituberculosis treatment recommended by the World Health Organization. Clinical examinations, assessements of micronutrient status, and anthropometric measurements were carried out before and after 2- and 6-months intervals of antituberculosis therapy. Anthropometry is concerned with comparative measurements in the human body.

"Vitamin A and zinc supplementation improved the effect of tuberculosis medication after 2 months of antituberculosis treatment, and results in earlier sputum amear conversion," the researchers said.

In addition to raw foods, fluids, alfalfa sprouts, garlic, yogurt, and kefir, Alternative Medicine recommends these supplements for tuberculosis:[11]

Vitamin A: 300,000 IU for the first 3 days; then 200,000 IU for the next 2 days; followed by 50,000 IU/day for several weeks.

Beta-Carotene: 25,000 to 50,000 IU/day.

Vitamin E: Increase up to 1,000 IU/day, unless premenopausal women with many premenstrual symptoms.

There appears to be a link between TB and being underweight, as it appears that being 10% below ideal body weight is a risk factor for the disease, reported Nutrition Week.[12]

In addition, one researcher reported that any nutritional impairment or compromise will increase the risk. And there may be several nutritional links to TB, especially in the elderly.

Low intakes of beta-carotene can depress the immune system, and protein malnutrition may be a factor as well, the publication added. Low zinc intake may depress cellular immune function, which may account for a resurgence in TB.

One researcher has wondered if the reactivation of TB among the elderly could be caused by today's overzealous cholesterol lowering diets.

Before drug therapies were developed in the 30s and 40s, therapies for TB utilized fresh air, lots of dairy products and carbohydrates, and a diet high in saturated fat and cholesterol. These were definitely weight-gaining types of diets, and they were favored in the sanitoria in the early 30s and 40s.

In his extensive Prescription for Nutritional Healing, James F. Balch, M.D., published a lengthy nutritional regimen for tuberculosis. Some of his recommendations:[13]

1. Garlic: 2 capsules 3 times daily, with meals.
2. Vitamin A: 25,000 IU/day. For those who are pregnant, do not exceed 10,000 IU/day.
3. Natural carotenoids: 25,000 IU/day.
4. Vitamin E: 400-800 IU/day.
5. Coenzyme Q10: 75 mg/day.
6. Selenium: 200 mcg/day.
7. B Complex: 100 mg of each 3 times daily. There are 8 vitamins in the B Complex and 3 vitamins B-like cousins.
8. Brewer's yeast: 1-2 tsp/day.
9. Zinc: 50-80 mg/day. Do not exceed 100 mg/day.

Tuberculosis remains the leading cause of infectious disease among adults worldwide, and, in recent years, drug-resistant TB has emerged as an expanding threat, with an estimated 489,000 new cases in 2006, according to N. Sarita Shah, M.D., of the Centers for Disease Control and Prevention in Atlanta, Georgia, and colleagues. Dr. Shah has since transferred to the Albert Einstein College of Medicine in Bronx, New York.[14]

Treatment of multidrug-resistant TB (MDR-TB) is over 100 times as costly as treatment for drug-susceptible TB, which requires intensive case management for its prolonged (18 to 24 months) and more toxic treatment course.

While treatment success rates of 40 to 80% have been observed in a number of settings, this remains lower than the 85 to 99% cure rate achievable for drug-susceptible TB, the researchers added.

"In 2005, a global survey of supranational reference laboratories defined a new TB disease category, termed extensively drug-resistant TB (XDR-TB), and determined that these cases had emerged in all regions of the world," the researchers said. "Initial reports found that treatment outcomes were poor among patients with XDR-TB, especially in settings of high HIV prevalence."

From 1993 through 2007, there have been 83 cases of XDR-TB, accounting for 0.04% of all culture-confirmed TB cases with reported drug susceptibility results that occurred in the United States, the researchers continued. Although the number of cases has declined since 1993, XDR-TB cases continue to occur each year.

Extensively drug-resistant TB, which is defined as tuberculosis that is resistant to rifampin, isoniazid, a fluoroquinolone, and a second-line injectable agent, poses a major challenge for global health, reported Edward D. Chan, M.D., and colleagues, in the August 7, 2008 issue of the New England Journal of Medicine.[15]

The researchers, from the National Jewish Medical and Research Center in Denver, Colorado, added that, "among a series of 205 consective patients who were referred to our specialty medical center for respiratory diseases, and treated between 1984 and 1998 for multidrug-resistant TB, the overall long-term success rate was 75%, and the rate of death from TB was 12%."

They went on to say that, "despite aggressive treatment at our referral center, extensively drug-resistant TB, as compared with multidrug-resistant TB, was associated with a significantly poorer initial treatment response and long-term outcome and a significantly lower survival rate."

Their data underscores the critical importance of optimal management of cases of multidrug-resistant TB, lest they develop into extensively drug-resistant tuberculosis, they added.

Tuberculosis is perhaps the most persistent human disease caused by an infectious bacterium, Mycobacterium tuberculosis, reported Jean-Emmanuel Hugonnet, M.D., of the Albert Einstein College of Medicine, Bronx, New York, and colleagues at various facilities.[16]

"The death toll remains extremely high, despite the

introduction of modern multidrug chemotherapy in the 1960s, with between 1.6 and 2 million deaths annually," they reported.

An increasing percentage of human clinical isolates are drug-resistant or multidrug-resistant strains that threaten the ability to treat the disease, they added. The continued use of multidrug therapy has caused an even more dire problem—strains of M. tuberculosis resistant to the first-, second-, and third-line agents. In a study from South Africa, 54 of 54 patients infected with such highly resistant strains died with a mean survival time from diagnosis of 16 days.

Since the discovery of penicillin in 1929, the beta-lactam class of antibiotics has included some of the most clinically important bacterial agents, they continued. The development of broad-spectrum derivatives of penicillin, such as the cephalosporins and olivanic acid, coupled with their low inherent toxicity, have made them the drugs of choice for the treatment of both Gram-negative and Gram-positive bacterial infections.

"However," they added," this class has never provided a compound useful in the treatment of TB, and beta-lactams are only rarely used in the treatment of this disease."

M. tuberculosis was observed and sterilization of aerobically grown cultures was observed within 14 days. The 2 drugs are approved by the Food and Drug Administration, and could possibly be used to treat patients with currently untreatable disease, the researchers said.

It is estimated that TB has been responsible for over 1 billion deaths, exceeding the 40 million deaths from the influenza pandemic of 1918, and the millions of deaths from bubonic plague, reported Jesse Roth, M.D., of Albert Einstein College of Medicine and Yeshiva University, Manhasset, New York.[17]

"The social deterioration and crowding that accompanied the industrial revolution, as well as major wars, ignited TB epidemics," he continued. "In 19th-century Europe, 25% of all deaths were attributed to TB. Human populations newly exposed to the bacillus were often decimated."

At one point in history, TB was recognized as the most dreaded disease of the human race, he said. Optimism about eradication, brought on by discovery of the first antituberculosis drugs, has been replaced by the sober recognition that TB-alone and in combination with drug resistance and AIDS—worldwide is second only to AIDS among the leading causes of death from infectious diseases.

"It is estimated that one-third of the world's population is infected with latent TB with about 9 million new cases and 1.6 million deaths occurring annually," he added.

Roth explores the possibility that TB epidemics during previous centuries generated selective pressure that intensified the metabolic syndrome and the inflammatory process now associated with obesity, and suggests a plausible, though hypothetical evolutionary process. Although these associations might be coincidental, it is important to recognize that theoretical constructs, no matter how logical, may yield conclusions that are not correct.

These proinflammatory devices—with immune systems that are especially robust and more easily triggered—in partnership with the metabolic syndrome, may have provided an advantage during the TB pandemic when food availability was limited and the average life span was short. Formerly called Syndrome X, metabolic syndrome is a complication of 5 conditions that are related to type 2 diabetes: glucose intolerance, obesity, high blood pressure, and high levels of cholesterol and triglycerides. Anyone with 3 of these 5 conditions may develop diabetes.

"One hypothesis for the obesity pandemic posits (assumes) that thrifty genes, mutations incorporated into the genome during millennia of lean times to protect against starvation, produce obesity in times of plenty," Roth continued. "If the evolutionary goal is to store extra calories to prevent death from starvation, the thrifty gene hypothesis fails to explain why obesity predisposes to the metabolic syndrome. Equally puzzling is the increase in circulating cytokine levels associated with obesity-related inflammation, despite the absence of a microbial threat."

In the preantibiotic era, physicians advised patients with TB to curtail severely physical activity, and to adhere to a calorie-protein-, and micronutrient-laden diet, meaneuvers now known to enhance proinflammatory processes, Roth said.

"Daily doses of cod-liver oil greatly augmented intake of (the then not yet discovered) vitamins A and D, which also boost immunity," he continued. "Sunshine, also prescribed, enhances the transformation in skin of endogenous precursors into fully active vitamin D. High altitudes were also recommended for patients with TB. Hypoxia, induced by high elevations, up-regulates hypoxia-inducible transcription factor, which in turn promotes a major proinflammatory cascade, another potential beneficial response against TB." Hypoxia means a lack of oxygen.

In 2007, 57.8% of the 13,293 new cases of TB in the United States were diagnosed in foreign-born people, and the TB rate among foreign-born people was 9; 9.8 times as high as that among U.S.-born people (20.6 vs 2.1 cases per 100,000 population), reported Yecai Liu, M.S., et al., of the Centers for Disease Control and Prevention in Atlanta, Georgia, and colleagues at other facilities.[18]

Annual arrivals of about 400,000 immigrants and 50,000 to 70,000 refugees from overseas are likely to contribute substantially to the TB burden among foreign-born people in the U.S.

TB is the second most common cause of death from infectious diseases in the world, the publication added. During 1990 through 2003, the incidence of TB increased globally.

"The World Health Organization reported that Asia and Sub-Saharan Africa accounted for 84.1% of the estimated 8.8 million new cases of TB worldwide in 2005," the publication continued. "Global migration has greatly affected the epidemiology of TB in developed countries. An estimated 27.5% of TB cases among foreign-born people are diagnosed within 2 years after their arrival in the U.S."

Overseas screening for TB, with follow-up evaluation in the U.S., is a high-yield intervention for identifying TB in the U.S.-bound immigrants and refugees, and could reduce the number of TB cases among foreign-born people in the U.S., the publication added.

"Improvements such as overseas use of myobacterial culture, drug-susceptibility testing, directly observed therapy, TB skin testing for children 2 to 14 years of age, and a shorter interval between screening and departure for the U.S., as well as use of CDC's Electronic Disease Notification system for data exchange among the CDC, state, and local health departments, and international partners, should increase the effectiveness of this intervention," the researchers said.

To further reduce and prevent TB, diagnosis and treatment of latent TB infection among U.S.-bound immigrants and refugees may be considered in the future, especially if shortened treatment regimens for latent TB infections are proved to be effective, the researchers concluded.

According to the 13th annual tuberculosis report of the World Health Organization, which was published on World Day on March 24, 2009, there were an estimated 9.27 million new cases of TB worldwide in 2007, reported Peter R. Donald, M.D., et al., in the June 4, 2009 issue of the New England Journal of Medicine.[19, 20]

While this figure is an increase from 9.24 million in 2006, the world population has also grown, making the number of cases per capita a more useful measure of the problem. This figure peaked in 2004 at 142 per 100,000 and fell to 139 per 100,000 in 2007.

"An estimated 1.32 million people who were not infected with HIV died of TB in 2007, as did an estimated 456,000 people who were HIV-positive," the researchers said.

They went on to say that prevalence and mortality rates appear to be falling in all 6 WHO regions, and the Americas, the eastern Mediterranean, and Southeast Asia appear likely to meet the Millennium Development Goal target, set in conjunction with the Stop TB Partnership, and the World Health Assembly, of halving TB prevalence and TB-related mortality between 1990 and 2015. However, this target will probably not be met by the African and European regions.

Some 22 high-burden countries account for 80% of the global TB burden, the researchers added. In 2007, the countries with the highest prevalence were India (with 2.0 million cases); China (1.3 million); Indonesia (530,000); Nigeria (460,000); and South Africa (460,000) of the estimated 1.37 million cases in HIV-positive people; 79% were in Africa, and 11% in Southeast Asia.

"Disturbingly," they continued, "there were an estimated 500,000 cases of multidrug-resistant (MDR) TB in 2007 (including 289,000 new cases). Of these, 131,000 were in India; 112,000 in

China; 43,000 in Russia; 16,000 in South Africa; and 15,000 in Bangledesh. By the end of 2008, 55 countries had reported cases of extensively drug-resistant TB.

"These last figures are reason for considerable concern, and highlight a potential threat to our ability to treat TB, both in individual patients and in the context of a treatment program," the researchers added.

The research team went on to say that in the absence of isoniazid, our most powerful bacterial agent, the rise of resistance to rifampin, the next-most-powerful bacterial agent increases, since neither pyrazinamide nor ethambutrol (nor streptomycin) is particularly effective in preventing resistance to companion drugs.

Once MDR TB has developed, there is little to stop the rapid acquisition of resistance to the remaining agents, the researchers added. Further progression of pre-XDR and XDR TB becomes only a question of time. Since this process takes place over months, or even years, the patient remains infectious, and it is not surprising that transmission of MDR and XDR TB occurs, especially in communities with a high incidence of HIV infection. XDR refers to extensively drug-resistant.

The Stop TB Partnership has established the Global Laboratory Initiative to promote the availability of new diagnostic tools in countries with high MDR burden, and country-specific budgets are being prepared, and funding could become available through the Global Fund and through UNITAID (an international facility for the purchase of drugs against HIV-AIDS, malaria, and TB).

"The tuberculosis tide has turned, but maintaining the momentum will require a financial and political commitment that may be beyond the capability of many struggling communities," the researchers concluded.

Tuberculosis is a leading cause of death from infectious disease, second only to HIV/AIDS, according to Andreas H. Diacon, M.D., of the University of Stellenbosch in Durban, South Africa, and colleagues at various institutions.[21]

In 2006, there were 9.2 million new cases of TB and 1.7 million deaths, with the burden of the disease occurring predominantly in the developing countries.

"It is estimated that one-third of the world's population is infected with latent M. tuberculosis, providing an enormous reservoir for future disease," the researchers said.

TB control is complicated by the synergy between TB and HIV/AIDS, they added, and by the emergence of multidrug-resistant strains of M. tuberculosis.

Multidrug-resistant TB-resistant to both isoniazid and rifampin—is prevalent in countries of the former Soviet Union, South Africa, and China, and it is currently responsible for an estimated 490,000 incident cases of TB and 110,000 deaths worldwide each year.

"Multidrug-resistant TB requires extended treatment with second-line drugs that are less effective and have more adverse effects than isoniazid-based and rifampin-based regimens," they added. "Furthermore, extensively drug-resistant TB, defined as multi-drug resistant TB plus resistance to a fluoroquinolone and an injectable second-line drug, has recently emerged as a public health threat."

They added that TMC 207 (formerly R207910) is an investigational diarylquinoline compound that offers a new mechanisms of anti-tuberculosis action by specifically inbiting mcycobacterial ATP synthase. Adenosine 5' triphosphate (ATP) is the primary energy of the cell.

In vitro, TMC 207 potently inhibits drug-sensitive and drug-resistant tuberculosis isolates, and it is also bactericidal against dormant (nonreplicating) tubercle bacilli.

"The safety and efficacy findings from our study clinically validate ATP synthase as a new target for anti-tuberculosis therapy," the researchers concluded. "The findings also confirm the earlier results obtained with TMC 207 in the murine (mouse) model of tuberculosis, and show the potential of TMC 207 in the treatment of patients with drug-resistant-TB."

A study has reported that most cases of drug-resistant tuberculosis among patients undergoing treatment for the disease may reflect new infections, not acquired resistance, reported Tracy Hampton, Ph.D., in the April 4, 2007, issue of the Journal of the American Medical Association.[22]

The findings run counter to the common suggestion that drug

resistance among treated patients is acquired through mutations in the infecting M. tuberculosis strain.

"By genotyping the initial and subsequent drug-resistant clinical isolates of M. tuberculosis collected from patients over a 5-year period, investigators at the Shanghai Medical College in China, found that 84% of patients—27 of 32—had primary drug resistance, indicating transmission of a drug-resistant strain of the bacterium," Hampton said. (Genotype is the genetic constitution of an individual).

The researchers added that only 16%—5 of 32—had acquired drug resistance because of a poor treatment regimen or nonadherence to an adequate regimen. Therefore, there were more than 5 times as many cases caused by reinfection than by genetic changes within the bacterium.

Extensively drug-resistant TB has been reported in 45 countries, including countries with limited resources and a high burden of TB, reported Carole D. Mitnick, Sc.D., and colleagues, at the Peruvian Ministry of Health in Lima.[23]

They added that extensively drug-resistant TB can be cured in HIV-negative patients through outpatient treatment, even in those who have received multiple prior courses of therapy for TB.

Patients with extensively drug-resistant TB were given daily, supervised therapy, including cycloserine, an injectable drug, and a fluoroquinolone. Of these, 29 (60.4%) completed treatment or were cured, as compared with 400 (66.3%) with multidrug-resistant TB.

"In spite of limited resources in Peru, aggressive regimens, as part of a comprehensive outpatient therapeutic approach, cured more than half of patients with extensively drug-resistant TB, who had previously been treated for TB" Mitnick said. "This strategy has now been integrated into the routine approach to treatment in Peru's National Tuberculosis Program."

However, their study underscores the importance of developing other interventions that will further improve treatment outcomes, as well as stem the development and spread of extensively drug-resistant TB, she concluded.

With the highest prevalence of multi-drug-resistant

tuberculosis (MDR-TB) ever reported in 13 years of global drug collection, the countries of the former Soviet Union face a serious and widespread epidemic of MDR-TB, reported Joan Stephenson, Ph.D., in the May 20, 2009 issue of the Journal of the American Medical Association.[24]

The findings, based on data gathered from more than 90,000 patients in 83 countries, between 2002 and 2007, indicate that former Soviet Union states reported the highest prevalence of resistance.

The percentage of TB cases that were MDR-TB ranged between 7% and 22% in some former Soviet states and citizens, including 19% in Moldova and 22% in Baku, Azerbaijan.

Two areas in China also had rates above 7%, Stephenson added. In high-income countries, the percentage of TB cases that were MDT-TB was 1% or less, of the half million MDR-TB cases estimated to have emerged in 2006, 50% were in China and India.

Currently, the world is far behind reaching the targets for MDR-tuberculosis diagnosis and management, reported the original research team in an online report in Lancet on April 15, 2009.

Of all the complications associated with the HIV virus disease, TB represents the greatest challenge, reported Diane V. Havlir, M.D., of the University of California at San Francisco, and colleagues at various facilities.[25]

"Tuberculosis results in enormous suffering and stigma, is a threat throughout the course of HIV disease, and it is a leading cause of death," they said. "TB is one of the few transmissible agents in the health care setting that poses a risk not only to patients seeking care, but also to the health care workforce in resource-limited settings, which is already short staffed."

There are currently an estimated 10,000 health facilities providing antiretroviral therapy (ART), including 4,200 in Africa. As HIV care expands further, there is both an opportunity and necessity for incorporation of TB control activities into these programs, the researchers added.

"Tuberculosis programs simply do not have the capacity to provide ongoing TB screening, prevention, and treatment for millions of people receiving HIV care," they said.

HIV case programs must take a bold approach to TB prevention, diagnosis, and treatment to successfully address the catastrophic and intersecting epidemics of HIV and TB, the researchers continued. HIV programs need to take advantage of new earmarked funds of HIV/TB activities from agencies such as PEPFAR and the Global Fund to Fight HIV, TB, and Malaria.

They added that they must push for access for rapid TB diagnostic tests, conduct operational research, and launch educational efforts in partnership with the community to reduce TB transmission. Shortages in the health care workforce and laboratory capabilities clearly represent the greatest obstacles.

"However," they concluded, "the possibility for progress has never been greater with the global commitment to health care infrastructure strengthening geared toward consolidating the momentum through disease-specific efforts such as those involving HIV and TB."

A Vitamin A deficiency is commonly observed in patients with TB, and this deficiency could be the result of loss of appetite, poor intestinal absorption, increased urinary loss of the vitamin, or acute phase reaction to the disease, reported the National Journal of India.[26]

As we know, a vitamin A deficiency lowers immunity, while vitamin A supplementation reduces morbidity and mortality, especially in measles and diarrhea. The vitamin also decreases mortality in HIV-infected children and delays the progression of HIV disease in infected people.

Some Holistic Therapies for TB

Garlic	2 capsules, 3 times daily with meals	Acts as a natural antibiotic and stimulates the immune system
Vitamin A	25,000 IU/day, if not pregnant	
Natural Carotenes	25,000 IU/day	
Vitamin E	400-800 IU/day	
pp. 508-510		

Balch, James F., M.D., and Balch, Phyllis A., CNC. Prescription for Nutritional Healing, 2nd edition. Garden City Park, NY: Avery Publishing Group, 1997.

References

1. Harvey, Jr., Edmund H., editor. Reader's Digest Book of Facts. Pleasantville, NY: The Reader's Digest Association, Inc., 1987, p. 203.
2. Altman, Lawrence K., M.D. "Rise in a Deadly TB Reveals a Global System in Crisis," The New York Times, March 20, 2007, pp. F1, F6.
3. Voelker, Rebecca. "Leaders Warn of Deadly HIV, TB Collision," JAMA 300(5): 491-492, 2008.
4. Cain, Kevin P., M.D., et al. "Tuberculosis Among Foreign-Born Persons in the United States," JAMA 300(4): 405-412, 2008.
5. Paralkar, Vikram, M.D. "Worlds Apart—Tuberculosis in India and the United States," New England Journal of Medicine 358: 1092-1095, 2008.
6. Chaisson, Richard E., M.D., and Martinson, Neil A., M.B. "Tuberculosis in Africa—Combating an HIV-Driven Crisis," *ibid*, pp. 1089-1092.
7. Karyadi, Elvina, et al. "A Double-Blind, Placebo-Controlled Study of Vitamin A and Zinc Supplementation in Persons with Tuberculosis in Indonesia: Effects on Clinical Response and Nutritional Status," American Journal of Clinical Nutrition 75: 720-727, 2002.
8. Department of Health, Republic of Indonesia. Proposed National Health Research Priorities: The View of National Institute of Health Research and Development. Jakarta, Indonesia: Ministry of Health, Republic of Indonesia, 1999.
9. Seha, K., et al. "Undernutrition in Lepromatous Leprosy. V. Severe Nutritional Deficit in Lepromatous Patients Co-Infected with Pulmonary Tuberculosis," European Journal of Clinical Nutrition 43: 117-128, 1989.
10. Orwubalili, J.K. "Malnutrition Among Tuberculosis Patients in Harrow, England," European Journal of Clinical Nutrition 42: 363-366, 1988.
11. Goldberg, I. Burton Group. Alternative Medicine. Tiburon, CA: Future Medicine Publishing, Inc., 1997, pp. 983-984.
12. "TB Surge: Diet Link Still Unclear," Nutrition Week, May 1, 1992, pp. 6-7.
13. Balch, James F., M.D., and Balch, Phyllis A., CNC. Prescription for Nutritional Healing, 2nd Edition. Garden City Park, NY: Avery Publishing Group, 1997, pp. 508-510.
14. Shah, N. Sarita, M.D., et al. "Extensively Drug-Resistant Tuberculosis in the United States, 1993-2007," JAMA 300(18): 2153-2160, 2008.

15. Chan, Edward D., M.D., et al. "Treatment Outcomes in Extensively Resistant Tuberculosis," New England Journal of Medicine 359-657-659, 2008.

16. Hugonnet, Jean-Emmanuel, M.D., et al. "Meropenem-Clavulante Is Effective Against Extensively Drug-Resistant Mycobacterium Tuberculosis," Science 323: 1215-1217, February 22, 2009.

17. Roth, Jesse, M.D. "Evolutionary Speculation About Tuberculosis and the Metabolic and Inflammatory Processes of Obesity," JAMA 301(24): 2586-2588, 2009.

18. Liu, Yecai, M.S., et al. "Overseas Screening for Tuberculosis in U.S.-Bound Immigrants and Refugees," New England Journal of Medicine 360: 2406-2415, 2009.

19. Donald, Peter R., M.D., et al. "The Global Burden of Tuberculosis—Combating Drug Resistance in Difficult Times," New England Journal of Medicine 360: 2392-2395, 2009.

20. "Global Tuberculosis Control: Epidemiology, Strategy, Financing: WHO Report 2009 (Publication No. WHO/HTM/TB. 209 411), Geneva: World Health Organization, 2009.

21. Diacon, Andreas H., M.D., et al. "The Diarylquinoline TMC 207 for Multidrug-Resistant Tuberculosis," New England Journal of Medicine 360: 2397-2405, 2009.

22. Hampton, Tracy, Ph.D., "Tuberculosis Resistance," JAMA 297(13): 1423, 2007.

23. Mitnick, Carole D., Sc.D., et al. "Comprehensive Treatment of Extensively Drug-Resistant Tuberculosis," New England Journal of Medicine 359: 563-564, 2008.

24. Stephenson, Joan, Ph.D "Drug-Resistant TB," JAMA 301(19): 1977, 2009.

25. Havlir, Diane V., M.D., et al. "Opportunities and Challenges for HIV Care in Overlapping HIV and TB Epidemics," JAMA 300(4): 423-430, 2008.

26. Mathur, M.L. "Role of Vitamin A Supplementation in the Treatment of Tuberculosis," National Medical Journal of India 20(1): 16-21, January/February, 2007.

20

ASTHMA

Asthma is characterized by inflammation of the air passages, resulting in the temporary narrowing of the airways that transport air from the nose and mouth to the lungs, according to the Asthma and Allergy Foundation of America in Washington, D.C.[1, 2]

Asthma symptoms can be caused by allergens or irritants that are inhaled into the lungs, which results in inflamed, clogged and constricted airways. Typical symptoms include difficulty breathing, wheezing, coughing, and tightness in the chest. In severe cases, asthma can be deadly.

The disease has a genetic component, the Foundation added. If 1 parent has asthma, chances are 1 in 3 that each child will have asthma. If both parents have asthma, it is more likely—7 in 10—that their children will have the disease.

These grim statistics have been released by the Foundation:

1. An estimated 20 million Americans—1 in 15—suffer from asthma, and 50% of asthma cases are "allergic-asthma." The prevalence of asthma has been increasing since the early 1980s across all age, sex, and racial groups.
2. Asthma is the most common chronic condition among children.
3. Asthma is more common among adult women than adult men.
4. Asthma is more common among male children than female children.

5. Nearly 5 million asthma sufferers are under the age of 18. It is the most common chronic childhood disease, affecting over 1 child in 20.
6. Asthma is slightly more prevalent among African-Americans than Caucasians.
7. Ethnic differences in asthma prevalence, morbidity, and mortality are highly correlated with poverty, urban air quality, indoor allergies, and lack of patient education, along with inadequate medical care.
8. Asthma accounts for one-quarter of all emergency room visits in the U.S. annually, with 2 million emergency room visits.
9. Each year, asthma accounts for more than 10 million outpatient visits and 500,000 hospitalizations.
10. The average length of stay for asthma hospitalization is 3 days.
11. Nearly half (44%) of all asthma hospitalizations are for children.
12. Asthma is the No. 1 cause of school absenteeism among children, accounting for more than 14 million total missed days of school.
13. Each day, 11 Americans die from asthma. There are more than 4,000 deaths due to asthma each year, many of which are avoidable with proper treatment and care. Asthma is also a contributing factor for almost 7,000 other deaths each year.
14. The annual cost of asthma is estimated to be nearly $18 billion. According to the Foundation, these are asthma triggers:

1. **Allergens** : Pollen from grasses, weeds, and trees; dust mites; mite proteins; animal dander; and mold spores are the culprits. Foods do not generally cause asthma, except as part of an anaphylactic reaction (peanuts).

2. **Tobacco Smoke** : The smoke carries various irritants, which when inhaled, create a series of biochemical events that results in asthma symptoms. Secondhand smoke can trigger asthma symptoms in those with the disease.

3. Exercise : A form of asthma called exercise-induced asthma is triggered by physical activity. When symptoms appear, it may mean the patient needs to adjust the medication. Asthma can also be triggered by laughing, crying, holding one's breath, and hyperventilating.

4. Weather Changes : Cold air, wind, rain, and sudden changes in the weather can sometimes trigger an asthma attack.

5. Medication : Over-the-counter and prescription medications can sometimes trigger symptoms. For example, ingestion of aspirin and aspirin-based products can increase asthma symptoms.

6. Illness : Viruses and bacterial infections related to colds, flu, and bronchitis can increase asthma symptoms. COPD, including emphysema and chronic bronchitis, may complicate the disease. Gastroesophageal reflux disease can also cause symptoms.

7. Environmental Factors : Perfume, paint fumes, cleaning solvents, and smog can also cause symptoms in susceptible people.

The erythrocyte, and all cells in the body, have several enzyme-catalyzed metabolic pathways that help to defend against oxidative stress, according to Lawrence S. Greene, Ph.D., of the University of Massachusetts at Boston.[3]

Vitamins with antioxidant activity function in a similar fashion, he continued. If oxidant stress from exogenous sources (pollution or chemicals), or endogenous sources (as a result of the inflammatory response) overwhelm the enzyme-catalyzed and vitamin-based antioxidant defense, then cellular damage may take place.

He went on to say that an exacerbated inflammatory response may lead to cell membrane and receptor damage and to the consequent predominance of bronchoconstrictive mechanisms. The chronic inflammatory process may also produce antigen modification of a number of macromolecules and secondary immune involvement that tends to dominate asthma symtomatology.

"I am arguing that the oxidant-induced inflammatory changes are the primary events in asthma etiology, and should be the focus of preventive strategies," he continued.

Increased free radical production due to elevated body stores of iron, dietary deficiency of selenium, which may compromise the last step of the glutathione pathway and lower cellular reducing capacity, and lowered dietary intakes of the antioxidant vitamins—vitamins C, E, and beta-carotene—are some of the factors that influence asthma.

"Minimizing lead exposure from household and water sources and excess iron intake from drinking water from rusting pipes would be beneficial in preventing asthma," he said.

For his own protocol, he takes 200 mcg/day of selenium; 200 IU/day of vitamin E; and he relies on his diet for adequate intakes of beta-carotene and vitamin C.

New research on asthma points to the antihistamine effects of vitamin C, and, in fact, the antioxidants—including vitamins A, C, and E—along with mixed carotenoids, zinc, and selenium, can help to reduce the inflammatory condition of asthma, according to Ronald L. Hoffman, M.D., in Intelligent Medicine. He operates the Hoffman Center, a well-known holistic facility in New York City, and he is the host of Health Talk on radio in that city.[4]

"Chief among nutrients important to people with asthma is magnesium, since intravenous infusions of magnesium can halt even some of the most severe exacerbations of emphysema under emergency room circumstances," Hoffman said.

Magnesium apparently acts as a natural bronchodilator, relaxing the smooth muscle that line the tiny tubules that bring air to the lungs so that doesn't go into spasm. Many people with chemical sensitivities turn out to have a magnesium deficiency, he added.

"Vitamin B6 is another important vitamin for asthma control, since, paradoxically, it is depleted by theophylline-type asthma drugs," Hoffman continued. "Vitamin B12 can provide relief to asthma sufferers through the ability to activate the body's chemical-detoxification pathways."

He went on to say that, "in my office, I sometime use an 'asthma drip,' and intravenous 'cocktail' of nutrients that are particularly helpful. It contains vitamin C, which acts as a natural antihistamine, pantothenic acid, a B vitamin that supports adrenal function, magnesium, which is helpful in patients with chemical sensitivities, zinc, and selenium."

The incidence of asthma worldwide is highest among inner-city children, but asthma strikes all racial, social, and economic classes, according to The Complete Guide to Pain Relief. The increase has been especially noticeable in China, Australia, and many Western countries.[5]

Some of the recommended remedies include exercise, herbal medicines, yoga, t'ai chi, and homeopathy.

"A recent study suggests that extra vitamin A may help to control asthma symptoms," the publication said. "Dosages up to 25,000 IU may be taken for short periods, such as when recovering from a lung infection."

For long-term use—over 3 months—the maximum safe dosage for adults is about 10,000 IU/day, the publication added. However, pregnant women should not exceed 8,000 IU/day, and children should not take vitamin A supplements without medical supervision.

In addition to eliminating allergic foods, Alan Gaby, M.D., recommends these supplements for asthma: vitamins C, B6, B12, niacinamide (B3), magnesium chloride, and calcium glycerophosphate, reported Alternative Medicine.[6]

For acute attacks, he supports an intravenous injection of these same vitamins and minerals, as well as the addition of quercetin, a flavonoid found in onions, beta-carotene, selenium, and manganese.

In a case-control study of 20 people with brittle asthma, 20 with non-brittle asthma, and 20 healthy controls, with a mean age of 49.5 years, of whom 27 were males, results showed that brittle asthmatics had statistically lower median dietary intakes of vitamins A and E than the other groups, reported Thorax.[7]

Blood levels of these antioxidants were within the normal range for each nutrient in all volunteers.

However, intakes less than the reference nutrient intakes (RNI) for magnesium and vitamins A and C and less than the safe intake (SI) for vitamin E, were more likely in patients with brittle asthma than in those with nonbrittle asthma, the researchers said.

Researchers at Nottingham University in England reviewed 40 studies over the past 30 years, which revealed that those with low intakes of vitamin C had a 12% increased risk of asthma, they reported in Thorax Journal.[8]

While less clear, there was still a significant association between asthma and a vitamin A deficiency.

Blood levels of vitamin A, retinol-binding protein—which transports vitamin A through the blood—and albumin-a simple protein—were evaluated in 35 asthmatic children. The study involved 24 males, ranging in age from 2 to 12 years, and 19 males acting as controls, according to Alternative Medicine Review.[9]

The research team found that there were low levels of vitamin A in the children with asthma in contrast to the controls. In fact, low blood levels of the vitamin were 4 times more in the study group than in the controls.

It was found that children with severe persistent asthma had markedly low blood levels of the vitamin.

Asthma Symptoms

* Severe cough or heavy wheezing.
* Difficulty talking; do not want to swallow or eat.
* Shoulders hunches for breathing; cannot lie down flat.
* Nostrils flare with breathing.
* Walking causes difficulty breathing.
* Skin is pale, gray.
* Lips or the area around the mouth are turning blue.
* Shoulders, ribs are expanding and contracting to help with work or breathing.
* Peak flow meter readings are in the danger zone.

Source: ''Asthma and Allergy Answers,'' Asthma and Allergy Foundation of America, Washington, D.C., 2006.

References

1. ''Asthma Facts and Figures.'' Asthma and Allergy Foundation of America, Washington, D.C., December 13, 2007.

2. "Asthma and Allergy Answers," *ibid*, 2006.
3. Hamilton, Kirk, PA.C. The Experts Speak. Sacramento, CA: I.T. Services, 1996, pp. 16-17. Also, Greene, Lawrence S., Ph. D. "Asthma and Oxidant Stress: Nutritional, Environmental, and Genetic Risk Factors," Journal of the American College of Nutrition 14(4): 317-324, 1995.
4. Hoffman, Ronald L., M.D. Intelligent Medicine. New York: Simon & Schuster, 1997, pp. 339ff.
5. Kalyn, Wayne, editorial director. The Complete Guide to Pain Relief. Pleasantville, NY: The Reader's Digest Association, Inc., 2000, pp. 114ff.
6. Goldberg, I. Burton Alternative Medicine. Tiburon, CA: Future Medicine Publishing, Inc., 1997, p. 819.
7. Baker, J.C., et al. "Dietary Antioxidants and Magnesium in Type I Brittle Asthma: A Case-Control Study," Thorax 54: 115-118, 1999.
8. "Vitamin Deficiency Asthma Link," BBC News, April 16, 2009.
9. Arora, P., et al. "Vitamin A Status in Children with Asthma," Alternative Medicine Review 13:223-226, October 2002.

21

HOW SAFE ARE VITAMIN A AND BETA-CAROTENE?

In countries where widespread endemic vitamin A deficiency results in large-scale morbidity and mortality, current public health programs and medical practice include the administration, once per 3 to 12 months, of 50,000 to 200,000 IU (15 to 60 mg) or more vitamin A to children, depending on age, to treat and prevent vitamin A deficiency, according to John N. Hathcock, Ph.D., in Vitamin and Mineral Safety.[1]

"Even though the dosage is high, it must be noted that this is not a daily dose, but is instead a periodic dose to target populations with very depleted liver stores of vitamin A and a large unused storage capacity," Hathcock said. "The situation is vastly different from daily intakes of high-potency vitamin A in a population that is nutritionally replete."

Being fat-soluble, vitamin A accumulates in the liver, but its absorption is not linear but is dependent on the vitamin A status of the individual. Very high intakes, however, can accumulate in the liver and other tissues. Thus, both the daily intake and the duration of consumption are important influences on the safety and actions of the vitamin."

Potential risk of a vitamin A toxicity is based on the ingestion of excessive amounts of preformed vitamin A in the forms of retinol or retinyl esters, but not from provitamin A forms such as beta-carotene or other provitamin A carotenoids, Hathcock added.

Consumption of 25,000 to 50,000 IU (7,500 to 15,000 mcg RE) of preformed retinol equivalents daily for periods of several months or more by women of child-bearing age can produce multiple adverse effects, including liver toxicity and possibly birth defects.

"The smallest daily supplement of vitamin A reported to be associated with liver cirrhosis in adults is 25,000 IU retinol equivalents (7,500 mcg RE) during 6 years," Hathcock continued. "The smallest daily supplement generally considered to generate any risk of birth defects is also 25,000 IU. However, one report concluded that there was a significantly increased risk of neural crest birth defects at maternal daily supplemental levels of more than 10,000 IU (more than 3,000 mcg RE)."

He went on to say that the average supplemental intake by this range group of women was 21,675 IU (6,500 mcg RE), but, unfortunately, the authors did not identify individual supplemental intakes in the seven cases associated with birth defects.

"Several issues have been raised about the validity of the defect classification scheme used and the resulting likelihood that the study overestimated the risk associated with vitamin A at the levels identified in the study," Hathcock added.

A few reports suggest the possibility that there may be some risk of vitamin A toxicity at supplementation levels below 20,000 IU (6,000 mcg RE/day). One report to the FDA suggested a characteristic birth defect in association with maternal supplementation at 18,000 IU (5,400 mcg RE/day). Another report found marginal indications in elderly people of adverse effects on the liver with chronic supplementation at levels of 5,000 to 10,000 IU (1,500 to 3,000 mcg RE/day), however, this observation has not been confirmed, and the same laboratory was unable to repeat this finding in later research, Hathcock said. No other reports have indicated adverse effects from vitamin A at these supplemented levels.

What About Beta-Carotene?

Beta-carotene is considered to be virtually non-toxic because humans tolerate high dietary dosages without apparent harm, and animal studies also fail to find any toxic effects, Hathcock added.

"Standard toxicological tests, including teratogenic, mutagenic, and carcinogenic assay, have been performed on beta-carotene without any evidence of harmful effects," Hathcock continued. "There is no evidence that conversion of beta-carotene to vitamin A contributes to vitamin A toxicity, even when beta-carotene is ingested in large amounts."

The only documented biological effects of high beta-carotene intakes has been discoloration of the skin related to hypercarotenemia, but this occurs only at extremely high intakes. Intakes as high as 180 mg/day have been given to humans for several months without observed adverse effects other than skin color change.

"Extensive data show that beta-carotene supplements at 50 mg every other day (equivalent to 25 mg/day) can be taken for more than a decade without harm," Hathcock said. "Skin coloration is harmless and self-correcting with intake reduction."

At the USDA Human Nutrition Research Center on Aging at Tufts University in Boston, Massachusetts, Elizabeth J. Johnson, Ph.D., and colleagues, evaluated 284 women, 40 to 70 years of age, concerning the relationship between dietary supplementation of vitamin A and biochemical markers of vitamin A toxicity.[2]

There was no difference in dietary vitamin A intake between users and nonusers of supplemental vitamin A. In the vitamin A supplements, the mean total vitamin intake was 952 IU/day.

For both supplementers and nonsupplementers, serum retinyl esters increased significantly over time, and the magnitude of increase was not different between the two groups.

The research team added that serum levels of retinol, retinyl esters, and retinol binding protein were not correlated with vitamin A intake in both supplemental and nonsupplemental groups. Biochemical measures of liver damage were not related to biochemical determinants of vitamin A status in both nonusers and users of supplemental vitamin A.

These results suggest that long-term supplementation with vitamin A in doses commonly found in multivitamin supplements, does not increase the risk for hypervitaminosis A, the researchers said.

A dose of 30,000 IU/day of vitamin A should be considered as nonteratogenic in humans, reported the International Journal of Vitamin and Nutrition and Research.[3]

Since elevated circulating retinyl ester levels have been correlated with vitamin A toxicity, a research team at the University of New Mexico School of Medicine at Albuquerque investigated the effects of long-term vitamin A supplementation on retinyl ester concentrations, liver damage, and risk of developing hypervitaminosis A.[4]

The researchers monitored dietary supplementation with vitamin A and biochemical symptoms of toxicity in 116 healthy elderly volunteers for 5 years.

Each year during the study, plasma retinol and retinyl ester concentrations, 7 liver-function tests, and dietary and supplemental vitamin A intakes were studied. The volunteers consumed between 2,528 IU/day and 23,032 IU/day of dietary vitamin A, and 0 to 47,000 IU/day of supplemental vitamin A during the trial.

The research team reported in the American Journal of Clinical Nutrition that supplemental intake of vitamin A was correlated with retinyl ester concentrations, but these levels remained constant throughout the study, regardless of supplemental dose. There were no signs of vitamin A toxicity.

The RDA for vitamin A ranges up to 5,000 IU/day, and the results of this study revealed that doses much greater than this extended over long periods apparently have no harmful effects, the researchers said.

Prolonged use of large amounts exceeding 50,000 IU as retinol can result in skin reshes, hair loss, and other skin effects that are reversible when the vitamin is withdrawn, according to Nestor W. Flodin, Ph.D., of the University of South Alabama College of Medicine in Mobile.[5]

There is concern that excessive intake of vitamin A during pregnancy could result in cleft plate and other birth defects, he added. If a supplement of vitamin A is taken during pregnancy, it should be in the form of beta-carotene, which does not lead to hypervitaminosis A, nor to birth defects.

"There is increasing interest in the supplemental use of beta-carotene because of its ability, independent of conversion to vitamin A in the body, to prevent free radical damage to cells," Flodin said.

He went on to say that epidemiological and laboratory studies indicate that beta-carotene protects against cancer and heightens immune response. The National Cancer Institute has sponsored long-term human studies showing that daily doses of 15 to 30 mg of beta-carotene may help in reducing cancer.

Doses of vitamin A as high as 300,000 IU/day for up to two years appear to be safer than previously thought, according to researchers at the Instituto Nazionale Tumori in Milan, Italy.[6]

Vitamin A supplementation in the prevention and treatment of cancer has gained increasing attention, since retinoids inhibit malignant transformation and reverse premalignant changes in numerous tissues and organs, the researchers reported in the Journal of Cancer Research.

In the study, 283 patients with Stage 1 lung cancer were randomized to receive either 300,000 IU/day of retinyl palmitate for 12 months or standard follow-up procedure. During the study, the patients received a physical examination, chest roentgenogram, blood chemistries and other tests.

Results showed that serum transaminase abnormalities were similar in both cases and controls, while gamma glutamyltransferase levels were elevated in the supplemented group. Triglycerides, serum retinol, and retinol binding protein levels were higher in the vitamin A group.

The research team added that pharmacological doses of vitamin A for the treatment of lung cancer can be used with reasonable safety for up to two years.

Emerging evidence suggests that subtoxicity without clinical signs of toxicity may be a growing concern, because intake from preformed sources of vitamin A often exceeds the recommended dietary allowance (RDA) for adults, especially in developed countries, according to Kristina L. Penniston and Sherry A. Tanumihardjo of the University of Wisconsin at Madison.[7, 8, 9]

"Assessing vitamin A status in those with subtoxicity or toxicity is complicated because serum retinol concentrations are nonsensitive indicators in this range of liver vitamin A reserves," the researchers said.

They added that the metabolism in well-nourished people of preformed vitamin A, provided by either liver or supplements, has been studied by several research groups. To control vitamin A deficiency, large therapeutic doses are administered in developing countries to women and children who are often malnourished.

Nevertheless, they continued, little attention has been given to the short-term kinetics (i.e., after absorption but before storage) of a large dose of vitamin A or to the short- or long-term effects such a dose given to lactating women on serum and breast-milk concentrations of retinol and its metabolites.

In addition, appropriate dosing regimens have not been systematically evaluated to ascertain the quantitative improvement in vitamin A status of the women and children who receive these supplements.

"The acute and chronic effects of vitamin A toxicity have been reported previously," the authors said. "However, further research is needed to ascertain the areas of the world in which subclinical toxicity exists, and to evaluate its effects on overall health and well-being."

They pointed out that vitamin A is obtained from preformed vitamin A (i.e., retinyl esters from animal foods, fortified foods, and pharmaceutical supplements), as well as from provitamin A carotenoids from plant sources.

"Preformed vitamin A is efficiently absorbed and utilized by humans at absorption rates of 70 to 90%," the authors said. "Up to 75% of dietary vitamin A in Europe, the United States, and other industrialized nations is preformed vitamin A, which is largely derived from multivitamins, fish liver oils, and the fortification of foods such as milk, butter, margarine, breakfast cereals, and some snack foods."

In the developing countries, however, 70 to 90% of vitamin A is obtained from provitamin A carotenoids in plant foods. These sources are absorbed much less efficiently, at ratios of 20 to 50%, depending on each person's vitamin A status and other dietary and nondietary factors.

"The cleavage of provitamin A carotenoids to retinol is a highly regulated step, and vitamin A toxicity from provitamin

A sources is largely impossible," the authors continued. "In contrast, absorption and hepatic (liver) storage of preformed vitamin A occurs very efficiently until a pathologic condition develops."

They added that most retinyl esters are hydrolyzed to retinol in intestinal lumen. Retinol is absorbed by intestinal epithelial cells, where it is reesterified to long-chain fatty acids and incorporated into chylomicra (which contains cholesterol, triglycerol, apolipoproteins, etc.), which circulate in the intestinal lymph before moving into the general circulation.

"As the chylomicra lose their triacylglycerol and other constituents, most of the retinol esters remain within, and the particiles become chylomicron remnants," the authors added. "Chylomicron remnants are cleared mainly by the liver, but extrahepatic uptake of the remnants may be important in the delivery of vitamin A to mammory tissue, bone marrow, adipose tissue, and spleen."

Ideally, vitamin A status is monitored as part of public health programs to prevent the occurrence of both subclinical deficiency and toxicity, the authors continued. The deleterious effects of vitamin A deficiency are known, but further research is needed to ascertain whether subclinical toxicity exists, and, if so, what are its effects on overall health and well-being.

In a letter in the October 2007 issue of the American Journal of Clinical Nutrition, Sam Newton and Seth Owusu-Agyei of the Kintampo Health Research Centre in Ghana, and Betty Kirkwood of the London School of Hygiene and Tropical Medicine in the United Kingdom, commented on an article, "Randomized Controlled Safety and Efficacy Trial of Two Vitamin A Supplementation Schedules in Tanzanian Infants," by Idindili, et al., in a previous issue of the magazine.[10, 11]

Idindili, et al., conducted a similar trial in Kintampo, Ghana, to the one discussed in Tanzania. Both were funded by the World Health Organization in 2002.

"Both studies assessed the effectiveness of a new maternal and young infant vitamin A dosing regimen, in which mothers and infants in the intravenous arm were given 400,000 IU of vitamin A within six weeks of delivery, and their infants were given 50,000 IU of vitamin A at 6, 10, and 14 weeks of age, as recommended by the Annency Acords," Newton, at al., reported.[12]

Mothers and infants in the control group were given the old regimen of 200,000 IU within 6 weeks of delivery, and their infants received 25,000 IU at 6, 10, and 14 weeks, along with diphtheria-pertussis-tetanus immunizations.

The effect of the 2 vitamin A recommendations on breast milk retinol concentrations, and on infant serum retinol concentrations, assessed by using modified-relative-dose response tests, were assessed at 6 weeks, 6 months, and 9 months of age. The incidence of side effects, such as bulging of the anterior fontanel (cranial bones of an infant), vomiting, and incidence of severe mortality, were also measured at these ages, the researchers continued.

Their results were similar to those of the Tanzinian study, but were only available for a small number of infants who were enrolled early in the trial, because the routine monitoring of capsule content showed degradation of some vitamin A capsules.

"The conclusion of both trials was that a regimen of 50,000 IU of vitamin A with early infant vaccines has no advantage over the previously recommended regimen of 25,000 IU, which has important policy implications," the Ghanan researchers added.

They went on to say that those trials, and the original WHO multicenter trials in Ghana, India, and Peru suggest no overall benefit of vitamin A supplementation in combination with vaccines in the first 5 months of life, and that it is no longer policy recommendation to do so. The emphasis remains on larger doses to older children.

Their other concern was that vitamin A supplements should be monitored to ensure that young children actually receive adequate amounts of the vitamin.

Replying to the letter by Newton, et al., in the May 2008 issue of the American Journal of Clinical Nutrition, Venkatesh Mannar of Micronutrient Initiative in Ottawa, Canada, and Alan Court UNICEF in New York City, said that the United Nations Children's Fund (UNICEF) and Micronutrient Initiative provide over 95% of the global supply of vitamin A capsules.[13]

Therefore, they added, they can confirm that over 95% of the 100,000 and 200,000 IU of vitamin A capsules manufactured, procured, and delivered through child survival programs and other public health programs to children less than 5 years of age in over 100 countries undergo rigorous quality assurance procedures.

"Despite the assurances of performance in the laboratory, we agree that it is very important to periodically assess on a larger scale the retinol stability of vitamin A capsules that have been exposed to real field conditions," Mannar and Court continued. "For this reason, Micronutrient Initiative, in collaboration with UNICEF, is in the process of systematically collecting samples of capsules that have been in the field since 2004 from 20 countries for independent laboratory analysis."

They went on to say that they are confident the quality assurance systems currently in place will continue to reinforce the current high level of confidence in vitamin A supplementation programs, and will allow them to focus on increasing the coverage of these life-saving supplements so that more children around the world have a chance to reach—and exceed—their fifth birthday.

References

1. Hathcock, John N., Ph.D. Vitamin and Mineral Safety. Washington, D.C.: Council for Responsible Nutrition, 1997, pp. 24ff.
2. Johnson, Elizabeth J., Ph.D., et al. "Lack of An Effect of Multivitamins Containing Vitamin A on Serum Retinyl Esters and Liver Function Tests in Elderly Women," Journal of the American College of Nutrition 11(6): 682-686, December 1992.
3. Wiegand, U.W., et al. "Safety of Vitamin A: Recent Results," International Journal of Vitamin Nutrition and Research 68: 411-416, 1998.
4. Stauber, P., et al. "A Longitudinal Study of the Relationship Between Vitamin A Supplementation and Plasma Retinol, Retinyl Esters, and Liver Enzyme Activities in a Healthy Elderly Population," American Journal of Clinical Nutrition 54: 878-883, 1991.
5. Flodin, Nestor W., Ph.D. "Antioxidant Vitamin Supplementation: How Safe?" The Nutrition Report 10(4): 25, 32, April 1992.

6. Infante, M., et al. "Laboratory Evaluation During High-Dose Vitamin A Administration: A Randomized Study on Lung Cancer Patients After Surgical Resection," Journal of Cancer Research 117: 156-162, 1991.
7. Penniston, Karistina L., and Tanumihardjo, Sherry A. "The Acute and Chronic Toxic Effects of Vitamin A," American Journal of Clinical Nutrition 83: 191-201, 2006.
8. Mehta, N.J. "Dietary Intervention with Dark Green Leafy Vegetables—Spinach (Spinacia oleracea) to Combat Subclinical Vitamin A Deficiency (SVAD) in Slum Children of Dharavi, Mumbai, India," Sight Life Newsletter 4: 32-33, 2001.
9. Olson, J.A. Vitamin A in: Ziegler, E.E., et al., editors. "Present Knowledge in Nutrition," 7th Edition. Washington, D.C.: International Life Sciences Institute Press, 2001, pp. 109-119.
10. Newton, Sam, Owusy-Agyei, S., and Kirkwood, B. "Is There Any Monitoring of the Quality of Vitamin A Capsules Used in Supplementation Programs?" American Journal of Clinical Nutrition 86(4): 1254, 2007.
11. Idindili, B., et al. "Randomized Controlled Safety and Efficacy Trial of 2 Vitamin A Supplementation Schedules in Tanzanian Infants," American Journal of Clinical Nutrition 85: 1312-1319, 2007.
12. Sommer, A., and Davidson, F.R. "Assessment and Control of Vitamin A Deficiency: The Annecy Accords," Journal of Nutrition 132: 2845S-2850S, 2002.
13. Mannar, V., and Court, A. "Ensuring the Quality of Vitamin A Capsules Used in Supplementation Programs," American Journal of Clinical Nutrition 87(5): 1539-1540, 2008.

22

ARE VACCINATIONS NECESSARY?

Vaccination became available in the latter part of the 18th century, when Edward Jenner (1749-1823), an English surgeon, noticed as a youth that when people were sick with the relatively benign disease cowpox they did not contract smallpox.[1]

In 1796, he innoculated a boy with matter taken from a dairymaid's fresh cowpox lesions. The boy caught cowpox, but when subsequently innoculated with smallpox, he did not contract it.

"Despite early difficulties," explained Merriam-Webster's Collegiate Encyclopedia, "the procedure spread and the death rate from smallpox fell. Jenner received worldwide recognition, although he was also subject to attacks and slander. He retired from public life in 1815, following the death of his wife."

In the early days, there was a rumor that vaccination would cause you to grow the horns and tail of a cow, added The Book of Health. With the advent of vaccination, smallpox became relatively rare in countries with high medical standards, although it killed 25 to 30% of the European population during the Middle Ages in a single epidemic.[2]

The area of the body chosen for vaccination most often is the upper arm or thigh. The area should be relatively free from friction by clothing or other parts of the body, the publication added.

Vaccination is usually done by placing a drop of vaccine upon the cleaned skin. The physician then rubs a needle against the skin underlying the drop of vaccine. Only the outermost layer of the skin is punctured, so that there is no bleeding, although lymph is exuded (oozed) from the wound and mixes with the vaccine. The lymph-vaccine mixture is allowed to dry on the skin. It is generally not necessary to bandage the vaccination unless the patient attempts to scratch the area, or that there is a possibility of irritation from clothing.

"A wheel, or slightly raised area, develops at the site of the vaccination almost immediately, but soon disappears," the publication continued. "A day or so later, the area becomes reddened and small blisters of pinpoint size appear within this reddish region. In the following days, the red area enlarges and the blisters fuse to form a single and larger blister. The fluid within the blister is clear at first, but gradually becomes cloudy and later pus-like."

During this period, the patient may exhibit a fever, and during the eight or ninth day following the vaccination, he may be ill. From the ninth to the twelfth day, the red area increases in size and the skin around it becomes hard and thickened.

After the twelfth day, the sore begins to heal and the blister disappears, leaving a black scab which begins to shrink. This scab becomes loose around the edges at first, and it eventually falls off. The skin under the crust is red and slightly pitted. The redness slowly disappears, and a slight scar may remain.

"The scratching of a fresh vaccination, followed by scratching of other parts of the body must be avoided," the publication continued. "That is because vaccination lesions can be transferred to any part of the skin in this way."

The immunity to say smallpox gained by vaccination is not permanent, consequently, vaccinations must be repeated, usually in 5 to 7 years, to insure continued safety.

"Doctors frequently recommend that vaccination be made during the first year of life," the publication said. "When the second or subsequent vaccinations do not 'take' that is, they heal in a few days, or do not form the customary lesion, the patient is said to have an immune reaction. This implies that the immunity from the previous vaccinations has not been lost. When an individual is vaccinated many years before but does not contract the disease, it is likely to be mild."

Certain precautions should attend smallpox vaccinations, the publication added. No one with general illness or extensive skin eruptions should be vaccinated, especially an infant or child with eczema or impetigo (7-year-itch). Also, any child with such a skin rash should be kept away from recently vaccinated people.

Eczema vaccinatum, which may follow such an exposure, is uncommon, but it carries a high mortality rate. Pregnant women should also avoid smallpox vaccination, unless there are compelling reasons, since fatal infection of the fetus sometimes occurs. Smallpox is especially hazardous to adults with cancer, who are being treated with steroids, nitrogen mustard, or radiation therapy. The therapeutic impairment of their natural immune system may allow the vaccine virus to multiply dangerously, to the point where the patient's life is threatened. Also, one should not receive yellow fever vaccination simultaneously, as both vaccines employ live viruses.

"It has been known for centuries that once a person has had smallpox, he is immune to the disease and will not contract it again," the publication added. "Vaccination is a deliberate infection of the patient with a disease—not actually smallpox itself, but one which is able to produce immunity to smallpox. The virus used may be obtained from lesions produced by calves or rabbits that have been infected with the smallpox virus. Such passage through one of these animals causes the virus to lose its ability to cause the natural disease in man."

However, when it is rubbed into the epidermis, the weakened virus causes a local sore, which lends immunity to the dangerous form of smallpox for 5 to 7 years. Cowpox virus, while causing a serious disease in cattle, may be used for vaccination of human beings. The material used for vaccination is called vaccine, and it is specially prepared so that it contains no infectious microorganisms, other than the particular virus, the publication said.

A vaccine works by sensitizing the body's immune system to a particular disease-causing bacterial toxin, virus, or bacterium, explained the American Medical Association Home Medical Encyclopedia. If the particular infectious agent invades the body at a later time, the sensitized immune system quickly produces antibodies that help destroy either the agent itself or the toxin it produces.[3]

"Most vaccines are preparations containing the very organisms (or parts of the organism) against which protection is sought" the publication said. "So that these organisms do not cause disease, they are killed or weakened. The term 'live attenuated organisms' describes strains of organisms that have been rendered harmless either by artificial alteration of their genes or by successfully infecting laboratory animals. This leads to changes in the organisms that considerably reduce their ability to cause disease without reducing their ability to induce immunity. Other vaccines contain chemically modified bacterial toxins."

Vaccines are available to protect against a variety of infectious diseases, the publication continued. Examples of live attenuated vaccines are those given to protect against measles, mumps, and rubella (often combined), yellow fever, Sabin's oral polio vaccine. Diphtheria and tetanus vaccines contain inactivated bacterial toxins. Cholera, typhoid fever, pertussis, rabies, viral hepatitis B, influenza, and Salk injected polio vaccines contain killed organisms or, in the case of hepatities B, only a part of the hepatitis B virus.

Oral polio vaccine is given on a sugar lump or by drops on the tongue, the publication added. Some vaccines require several doses, spaced some weeks apart, while others require only one dose. (The vaccine being developed against Swine Flu reportedly requires 2 doses).

"Although diseases such as diphtheria, measles, mumps, rubella (German measles), poliomyelitis, and pertussis (whooping cough) are today rare in the United States, routine immunization against them must continue," the publication added. "If a large proportion of the population were nonimmunized, there would be a risk of a new epidemic because there is still a steady flow of infectious diseases, many of which are imported."[4]

Immunization may be active or passive. The terms vaccination and active immunization are used interchangeabiy, and the word vaccination is derived from the vaccina virus—which is similar to the smallpox vaccine—which was used for vaccination against smallpox.

"Although most modern vaccines provide a reliable method of preventing disease, they do not all provide 100% protection," the publication said. "Cholera and typhoid fever vaccinations give only partial protection, so other precautions—principally food and water hygiene—must be observed during travel to areas where there is a risk of these diseases."

Vaccination is ranked as one of the 10 greatest public health achievements of the last century, and it is the number one contribution to decreased global morbidity and mortality, reported Yvonne A. Maldonado, M.D., of the Stanford University School of Medicine in Palo Alto, California.[5]

"Pediatric vaccinations have had the most profound impact on any intervention on increasing global child survival, accounting for 3 million pediatric lives saved annually," she said.

However, even in the 21st century, vaccine-preventable infectious diseases remain important causes of illness and death in many parts of the world.

Globally, she continued, tetanus, measles, and pertussis are the main vaccine preventable causes of death in children, while septicemia and influenza-related pneumonia are among the top 10 causes of death in adults and children worldwide, including the United States. Formerly called "blood poisoning", septicemia is systemic disease caused by microorganisms and their toxins circulating in the blood.

"Although U.S. pediatric vaccination rates remain high, there is a small but vocal antivaccine movement concerned about vaccine safety that may affect vaccination efforts in the United States and elsewhere," Maldonado added.

In adults, vaccine preventable diseases result in $10 billion in health care costs, and more than 30,000 preventable deaths annually, but vaccination rates among adults remain poor and recommended vaccine schedules for U.S. adults are markedly underutilized, she added.

These local reactions are common and may occur in up to 50% of vaccines, but symptoms such as fever, headache, irritability, or diminished activity are less common. Rarely, moderate to severe reactions to vaccines, such as febrile seizures and allergic reactions, occur at a frequency of 1 reaction per thousands or millions of doses administered. A full listing of vaccine-associated adverse events is available online at http://www.cdc.gov/nip.

Misconceptions regarding vaccinations prevent many children and adults from getting the protection they need, but these views are often based on anecdotal reports or data not stringent to support the association, she continued.

As an example, there is the claim that diabetes mellitus is due to increased exposure to vaccine antigens in childhood, but scientifically rigorous studies have refuted this hypothesis.

"Another hypothesis linking measles immunization to autism has been the subject of intense international controversy," Maldonado continued. "However, rigorous analysis of the incidence of autism relative to the timing of introduction of measles vaccine into populations has failed to demonstrate any temporal association between the 2 events, and no biologically plausible hypothesis has yet been developed to support an association."

Increasing public awareness of the controversies surrounding vaccine safety, and the need to maintain the achievements of vacination programs have resulted in creation of a variety of vaccine information services.

In the private sector, the National Network for Immunization Information has a website—http://www.immunizationinfo.org.

"These sites can serve as rapid, accurate, and objective sources of current information on vaccine recommendations, risks, benefits, and frequently asked questions regarding vaccines," she continued. "Timely and accurate information regarding vaccine safety issues will facilitate continued implementation of safe and effective immunization programs."

In 2009, 3 special masters of the U.S. Court of Federal Claims issued carefully reasoned, strongly worded opinions rejecting claims that medical and scientific evidence could demonstrate causal links between thimerosal-containing vaccines or measles-mumps-rubella (MMR) vaccinations and the development of chronic health conditions such as autism, immune dysfunction, and gastrointestinal dysfunction, reported Ross D. Silverman, J.D., M.P.H., in the June 11, 2009 issue of the New England Journal of Medicine.[6]

The 3 cases were test cases drawn from over 5,000 similar claims filed under the National Vaccine Inquiry Compensation

Program (VICP), which was established in 1988, in response to concerns that injury lawsuits against vaccine manufacturers and administrators were threatening the nation's childhood-vaccine supply.

"Because the injuries claimed in these cases were not listed in the VICP's Vaccine Injury Table, in order to receive compensation under the program, the families had to demonstrate through medical or scientific evidence that it is more likely than not that vaccination played a significant role in causing such injuries," Silverman said.

The special masters informed their decisions by reviewing an extraordinary amount of scientific and medical evidence, including the testimony of 28 medical experts, 50 expert reports, and over 5,000 pages of proceedings, transcripts, and briefs that included over 900 scientific articles.

"The concerns the special masters felt for the families who must cope with the daily challenges of caring for children with devastating chronic illness of as yet unknown origin is evident throughout the over 600 pages of legal decisions," Silverman added.

In addition, the special masters were convinced that the parents had filed their claims in good faith. However, they were far less sympathetic toward both the evidence proffered by the claimants and the physicians who testified and offered research in support of the claims.

Special Master George Hastings, in referring to one case, said that, "unfortunately, the Cedillos have been misled by physicians who are guilty, in my view, of gross medical misjudgement."

He added that, "absent significant and dramatic new scientific findings, future litigation attempts to tie autism to vaccination is likely to meet a similar fate."

The success of the childhood immunization program can in part be traced to state laws requiring parents to provide evidence that their children have been vaccinated as a prerequisite for enrolement in schools and day-care centers.

"Most states permit exemptions on religious grounds, and a growing number of states permit exemption claims based on broader philosophical or personal objections,'' Silverman continued. ''States also have widely varied administrative structures for approving exemption requests.''

Not surprisingly, he said, states with expansive bases for exemptions and more limited administrative requirements for fulfilling exemption requests have more parents opting out of vaccinating their children—a trend that increases the likelihood of outbreaks of vaccine-preventable diseases, and creates potential geographic ''hot spots'' where high concentrations of exempted children may compromise community-wide protection. (There are occasional outbreaks of measles in the United States, although the disease was thought to have been erradicated).

''While continuing to support the rights of parents to choose to refuse vaccinations for their children, states should explore strengthening their administrative process for approving exemptions to ensure that they are limited to families with deeply held beliefs,'' Silverman said.

He went on to say that the benefits of vaccination to the child and the public are widely known and may be demonstrated with the use of scientific data. A failure to ensure adequate public participation can lead to a potentially damaging backlash against such public health interventions, as was seen in the extremely negative response to the decision by the governor of Texas to circumvent the legislature and issue an executive order mandating the vaccination of adolescent girls against the human papilloma virus (HPV), as well as the reaction to the news that the HPV vaccine manufacturer was lobbying hard to get the shot added to the list of mandatory immunizations.

''I would also argue that public health officials should explore options in lieu of mandates to encourage the uptake of new vaccinations, such as public education programs or public funding for immunization, and as others have, I would encourage states to consider limiting mandates to illnesses that can reasonably be tied to school attendance,'' Silverman added.

He said that as national health care reform efforts move forward, policymakers should be encouraged to support the restructuring of the reimbursement system in order to enhance the opportunity for physicians to engage in preventive care interventions, including efforts to educate patients and vaccine distribution.

Autism is a condition in which children fail to form relationships with others, according to the American Medical Association Home Medical Encyclopedia. It occurs in about 2 to 4 out of every 10,000 children. Almost 3 times more boys than girls are affected. It is usually apparent in the first year of life.[7]

While the precise causes of autism are not known, evidence points to a physical basis. Since about one-fourth of the autistic children have signs of a neurological disorder, and epileptic seizures develop in almost one-third of the children in adolescence, it is likely that there is a subtle form of brain damage.

The child often remains normal for the first few months before becoming increasingly unresponsive to parents or other stimuli. The first sign may be resistance to being cuddled with the child screaming to be put down when picked up, even if hurt or tired.

Writing in Autism Research Review International in 1996, Bernard Rimland, Ph.D., said that 18 studies have been published since 1963 on the role of high doses of vitamin B6 (pyridoxine) in autism, which show that benefit may occur in about half of the autistic children and adults.[8]

In 8 of the experiments, abnormal substances that appeared in the urine of autistic children were normalized by vitamin B6. In other studies, brain waves were normalized with the vitamin.

Eighteen consecutive studies showed vitamin B6 to be effective and no studies showed that megadoses of the vitamin failed. None of the studies reported significant adverse effects, he said.

Magnesium and the other B vitamins may help prevent reversible toxicity of vitamin B6 when taken at doses of 2,000 to 6,000 mg/day.

Rimland, who had followed thousands of autistic children and adults on megadoses of B6 for over 30 years has only encountered cases of peripheral neuropathy. When B6 was discontinued or the dosage reduced, these symptoms went away quickly and completely.

Rimland's son, who was 40 at the time of the article, had been taking 1 gram (1,000 mg) of B6 along with 400 mg of magnesium and other nutrients daily for over 30 years.

Rimland added that vitamin B6 at 100 to 300 mg/day taken for several years has shown a 27% reduction in the risk of heart disease in the elderly, and at 300 mg/kg/day (18 times the dose used in autism) was superior to seizure drugs in epileptic children.

Vitamin A supplementation (VAS) to children over 6 months of age in low-income countries has been estimated to reduce overall mortality by 23 to 30%, reported Christine S. Benn of the Studens Serum Institut in Copenhagen, Denmark, and colleagues at other facilities.[9, 10, 11, 12]

Estimates are based on several meta-analysis (a compilation of trials) of VAS trials conducted in the 1980s and early 1990s.

"Currently, the World Health Organization recommends administration of VAS at vaccination contacts after 6 months of age," the researchers said. "However, none of the trials that found reduced mortality after VAS examined the link with vaccination status. Hence, it is unknown whether the effect of VAS on mortality is independent of vaccinations."

They went on to say that VAS clearly reduced the risk of developing xerophthalmia in boys and girls with and without a health card. Hence, vitamin A deficiency was present and prevented or treated by means of VAS. In spite of this, VAS had no effect on mortality in children who were vaccinated, and it was associated with increased mortality among measles-vaccinated girls who were likely to have received diphtheria-tetanus-pertussis (DTP) vaccine during follow-up. Xerophthalmia is a dry, thickened condition of the conjunctiva and cornea. It can be the result of chronic inflammation, a disease of the tear-producing appeartus, or a vitamin A deficiency.

"Note that the first large randomized VAS studies, which led to the current VAS policy, took place when the global vaccination program was in its initial phase," they added. "The present study adds to an accumulating number of studies suggesting that the effect of VAS is not independent of routine vaccines and may be harmful in some situations."

They went on to say that this is potentially problematic because the official policy is to give VAS at vaccination contacts. Because the current VAS policy is not based on specific studies, there is an urgent need to reassess interactions between VAS and vaccines in data from previously conducted studies if data on vaccination status were collected and to test the effect of VAS and different vaccination practices in future randomized trials.

Commenting on the Benn, et al. article, Charles B. Stephenson and Kimberly A. Livingston, of the University of California at Davis, said that, whereas preventing vitamin A deficiency is the only approach to peventing xerophthalmia, there are many options for preventing death from infectious diseases, including vaccination, environmental intervention to decrease transmission, and health care initiatives to increase diagnosis and treatment of serious infections.[13]

In the just-named study, the children did not enter the trial until 6 months of age, and they should have received the bacille Calmette-Guerin vaccine at birth and DTP and oral polio vaccine by 14 weeks of age, but many did not.

"Whereas vaccines are not available for all potential lethal pathogens, and children who receive vaccines may still succumb to fatal infections, the result makes intuitive sense because it suggests that the mortality-reducing benefits of vitamin A supplementation accrue to those at greatest risk, in this case those who did not receive regularly scheduled vaccines," the authors said.

They added that a caveat to this conclusion is that we do not know the causes of death from this study, so concluding that the excess deaths in the less-vaccinated children were vaccine-preventable is an implicit assumption.

Among the children who had received vaccines, Benn, et al., report that the boys benefited by reduced mortality, whereas the girls did not.

"An obvious explanation," they added, "would be that the vitamin A status of the boys was worse than that of the girls. Therefore, the boys had a greater need for the supplements.

While adults have different serum retinol concentrations, this sex difference has not been reported in infants."

They went on to say that the nutritional status data on individual subjects in the Benn, et al. study are lacking, and, therefore, we cannot evaluate that possibility.

"Another observation is that vitamin A supplementation was associated with increased mortality in girls who did not receive all 3 of the DTP injections at the appointed times early in infancy and 14 weeks of age, but received them later in infancy after the measles vaccine was given at 9 months of age," the authors continued.

This observation is puzzling, the authors added, and it could be attributed to a sex difference in immunity, because some differences have been reported in immune measures between sexes, even infants.

Benn, et al., speculate that vitamin A interacts with the vaccine at the level of the immune system to create a susceptibility to other infections, the authors said. One possibility is that the high-dose vitamin A supplements—200,000 IU; 100,000 IU 6-11 months of age—bypass the normal physiologic controls on the availability of vitamin A in the immune system. Iron supplementation regimens face a similar conumdrum with regard to adverse interactions with malaria infection.

"Perhaps the broader question for nutritionists is whether high-dose supplements have risks not seen for low-dose supplementation or fortification under certain situations, for example, some infections," the authors added. "Most data on nutrition-immune function interactions are derived from mouse models."

Perhaps a logical way forward to examine these questions is to carry out more functional studies in humans on the effect of nutritional interventions on the immune response to immunization, infection, or other challenges to the immune system, the authors concluded. Such studies are challenging, especially in infants and young children, but should help provide answers to questions that are currently problematic for the international health community.

Risk from Disease vs Risk from Vaccines
Measles-Mumps-Rubella (MMR)
Risk from Disease

Measles

Pneumonia: 1 in 20

Encephalitis: 1 in 2,000

Death: 1 in 3,000

Mumps

Encephalitis: 1 in 300

Rubella

Congenital Rubella Syndrome:

1 in 4 (if women infected during first trimester)

Risk from MMR Vaccine

Encephalitis or severe allergic reaction: 1 in 1,000,000

Source: JAMA 288(24): 3158, 2002.

References

1. Stevens, Mark A., editor. Merriam-Webster's Collegiate Encyclopedia. Springfield, MA: Merriam-Webster, Inc., 2000, p. 842.
2. Clark, Randolph Lee, M.D., and Cumley, Russell W., Ph.D., editors. The Book of Health. New York: Van Nostrand Reinhold Co., 1973, p. 263ff.
3. Clayman, Charles B., M.D., medical editor. The American Medical Association Home Medical Encyclopedia. New York: Random House, 1989, p. 1034.
4. *Ibid*, pp. 571ff.
5. Maldonado, Yvonne A., M.D. "Current Controversies in Vaccination," JAMA 288(24): 3155-3158, 2002.
6. Silverman, Ross D., J.D., M.P.H. "Litigation, Regulation, and Education—Protecting the Public's Health Through Childhood Immunization," New England Journal of Medicine 360(24): 2500-2501, 2009.
7. Clayman, Charles B., M.D., editor. *ibid*, p. 145.
8. Rimland, Bernard, Ph.D. "Vitamin B6 in Autism: The Safety Issue," Autism Research Review International 10(3): 3, 1996.

9. Benn, Christine S., et al. "Does Vitamin A Supplementation Interact with Routine Vaccinations? An Analysis of the Ghana Vitamin A Supplementation Trial," American Journal of Clinical Nutrition 90: 629-639, 2009.

10. Beaton, G.H., et al. "Effectiveness of Vitamin A Supplementation in the Control of Young Child Morbidity and Mortality in Developing Countries." Toronto, Canada: University of Toronto, 1993.

11. Fawzi, W.W., et al. "Vitamin A Supplementation and Child Mortality: A Meta-Analysis," JAMA 269: 898-903, 1993.

12. Mahalaanbis, D., et al. "Vitamin A Megadoses During Early Infancy on Serum Retinol Concentrations and Acute Side Effects and Residual Effects on 6 Months Follow-Up," Nutrition Reviews 17: 649-659, 1997.

13. Stephenson, Charles B., and Livingston, Kimberly A. "Vitamin Supplements and Vaccines: Maximize Benefits, Evaluate Potential Risks," American Journal of Clinical Nutrition 90: 457-458, 2009.

INDEX

D